The Nurse Practitioner's Guide to Nutrition

Second Edition

The Nurse Practitioner's Guide to Nutrition

Editors

Lisa Hark, PhD, RD

Director
Department of Research
Wills Eye Institute
Associate Professor
Jefferson Medical College

Kathleen Ashton, PhD, RN, ACNS-BC

Professor
School of Nursing
Thomas Jefferson University

Darwin Deen, MD, MS

Medical Professor
Sophie Davis School of Biomedical Education
City College of New York

SECOND EDITION

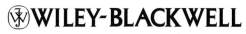

A John Wiley & Sons, Inc., Publication

This edition first published 2012 © 2012 by John Wiley & Sons, Inc.

Wiley-Blackwell is an imprint of John Wiley & Sons, formed by the merger of Wiley's global Scientific, Technical and Medical business with Blackwell Publishing.

Editorial Offices

2121 State Avenue, Ames, Iowa 50014-8300, USA

The Atrium, Southern Gate, Chichester, West Sussex, PO19 8SQ, UK

9600 Garsington Road, Oxford, OX4 2DQ, UK

For details of our global editorial offices, for customer services and for information about how to apply for permission to reuse the copyright material in this book please see our website at www.wiley.com/wiley-blackwell.

Library of Congress Cataloging-in-Publication Data

The nurse practitioner's guide to nutrition / editors-in-chief, Lisa Hark, Kathleen Ashton, Darwin Deen. – 2nd ed.
  p. ; cm.
  Guide to nutrition
  Includes bibliographical references and index.
  ISBN 978-0-470-96046-2 (pbk. : alk. paper)
I. Hark, Lisa. II. Ashton, Kathleen. III. Deen, Darwin. IV. Title: Guide to nutrition.
[DNLM: 1. Nursing Care. 2. Nursing Assessment. 3. Nutrition Assessment.
4. Nutrition Therapy–nursing. 5. Nutritional Physiological Phenomena. WY 100]
  610.73–dc23
                                    2012005068

A catalogue record for this book is available from the British Library.

Cover design by Modern Alchemy LLC

Set in 10/12.5pt Minion by SPi Publisher Services, Pondicherry, India
Printed and bound in Malaysia by Vivar Printing Sdn Bhd

1   2012

Contents

Chapter 9 Endocrinology Care of the Diabetic Patient, 184
Neva White, Rickie Brawer, and Cheryl Marco

Chapter 10 Digestive Disorders and Gastrointestinal Care, 207
Julie Vanderpool and Beth-Ann Norton

Chapter 11 Renal Care, 235
Jean Stover and Lauren Solomon

Chapter 12 Cancer Prevention and Oncology Care, 261
Tamara B. Kaplan, Maureen Huhmann, and Theresa P. Yeo

Chapter 13 Enteral and Parenteral Nutrition Support, 289
Jennifer M. Dolan, Nancy Sceery, and Nancy Stoner

About the Editors

Lisa Hark, PhD, RD, is Director of the Department of Research at the Wills Eye Institute and an Associate Professor at Jefferson Medical College in Philadelphia. She was previously Director of Nutrition Education and Prevention Program at the University of Pennsylvania School of Medicine from 1995 to 2009. Dr. Hark has broad experience in teaching nutrition to nurse practitioners and medical students and is a nationally known nutrition educator. She co-edited four editions of the most popular nutrition textbook for medical students, ***Medical Nutrition and Disease*** (Wiley-Blackwell), published in 1995, 1999, 2005, and 2009. She also co-edited several other Wiley-Blackwell books including: ***The Complete Guide to Nutrition in Primary Care*** in 2006 and ***Achieving Cultural Competency: A Case-Based Approach to Training Health Professionals*** in 2009. Dr. Hark is also co-editor of ***Cardiovascular Nutrition: Disease Management and Prevention***, published by the American Academy of Nutrition and Dietetics in 2004. In addition, Dr. Hark is the author of ***Nutrition For Life*** and ***The Whole Grain Diet Miracle***, published by Dorling Kindersley in 2005 and 2007. Aimed at consumers, these books have been translated into 15 languages and are available in paperback.

Kathleen Ashton, PhD, RN, ACNS-BC holds a Baccalaureate in Nursing from Coe College, a Masters in Nursing from the University of Maryland, and a Doctorate in Health Education from Temple University. She has taught nursing at the undergraduate and graduate levels for over 30 years and currently holds the rank of Professor of Nursing at Thomas Jefferson University, Jefferson School of Nursing in Philadelphia. Dr. Ashton's area of practice is adult health with a specialty in cardiovascular nursing. Over the past 20 years, she has conducted numerous funded research studies on women and heart disease. Dr. Ashton has won local, state, and national awards for her research, teaching, advanced nursing practice, and public service, including the 2003 New Jersey Governor's Merit Award for Advanced Nursing Practice. She recently served as a co-editor for the 4th edition of the book, ***Nursing Malpractice***, and regularly reviews for the ***Journal of Clinical Nursing*** and the ***Journal of Legal Nurse Consulting***.

Darwin Deen, MD, MS, is a Medical Professor at the Sophie Davis School of Biomedical Education at the City College of New York. A board certified family physician, Dr. Deen also holds a Masters in Human Nutrition and has been teaching nutrition to health professionals for more than 30 years. He is the author of numerous papers in peer-reviewed journals and has served as a journal contributing editor and manuscript reviewer for family medicine and nutrition journals as well as a popular nutrition text. Dr. Deen is co-editor of *The Complete Guide to Nutrition in Primary Care* published by Wiley-Blackwell in 2006 and co-author of *Nutrition For Life* and *The Whole Grain Diet Miracle*, published by Dorling Kindersley in 2005 and 2007. He has also served as associate editor of four editions of *Medical Nutrition and Disease* (Wiley-Blackwell) and the first edition of *Achieving Cultural Competency: A Case-Based Approach to Training Health Professionals* (Wiley-Blackwell).

Contributors

Editors

Lisa Hark, PhD, RD
Director, Department of Research
Wills Eye Institute
Associate Professor, Jefferson Medical College
Philadelphia, PA

Kathleen Ashton, PhD, RN, ACNS-BC
Professor
School of Nursing
Thomas Jefferson University
Philadelphia, PA

Darwin Deen, MD, MS
Medical Professor
Sophie Davis School of Biomedical Education
City College of New York
New York, NY

Associate Editors

Michael Clark, CRNP, DRNP, CNL
Assistant Professor, Department of Nursing
College of Health Professions and Social Work
Temple University
Assistant Director of Nursing Research
Temple University Hospital
Philadelphia, PA

Carlene McAleer, RN, MS, MSN, CRNP
Assistant Professor, Department of Nursing
College of Health Professions and Social Work
Temple University
Philadelphia, PA

Diana Orenstein, RD, MsEd
Clinical Dietitian
Hartford Hospital
Hartford, CT

Frances Ward, PhD, RN, CRNP
Executive Director
Pennsylvania Action Coalition
Harrisburg, PA

David Weiss, BA
Research Manager
Department of Research
Wills Eye Institute
Philadelphia, PA

Managing Editors

Deiana M. Johnson, BS
Research Assistant and Community Health
    Educator
Department of Research
Wills Eye Institute
Philadelphia, PA

Bianca Collymore, MS
Project Manager
Department of Research
Wills Eye Institute

Contributors

Virginia Biddle, PhD, RN, PMHNP-BC, CPNP (Counseling)
Pediatric Nurse Practitioner
Family Psychiatrist/Mental Health Nurse
    Practitioner
Department of Psychiatry and
    Human Behavior, Division of Child and
    Adolescent Psychiatry
Thomas Jefferson University
Jefferson University Physicians
Philadelphia, PA

Cecilia Borden, EdD, MSN, RN (Elderly)

Assistant Professor, School of Nursing
Thomas Jefferson University
Jefferson College of Health Professions
Philadelphia, PA

Rickie Brawer, PhD, MPH, CHES (Endocrine)

Associate Director, Center for Urban Health
Assistant Professor
Department of Family and Community Medicine
Thomas Jefferson University Hospital
Philadelphia, PA

Frances Burke, MS, RD (Cardiology)

Clinical Dietitian
Perelman Center for Advanced Medicine
Hospital for the University of Pennsylvania
Philadelphia, PA

Christine Conner, MPA-HAS, BSN, RN (Elderly)

Director of Nursing
Manor Care Health Services
Skilled Nursing and Rehabilitation Facility
Walnut Creek, CA

M. Elayne DeSimone, PhD, NP-C, FAANP (Assessment)

Professor, Department of Nursing
College of Health Professions and Social Work
Temple University
Philadelphia, PA

Patricia Digiacomo, MSN, RNC (Pregnancy)

Assistant Professor
College of Health Professions and Social Work
Temple University
Philadelphia, PA

Dara Dirhan, MPH, RD, LDN (Counseling)

Dietetic Intern
Corporate Wellness Dietitian
Private Practice Consulting
Philadelphia, PA

Jennifer M. Dolan, MS, RD, CNSC (Nutrition Support)

Advanced Clinical Dietitian Specialist
Clinical Nutrition Support Service
Hospital of the University of Pennsylvania
Philadelphia, PA

Dory Ferraro, MS, APRN-CS (Obesity)

Clinical Director of Bariatric Services
Stamford Hospital
Stamford, CT

Susan Breakell Gresko, MSN, CRNP, PNP-BC (Pediatrics)

Assistant Professor in Nursing
Department of Nursing
College of Health Professions and Social Work
Temple University
Philadelphia, PA

Maureen Huhmann, DCN, RD, CSO (Oncology)

Manager, Clinical Sciences
Nestle Healthcare Nutrition
Florham Park, NJ

Tamara B. Kaplan, MD (Oncology)

Neurology Resident
Joint Partners Neurology Resident Program
Massachusetts General Hospital
Brigham and Women's Hospital
Boston, MA

Kathleen Larkins, MSN, CNS, RNC-OB (Pregnancy)

Instructor
Roxborough Memorial Hospital
School of Nursing
Philadelphia, PA

Cheryl Marco, RD, LDN, CDE (Endocrine)

Clinical Dietitian and Diabetes Educator
Department of Medicine, Division of Endocrinology, Diabetes and Metabolic Diseases
Thomas Jefferson University
Philadelphia, PA

Amy McKeever, PhD, CRNP (Pregnancy)

Women's Health Nurse Practitioner
Assistant Professor in Nursing
Villanova University,
College of Nursing
Villanova, PA

Beth-Ann Norton, MS, RN, ANP-BC (Gastrointestinal)

Nurse Manager
Inflammatory Bowel Disease Center
Mt. Sinai Medical Center
Division of Gastroenterology/IBD
New York, NY

Nancy Sceery, LD, RD, CNSC (Nutrition Support)

Nutrition Support Team
Massachusetts General Hospital
Boston, MA

Lauren Solomon, MSN, ANP-BC, GNP-BC (Renal)

Nephrology Nurse Practitioner
Hospital of the University of Pennsylvania
Department of Renal, Electrolytes, and
    Hypertension
In conjunction with DaVita Dialysis
Philadelphia, PA

Nancy Stoner, RN, MSN, CNSC (Nutrition Support)

Clinical Nurse Specialist
Clinical Nutrition Support Service
Hospital of the University of Pennsylvania
Philadelphia, PA

Jean Stover, RD, LDN (Renal)

Nephrology Dietitian
Hospital of the University of Pennsylvania
Department of Renal, Electrolytes, and Hypertension
In conjunction with DaVita Dialysis
Philadelphia, PA

Bridget S. Sullivan, MSN, MS, CRNP, RD (Pediatrics)

Pediatric Nurse Practitioner, Registered Dietitian
Mt Airy Pediatrics, LLC
Philadelphia, PA

Julie Vanderpool, RD, MPH, RN, MSN, ACNP (Gastrointestinal)

GI Nurse Practitioner, Registered Dietitian
Nashville Gastroenterology Associates
Nashville, TN

Neva White, DNP, MSN, CRNP, CDE (Endocrine)

Diabetes Nurse Practitioner
Senior Health Educator
Center for Urban Health
Thomas Jefferson University Hospital
Philadelphia, PA

Theresa P. Yeo, PhD, MPH, MSN, AOCNP

Associate Director, Jefferson Pancreas Tumor
    Registry
Department of Surgery
Thomas Jefferson University Hospital
Adjunct Associate Professor
Jefferson School of Nursing
Philadelphia, PA

Reviewers

Kellie Smith, EdD, RN

Assistant Professor
School of Nursing
Thomas Jefferson University
Philadelphia, PA

Sharon Rainer, MSN, CRNP

Instructor, School of Nursing
Thomas Jefferson University
Philadelphia, PA

Pat Iyer, MSN, RN, LNCC

Legal Nurse Consultant
Med League Support Services
Flemington, NJ

Section 1
Introduction to Nutrition Concepts

1 The Role of Nurse Practitioners

Kathleen C. Ashton, PhD, RN, ACNS-BC

OBJECTIVES

- Discuss the role of nutrition as a component of practice for Nurse Practitioners.
- Describe the relationship between nutrition and commonly occurring problems such as obesity.
- Identify effective methods for integrating concepts of sound nutrition into areas of practice for Nurse Practitioners.

Nurses have outranked all professions in Gallup's annual Honesty and Ethics Survey[1] every year since 1999 (Gallup Poll). This vote of confidence from 81% of Americans participating in the survey comes with the responsibility to provide the best care to those who turn to us for information and advice to prevent disease and maintain health. Given this trust for nurses, we play a pivotal role in educating individuals about nutrition. Research findings demonstrate that consistent, intensive, lifestyle-based interventions can effectively reduce the risk of chronic disease.[2–4]

Practitioners cite barriers to providing nutrition and lifestyle counseling such as lack of time, lack of nutrition knowledge and confidence, poor patient adherence, low levels of patient health literacy, and lack of teaching materials.[5] A major key is consistency, addressing the lifestyle changes at every patient encounter where appropriate. The nutrition objectives for *Healthy People 2020* state that 75% of primary care clinician office visits should include nutrition counseling for individuals with diabetes, hyperlipidemia, and hypertension.[6] In addition, it may be difficult to translate nutrition science into practical dietary advice. We created *The Nurse Practitioner's Guide to Nutrition* to address many of these barriers and to assist Nurse Practitioners in providing useful nutrition education and interventions to those who most stand to benefit.

As healthcare practices and regulations change, nursing practices must evolve to keep abreast of those changes. The Patient Protection and Affordable Care Act of 2010 will provide healthcare coverage to an increased number of individuals. This presents an opportunity to address health disparities and provide resources to

---

The Nurse Practitioner's Guide to Nutrition, Second Edition. Edited by Lisa Hark, Kathleen Ashton and Darwin Deen.
© 2012 John Wiley & Sons, Inc. Published 2012 by John Wiley & Sons, Inc.

many for whom this has not previously been a possibility. Partnerships with nurses and other professionals can help to effect change at the individual and community levels. In whatever setting Nurse Practitioners are working (outpatient, home-based, hospital, nursing home, or community), whatever the reason for the encounter (acute problem vs chronic disease management vs health maintenance), and whatever the patient's life-cycle stage, we have the opportunity to improve health outcomes. For example, when patients seek care in the office setting, we have an opportunity to identify nutrition-related risks associated with their usual dietary intake. In the hospital, we must ensure that a patient's diet orders promote restoration of health while minimizing the potential for further deterioration. In nursing homes, where the risk of malnutrition is common, screening and monitoring caloric intake are para-mount. Home visits are a unique opportunity to assess how diet and lifestyle informa-tion is actually practiced. The community affords opportunities to model healthy nutritional choices and impact population health.[5]

When patients present for an acute problem we should assess the potential impact of that problem on their ability to maintain healthy eating and activity patterns and identify potential nutrition-related problems. Patients seeking health maintenance need routine dietary screening and appropriate patient education. Those with identi-fied nutrition-related problems require a plan to address those problems, part of which should include a follow-up visit to initiate and monitor behavior changes. Assessing patients' readiness to change is a critical component in this process (Chapter 3). Patients being seen for chronic disease follow up may require significant change to their routine dietary intake and often will benefit from a referral to a registered dietitian for more in-depth dietary counseling.[5]

The Nurse Practitioner's involvement does not cease with referral to a dietitian, as is the case with referral to any specialist. We must follow-up on the nutrition consult, support the plan, provide on-going guidance, evaluate the patient's ability to adhere to the diet, and revise the plan as needed. The overarching goal is establishing an eating pattern that provides an array of options that incorporate ethnic, cultural, traditional, and personal preferences while considering food cost and availability. Interventions are indicated across the lifespan. With an infant or toddler, we can teach parents a healthy eating pattern to help maximize their child's growth and development while minimizing the impact of their genetic predisposition for disease (Chapter 4). We can help adults to identify their potential disease risk and educate them about eating properly to minimize that risk or to maximize wellness. As adults age, metabolism slows and small, nutritionally-dense meals are beneficial to minimize the calories consumed and prevent obesity (Chapter 7). In older adulthood we need to screen for nutrition-related problems which affect ongoing health and address the need for a meal plan designed to mitigate the impact of chronic disease (Chapter 6).[5]

Nutrition for Life

What is the best eating pattern for life? How does one sift through all of the recom-mendations and fads? And of what benefit is the best nutrition advice if it is not followed? The *US Dietary Guidelines for Americans, 2010* was updated amid concern for the growing epidemic of overweight and obese Americans (Table 1-1).[7]

Table 1-1 Dietary Guidelines for Americans 2010[7] Key Recommendations

---

Balancing Calories to Manage Weight

- Prevent and/or reduce overweight and obesity through improved eating and physical activity behaviors.
- Control total calorie intake to manage body weight. For people who are overweight or obese, this will mean consuming fewer calories from foods and beverages.
- Increase physical activity and reduce time spent in sedentary behaviors.
- Maintain appropriate calorie balance during each stage of life – childhood, adolescence, adulthood, pregnancy and breastfeeding, and older age.

Foods and Food Components to Reduce

- Reduce daily sodium intake to less than 2300 mg and further reduce intake to 1500 mg among persons who are 51 and older and those of any age who are African American or have hypertension, diabetes, or chronic kidney disease. The 1500 mg recommendation applies to about half of the US population, including children, and the majority of adults.
- Consume less than 10% of calories from saturated fatty acids by replacing them with monounsaturated and polyunsaturated fatty acids.
- Consume less than 300 mg per day of dietary cholesterol.
- Keep *trans* fatty acid consumption as low as possible by limiting foods that contain synthetic sources of *trans* fats, such as partially hydrogenated oils, and by limiting other solid fats.
- Reduce the intake of calories from solid fats and added sugars.
- Limit the consumption of foods that contain refined grains, especially refined grain foods that contain solid fats, added sugars, and sodium.
- Consume alcohol, if at all, in moderation – up to one drink per day for women and two drinks per day for men – and only by adults of legal drinking age.

Foods and Nutrients to Increase

Individuals should meet the following recommendations as part of a healthy eating pattern while staying within their calorie needs:

- Increase vegetable and fruit intake.
- Eat a variety of vegetables, especially dark green, red and orange vegetables and beans and peas.
- Consume at least half of all grains as whole grains. Increase whole-grain intake by replacing refined grains with whole grains.
- Increase intake of fat-free or low-fat milk and milk products, such as milk, yogurt, cheese, or fortified soy beverages.
- Choose a variety of protein foods, which include seafood, lean meat and poultry, eggs, beans and peas, soy products, and unsalted nuts and seeds.
- Increase the amount and variety of seafood consumed by choosing seafood in place of some meat and poultry.
- Replace protein foods that are higher in solid fats with choices that are lower in solid fats and calories and/or are sources of oils.
- Use oils to replace solid fats where possible.
- Choose foods that provide more potassium, dietary fiber, calcium, and vitamin D, which are nutrients of concern in American diets. These foods include vegetables, fruits, whole grains, and milk and milk products.

Recommendations for Specific Population Groups

Women capable of becoming pregnant:

- Choose foods that supply heme iron, which is more readily absorbed by the body, additional iron sources, and enhancers of iron absorption such as vitamin C-rich foods.
- Consume 400 micrograms (µg) per day of synthetic folic acid (from fortified foods and/or supplements) in addition to food forms of folate from a varied diet.

(Continued)

Table 1-1 (*Continued*)

Women who are pregnant or breastfeeding:
- Consume 8–12 ounces of seafood per week from a variety of seafood types.
- Due to their high methyl mercury content, limit white (albacore) tuna to 6 ounces per week and do not eat the following four types of fish: tilefish, shark, swordfish, and king mackerel.
- Take an iron supplement, as recommended by your health care provider.

Individuals Ages 50 Years and Older:
- Consume foods fortified with vitamin B_{12}, such as fortified cereals, or dietary supplements.

Building Healthy Eating Patterns
- Select an eating pattern that meets nutrient needs over time at an appropriate calorie level.
- Account for all foods and beverages consumed and assess how they fit within a total healthy eating pattern.
- Follow food safety recommendations when preparing and eating foods to reduce the risk of food-borne illnesses.

Source: Dietary Guidelines for Americans 2011.

Approximately one-third of American adults are obese and 72% of men and 64% of women are overweight or obese.[8]

Despite the fact that patients accept the old adage "You are what you eat", they do not seem able to apply this to their day-to-day dietary intake.[5] While many of our patients recognize how important it is to "eat right and exercise", a study from the Pew Research Center found that Americans see weight problems everywhere but in the mirror. According to this report, 90% of American adults say most of their fellow Americans are overweight, but only 70% say this about "the people they know", and 40% say they themselves are overweight.[9]

Approximately 75% of adults are not eating enough fruits and vegetables.[10] Our culture supports convenience, our policies favor junk food, our restaurants have huge portion sizes to increase the perception of value, and our TV viewing habits demonstrate avoidance of exercise. Convenience foods, ever more popular, are typically not healthy choices. When attempting to counsel a patient about nutrition, the Nurse Practitioner faces the barriers of time, money, taste preference, culture, family, and habit. Health is unfortunately far down on the list of factors that are considered when food choices are made.[5]

The typical American diet is too high in calories, sugar, saturated fat, and salt, and limited in fruits, vegetables, and low-fat dairy foods. Fewer than 25% of Americans get five servings of fruits and vegetables daily. Even among children, calcium intake is inadequate in almost half of 3–5 year olds, and 70% of 12–19 year olds.[11] Whether it is the phosphates in soda that may leach out calcium or the displacement of dairy intake, many teens are losing calcium instead of storing it up during this critical time for building strong bones. Osteoporosis later in life is one complication that may result from over-consumption of soda over many years.[12]

To correct these imbalances, we need to encourage patients to reduce portion sizes to reduce calories; choose healthy snacks (fruits and vegetables, not candy bars or chips); and reduce the consumption of products made with sugar (cakes, cookies, and pastries) or high fructose corn syrup (soda and sweetened fruit or sports drinks).[5] Sugar and other sweeteners hide in baked goods and beverages. Using more herbs and spices can enhance flavor in foods while providing less salt and more health-promoting antioxidants. Low-fat milk and other low-fat dairy foods, lactose-free and soy products supplemented with calcium, and calcium-fortified products (like orange juice) are good alternatives, yet many of these products may also contain sugar.[5] Prescribing a calcium supplement will help address a chronic inadequate calcium intake that is prevalent in our population and may reduce the risk of osteoporosis in the elderly (See Chapters 6, and Appendices G and H).

Case 1

Joey is a 16-year-old boy who comes in for a school physical. He is 5′ 9″ and weighs 200 lb. He loves junk food and hates vegetables. His mom says he watches a lot of television and when questioned, he reports playing video games for at least 3 hours every day. He is on the honor roll in school, but doesn't have many friends. You identify the following problems:
- BMI: 30 (>95th percentile diagnostic of obesity).
- No exercise with highly sedentary activities.
- Excessive fat and sugar from junk food and sweets.
- Avoids vegetables.

APPROACH: This common case can be overwhelming and it is hard to know where to start. First ask Joey if he likes any kind of exercise and encourage those activities, including walking, biking, or weight lifting. A teenage boy with few friends may find it harder to engage in team activities such as playing street hockey or those that require a partner such as tennis. Quantify the number of hours he plays video games and negotiate that this should be reduced and daily physical activity increased. Discuss the importance of reducing junk food, avoiding candy, cookies, and chips, and emphasize healthier snacks. Always include at least one parent, grandparent or guardian in the discussion and be sure to emphasize that the parent's role is to stop buying junk food and offer healthier snacks and vegetables when the teenager is most hungry, such as after school. Often overweight children and teenagers have at least one overweight parent and the entire family's dietary choices and lifestyle need to be addressed. It's important not to expect rapid results and parents should be discouraged from criticizing. Lifestyle change is hard and changes need to be sustainable! Praise any change in a positive direction.

Assessment and Diagnosis

Successful nutrition interventions begin with careful assessment of the individual including a family history of risk factors, such as obesity, cardiovascular disease or diabetes (Chapter 2). The patient's meal and exercise patterns can be ascertained through directed questioning and perhaps keeping a food diary to prevent the pitfalls of recall and perception. Body mass index (BMI) should be calculated for everyone, including children and teenagers, followed by a discussion of how the patient's weight compares with norms (Chapter 7). Use prevention visits as an opportunity to educate patients regarding the deleterious effects of a sedentary lifestyle and unnecessarily large portion sizes.

Food insecurity is a mounting problem in the current economic climate. Research shows that almost 15% of American households do not consume adequate food to

---

Case 2

Abby is a 30-year-old consultant who comes in for a check-up. She travels a lot for work and eats most meals out. She likes to exercise but says that she is often too busy. She is 5'4" and weighs 165 lb. She played field hockey in college but has gradually gained weight since that time. You identify the following issues:

- BMI: 29 (diagnostic of overweight).
- Eats a lot of restaurant meals.
- Not enough exercise.

APPROACH: Abby's current BMI places her close to the diagnosis of obesity and if she continues her current lifestyle, it is likely that her weight will reach a BMI of 30, increasing her risk of chronic diseases. Discussing how to eat healthily in restaurants would be most useful. Suggest strategies such as skipping bread, limiting wine to one glass, ordering salad dressing on the side, ordering broiled, grilled or baked fish or chicken, and limiting portion sizes, especially if she orders a high fat cut of meat. While sharing dessert may not be possible during business dinners, it may be on social occasions. Brainstorm with her regarding ways to increase exercise and suggest she use weight rooms at hotels, climb stairs when possible, and walk instead of taking taxis. Recommend follow-up in 3 months.

---

meet dietary needs due to lack of sufficient funds or other food resources.[12] A thorough dietary assessment includes information on income and resources for obtaining food in addition to food intake and eating patterns.

Help patients who need to change eating patterns by identifying community resources including websites such as www.choosemyplate.gov and offer advice, encouragement, and referral when indicated.[6,14] Start the discussion of healthy eating with everyone, but especially focus on those with hypertension, diabetes mellitus, and hyperlipidemia who stand to benefit the most from improved nutrition. It is important to help those who are not eating what they should or not exercising regularly to begin doing so before they develop the health problems that result from poor lifestyle habits. Small changes are the best way to begin and then monitor progress towards a goal.

Effecting Change

Motivating clients starts with Nurse Practitioners. Patients are likely to take note of, and perhaps even be motivated by, a busy professional who practices what he or she preaches. Following the lifestyle and eating pattern we recommend bolsters our credibility with our patients. Certainly this is a win–win situation for us and our patients, and can be accomplished in various ways. Become knowledgeable about exercise options available in your community, advertise fundraising walks and races where you see patients, join them when you can, and be seen where good nutrition is being promoted. Participate in physical activity yourself, encourage your children's involvement in team sports, get involved in your local school or community, and be a voice for more physical activity and healthier food choices. Encourage your colleagues to eat healthy and to exercise regularly. If clinicians don't promote work-site health, who will? The internet, used judiciously, has good nutrition information and can be an excellent resource. When your patients see you living the lifestyle, they will be more inclined to seek out and follow your advice when they need help. Become a resource in your community: volunteer to speak about promoting good nutrition at school and business events, town hall meetings, or church functions. Help your neighbors to identify ways to eat healthier and increase physical activity. The more experience you have with these lifestyle challenges, the more of a resource you will be for those who look to you for assistance.[5] Unfortunately, the literature does not provide us with models that have been shown to be universally effective, so it is up to each of us to develop our own approach to addressing eating patterns and activity counseling for our patients. Examples of models that have been developed are described in Chapter 3.

Food is much more than nutrition for every individual. It represents nurturing, love, sociability, and even entertainment (as evidenced by the popularity of the Food Network). For many Americans, a chubby baby is a healthy baby and attempts to direct parents toward a more appropriate feeding style will not be appreciated. The news media is not helping. Each new dietary study is trumpeted with the fanfare of a newly discovered scientific fact. So when contradictory results are found (which happens often in science), patients (and their clinicians as well) are left confused about what to believe and what to include in a "healthy diet".[5]

Cultural factors and diet-related attitudes and behaviors strongly influence health.[15,16] The cultural milieu that affects a person's diet includes: the rules surrounding the person's upbringing, whether or not the person immigrates to a new society, the degree of acculturation to the new society, and the degree to which traditional foods in the culture of origin are available in the new society.[15,17] The meanings and uses ascribed to foods in any particular culture may be unique to that culture, even though the foods themselves are commonly available and may have different or no special meaning in other cultures.[18-20] Culture influences many food-related behaviors including food choice, food purchasing, preparation, where and with whom food is eaten, health beliefs related to food, and adherence to dietary recommendations.[16,21-23]

Culturally competent health care builds upon the understanding of these cultural influences and facilitates the development of stronger patient–provider relationships with higher levels of trust. This has been shown to be associated with increased use of recommended preventive services in ethnic minority patients.[20] Therefore, understanding the sociocultural context of health for individual patients is very important for effective health care, as culture may influence health knowledge, attitudes, and behaviors, including diet.

At the community level, providers trying to address the behaviors that lead to obesity face a similar unsupportive environment that we had trying to help patients quit smoking in the 1950s. Policy changes currently being considered that may help move our patients from where they are to where they need to be include: requiring fast food restaurants to include nutritional information on their packages, taxing sweetened beverages, and developing devices that monitor television viewing and video game use by our children.[5] Change begins with one small step and gains momentum. *The Nurse Practitioner's Guide to Nutrition* is a key resource to effectively begin the journey to provide optimal nutrition therapy for patients in order to reduce chronic disease and change diet and lifestyle.

References

1. Gallup Poll. Available at http://www.gallup.com/poll/145043/Nurses-Top-Honesty-Ethics-List-11-Year.aspx
2. Centers for Disease Control and Prevention. National Diabetes Fact Sheet, 2007. Available at http://www.cdc.gov
3. National Cancer Institute. Surveillance Epidemiology and End Results (SEER) Stat Fact Sheets: All Sites. Available at http://seer.cancer.gov/statfacts/html/all.html
4. Appel LJ, Brands MW, Daniels SR, et al. Dietary approaches to prevent and treat hypertension: a scientific statement from the American Heart Association. *Hypertension* 2006;47: 296–308.
5. Deen D, Margo K. Nutrition and the Primary Care Clinician. In: Deen D., Hark L (Eds), *The Complete Guide to Nutrition in Primary Care.* Wiley-Blackwell, Malden MA, 2007.
6. *Healthy People 2020.* Department of Health and Human Services, Washington, DC. www.healthypeople.gov
7. *Dietary Guidelines for Americans, 2010.* Available at http://www.health.gov/dietaryguidelines/dga2010/DietaryGuidelines2010.pdf
8. Flegal KM, Carroll, MD, Ogden, CL, et al. Prevalence and trends in obesity among US adults, 1999–2008. *JAMA* 2010;303:235–241.
9. Taylor P, Punk C, Craighill P, for Pew Research Center, 2006. *Americans See Weight Problems Everywhere But In the Mirror.* http://pewresearch.org/assets/social/pdf/Obesity.pdf. Report Published April 11, 2006.
10. National Health and Nutrition Examination Survey (NHANES) III. www.cdc.gov/nchs/nhanes.htm. Accessed 2012.
11. Greer FR, Krebs NF; American Academy of Pediatrics Committee on Nutrition. Optimizing bone health and calcium intakes of infants, children, and adolescents. *Pediatrics* 2006;117: 578–585.
12. Tucker KL. Osteoporosis prevention and nutrition. *Current Osteoporosis Reports* 2009;7: 111–117.
13. Nord M, Coleman-Jensen A, Andrews M, et al. Household food security in the US. 2009, Washington, D.C. US Department of Agriculture, Economic Research Service, 2010, Nov. Economic Research Report Number ERR-108. Available at http://www.ers.usda.gov/publications/err108
14. *USDA's MyPlate.* http://www.choosemyplate.gov
15. Gans K, Eaton C. Cultural considerations. In: Deen D, Hark L. (Eds), *The Complete Guide to Nutrition in Primary Care.* Wiley-Blackwell, Malden, MA, 2007.
16. James DC. Factors influencing food choices, dietary intake, and nutrition-related attitudes among African Americans: application of a culturally sensitive model. *Ethn Health* 2004;9:349–367.
17. Curry KR, Jaffe A (Eds). *Nutrition Counseling and Communication Skills.* WB Saunders Company, Philadelphia, PA, 1998.
18. Airhihenbuwa CO, Kumanyika S, Agurs TD, et al. Cultural aspects of African American eating patterns. *Ethn Health* 1996;1:245–260.
19. Karmali WA. Cultural issues and nutrition. In: Carson J, Burke F, Hark L. (Eds), *Cardiovascular Nutrition: Disease Management and Prevention.* American Dietetic Association, Chicago, IL, 2004.

20. Hark L, Delisser H. *Achieving Cultural Competency: A Case-Based Approach.* Wiley-Blackwell, Malden, MA, 2009.

21. Kittler PG, Sucher KP. *Food and Culture in American: A Nutrition Handbook.* 2nd edition. West/Wadsworth Publishing, Belmont, CA, 2001.

22. Burrowes JD. Incorporating ethnic and cultural food preferences in the renal diet. *Adv Ren Replace Ther* 2004;11:97–104.

23. Graves, DE, Suitor, CW. *Celebrating Diversity: Approaching Families Through Their Food.* National Center for Education in Maternal and Child Health, Arlington, VA, 1998.

2 Nutrition Assessment for Nurse Practitioners

M. Elayne DeSimone, PhD, NP-C, FAANP
Lisa Hark, PhD, RD

OBJECTIVES

- Discuss the value of nutrition assessment in the comprehensive care of ambulatory and hospitalized patients.
- Integrate relevant components of the nutrition history into both the comprehensive and episodic evaluation of patients.
- Demonstrate how to conduct an appropriate physical examination, calculate body mass index, measure waist circumference, evaluate growth and development, and recognize signs of nutritional deficiency or excess.
- Identify the most common physical findings associated with altered nutritional status including vitamin/mineral deficiencies or excesses.
- Interpret the laboratory measurements commonly used to assess the nutritional status of patients.
- Synthesize nutrition assessment data to formulate comprehensive treatment plans.

Integrating Nutrition into the Assessment

The value of incorporating nutrition into the Nurse Practitioner assessment cannot be overstated. Dietary intake affects all body systems and as such, manifests in both subtle and obvious signs and symptoms that may be appreciated through a careful history and physical examination, along with appropriate diagnostic tests. Regardless of the type of encounter or setting, the effective Nurse Practitioner will include relevant aspects of nutrition assessment prior to making treatment decisions. This chapter outlines how a comprehensive nutrition assessment should be an integral part of all initial evaluations, with questions tailored to the specific patient's medical problems. In the initial assessment the nutrition history is expanded, and explored fully in the context of both health and disease. Nutrition assessment requires that the Nurse Practitioner go beyond the disease model to examine influencing factors, such as social and environmental determinants, food security, motivation, adherence, literacy, numeracy, food knowledge, and skills. Given the time constraints in a busy practice or hospital setting, these data may need to be collected over time in

The Nurse Practitioner's Guide to Nutrition, Second Edition. Edited by Lisa Hark, Kathleen Ashton and Darwin Deen.
© 2012 John Wiley & Sons, Inc. Published 2012 by John Wiley & Sons, Inc.

multiple encounters. The use of an electronic health record helps to simplify data collection if valid and reliable assessment tools are used. Patients can complete data entry on their own for later review with the Nurse Practitioner. It is important to note that nutrition-related treatment goals that take into consideration the patients' environment will be more likely to succeed. For some patients with complex nutrition-related problems, a timely referral to a registered dietitian is beneficial, as it fosters a team approach to assessment and follow-up care. Treatment for many dietary-related disorders often requires repeated nutrition assessment to monitor a patient's progress. Eligibility for outcomes-based health care reimbursement requires that initial and ongoing nutritional data be analyzed. Nurse Practitioners who are able to integrate relevant nutrition information into all patient assessments will be more likely to help patients achieve desired goals. The purposes of nutrition assessment are to:

- Evaluate accurately a patient's dietary intake and nutritional status.
- Monitor changes in nutritional status.
- Determine if nutrition therapy and/or counseling is needed.
- Evaluate the effectiveness of nutritional interventions.

Patient History
Chief Complaint and History of Present Illness
Nutrition assessment can be woven into most of the standard categories of a patient's history. When considering potential questions relating to individual chief complaints, Nurse Practitioners should think about nutrition-related factors, especially if the symptoms reflect possible systemic disease. A complete history of present illness will contain specific questions about either a nutritional cause or effect of the presenting symptom(s). Complaints such as fatigue, weight gain, weight loss, or changes in appetite should prompt a thorough nutritional evaluation at the outset of the patient history. Disorders of most body systems can manifest in nutritional abnormalities, especially those that affect the head and neck, cardiovascular, gastrointestinal (GI), endocrine, and renal systems. Pregnancy, lactation, chronic pain, addiction, and other psychiatric illnesses should prompt Nurse Practitioners to investigate further.

Past Health History
A history of hospitalizations, surgeries, major injuries, chronic illnesses, prolonged immobility, and significant acute illnesses can have nutritional implications. Ask if the patient's weight has been stable. If not, have the patient describe his/her weight history over time and detail attempts at dieting (year, type of diet, weight lost/gained). Inquire about current or recent prescription medications, use of vitamins, minerals, laxatives, topical medications, over-the-counter medications, and products such as nutritional or herbal supplements that patients frequently do not recognize as medications. It is helpful to have patients bring all of their supplements and medicines to a visit for review. Important information about the specific components of over-the-counter supplements, as well as the patient's level of knowledge can be obtained by this strategy. Nutritional supplements include

any products that patients use to increase caloric, vitamin, or protein intake. Information about food allergies and lactose intolerance should include symptoms and self-care practices.

Family History
Familial occurrences of certain disease states should prompt Nurse Practitioners to investigate further. Common familial diseases with nutritional implications include diabetes, heart disease, hyperlipidemia, hypertension, obesity, thyroid disease, chronic kidney disease, and osteoporosis. Knowing the risk status for certain disease states may help patients make necessary preventive lifestyle alterations. The health of family members, as well as causes of death may reveal important information about the nature of disease. Specific conditions such as food allergies, eating disorders, alcoholism, and addiction often are seen in constellations in families. During the family history, ask specifically about height loss in a family member, as this may indicate a risk for osteoporosis.

Social History
The social history is often where the patient's diet history is explored. Information obtained in this section helps to understand patients in the context of their environment and is used to tailor treatment strategies that not only address the medical diagnoses, but are specific to the patient. Economic limitations that influence access to an adequate diet, difficulties shopping for or preparing food, and participation in feeding programs (e.g. Women, Infants, and Children (WIC), Meals on Wheels) are relevant. Unmet needs regarding access to healthy food and food safety or security are explored at this point. Can the patient afford adequate food? Is there a local source of healthy food? Where does the patient most often obtain food? These quick questions are used to screen for societal factors which can impact nutritional status.

Knowledge of the patient's educational level, along with his/her level of health literacy and numeracy are needed to make treatment plans that are easily understood and followed. Food-related knowledge and cooking and shopping skills both impact a patient's ability to adhere to a diet plan and should be documented in the social history. An exploration of the patient's motivation to change behavior and ability to adhere to a diet prescription will help to refine mutually set goals. Knowledge of culture-bound food practices will enable Nurse Practitioners to ask individualized questions about food preferences and practices, family role responsibilities, and other factors that may impact the nutrition plan. Details concerning the duration and frequency of the patient's use of substances such as alcohol, tobacco, illicit drugs, and caffeine are also documented. Lastly, the patient's level of activity and exercise patterns should also be included.

Diet History
Dietary information may be collected using any of the methods described in this section.[1] In addition, the patient's current food intake patterns, such as vegetarian or kosher dietary practices, cultural background, and social situations should be considered during the interview. Family members who assist with purchasing and preparing foods should also be involved in the interview process whenever possible. Key diet

Table 2-1 Key Diet History Questions for Brief Intervention

Questions for All Patients
- How many meals and snacks do you eat every day?
- Describe your pattern of eating — do you ever skip meals?
- What is your largest meal of the day?
- Do you feel that you eat a healthy, balanced diet? Why or why not?
- What do you like to drink during the day?
- Do you drink alcohol? What kind and how much?
- How many servings of fruits and vegetables do you eat every day?
- How many servings of dairy products do you eat every day? Low-fat or regular type?
- What type of protein do you eat? Meat, fish, poultry, vegetarian, vegan?
- How often do you eat out? What kinds of restaurants?
- Do you usually finish what is on your plate or do you leave food?
- How often do you exercise, for how long and what type?
- Is your job sedentary?
- Who obtains and prepares the food in your family?
- Do you eat alone or with others?

In addition to the questions above
Questions for Patients with Hyperlipidemia
- How often do you eat fatty meats (hot dogs, bacon, sausage, salami, pastrami, corned beef)?
- How often do you eat fish? How is it prepared?
- What types of fats do you use in cooking and bakig?
- What do you spread on your bread?
- What type of snacks and desserts do you eat?

Questions for Patients with Hypertension
- Do you use salt at the table or in cooking?
- Do you read food labels for sodium content? (<400 mg/serving permitted)
- How often do you eat canned, smoked, frozen, or processed foods?
- Are you familiar with the DASH diet recommendations?

Questions for Patients with Diabetes
- What times do you take your diabetes medication (including insulin)?
- What times do you eat your meals and snacks?
- Do you ever skip meals during the day?
- How many servings of starchy foods such as breads, cereals, rice, pasta, corn, peas, or beans do you eat during a typical day?
- Have you been prescribed a particular diet to follow?
- How do you change your diet and medication during a minor episodic illness?
- Do you know what sick day rules are?

Source: Lisa A. Hark, PhD, RD, 2012. Used with permission.

history questions should ideally take only a few minutes, if properly directed (see Table 2-1). The information obtained in a diet history may prompt a referral to a registered dietitian who will gather more detailed information and analyze the nutritional content of the patient's dietary records in order to determine total calories, fat, protein, sodium, fiber, and adequacy of vitamin and mineral intake. The results of such analyses prove invaluable when it is necessary to prescribe specific diets and supplements.

24-Hour Recall

Purpose This informal, retrospective method elicits all foods and beverages the patient has consumed in the preceding 24 hours. This method is recommended because of the ability to assess the timing of meals and snacks. For patients with diabetes, the relationship of food intake to diabetes medications, especially insulin can also be obtained. As with other self-reported measures, it is important to stress that there are no correct or incorrect responses. Patients who understand that the basis for collecting these data is not to judge, but to prepare the most effective dietary intervention, may be more likely to respond accurately. Family members are usually consulted if the patient is a child or is unable to convey adequate information.

Questions "Please describe everything that you ate and drank within the past 24 hours (meals and snacks), including quantities, and how you prepared these foods." Begin with the last meal eaten and work backwards or ask for a description of everything that the patient ate the day before. Ambulatory patients can be asked to complete the 24-hour diary either prior to their appointment or while they are waiting to be seen. Hospitalized patients can be monitored through calorie counts reported by the nursing or dietary staff, who record the daily amounts of food and drink the patient consumes. Keep in mind that the 24-hour recall method, when used alone, may underestimate or overestimate a patient's usual caloric intake since the patient's most recent intake may not reflect long-term dietary habits.

Usual Intake/Diet History

Purpose Similar to the 24-hour recall, a usual intake/diet history is a retrospective method to obtain dietary information by asking the patient to recall his or her normal daily intake pattern, including amounts of foods consumed. This method is suggested for older adults who frequently skip meals, and for those interviewing pediatric patients whose diets may not be varied. This approach provides more information than others about usual intake patterns and tends to reflect long-term dietary habits with greater accuracy.

Questions "What do you usually eat and drink during the day for meals and snacks?" As a busy Nurse Practitioner, this question may be all that you typically have time to ask, but it can serve as a screening mechanism to identify patients who need further assessment. When using this approach it is important to be flexible. Begin by asking patients to describe their usual intake and if they cannot recall their usual diet, ask what they ate and drank the day before (a switch to the 24-hour recall method). You can then ask if these 24 hours are typical. Again, bear in mind that some patients tend to report having eaten only those foods that they know are healthy and may underestimate their use of unhealthful foods or alcohol.

Food Frequency Questionnaire

Purpose The food frequency questionnaire is another retrospective approach used to determine trends in a patient's frequency of consumption of specific foods.

Questions The patient is asked several key questions regarding the frequency of intake of particular foods. Frequencies can be listed to identify daily, weekly, or monthly consumption patterns. These results are then compared with evidence-based dietary recommendations and national guidelines to determine risks for disease. This is commonly the method used to estimate alcohol intake, but can be used to assess other aspects of the diet as well. For example, by asking patients to describe how much milk, cheese, and yogurt they consume each day, it is possible to compare this to the 3-A-Day dairy recommendations. Questions can be geared toward the patient's existing medical conditions, which is why this method is suitable for patients with diabetes, heart disease, hypertension, or osteoporosis.

Standardized Assessment Tools

Numerous questionnaires have been developed for brief diet assessment. Several examples include the "Mini Nutritional Assessment" (MNA), which is particularly useful with geriatric patients, the "Rapid Eating Assessment for Patients" (REAP), Quick "Weight, Activity, Variety and Excess Screener" (WAVE) for adults and adolescents, and "Rate Your Plate".[2-8] These valid and reliable instruments are specifically designed to be used as a baseline for further evaluation and are particularly useful if there are different Practitioners who may evaluate the patient over time.

Percent Weight Change

Weight loss is very common in hospitalized and nursing home patients. Weight loss is also frequently seen in older adults or those with significant appetite changes due to chronic illnesses such as cancer, GI problems, or to surgery, chemotherapy, or radiation therapy. If weight loss is identified in the medical history or review of systems, it is essential to determine the percent weight change over a period of time using the patient's current body weight and usual weight. Severity of weight loss is defined by percent change in a defined period of time as shown in Table 2-2.

$$\text{Percent weight change} = \frac{\text{Usual Weight} - \text{Current Weight}}{\text{Usual Weight}} \times 100$$

Table 2-2 Interpretation of Percent Weight Change

Time	Significant Weight Loss (%)	Severe Weight Loss (%)
1 week	1–2	>2
1 month	5	>5
3 months	7.5	>7.5
6 months	10	>10
1 year	20	>20

Source: Blackburn 1977.[9]

Review of Systems

The review of systems is typically done at the end of the health history. Its purposes are to elicit any additional health problems, review potential symptoms related to each system, determine health promotion practices, and evaluate self-management of

Table 2-3 Review of Systems with Nutritional Implications

General Health: energy levels, fatigue, activity tolerance, weight changes, clothing fitting looser or tighter, and night sweats.

Skin: coarse or silky skin, changes in hair or nails.

Head: dentition (condition of teeth and gums, caries, extractions, dentures, caps, bleeding gums, pyorrhea), difficulty chewing, sore tongue, taste changes, date of last dental exam, difficulty swallowing, changes in voice quality, olfactory changes, headache.

Neck: goiter or lymphadenopathy.

Cardiorespiratory: weight gain, shortness of breath, activity intolerance.

GI: changes in appetite, dysphagia, lactose intolerance, dehydration, food intolerance, symptoms of reflux, abdominal pain, nausea, vomiting, hematemesis, excessive belching, flatus, change in bowel habits, diarrhea, constipation, frequency of bowel movements, hemorrhoids, melena, mucous in stool, hernia, jaundice, disordered eating patterns.

Genitourinary: amenorrhea, polyuria, calculi, age of menarche, last menstrual period, currently pregnant or lactating?

Endocrine: thyroid disease, goiter, heat or cold intolerance, change in voice, excessive sweating, polyuria, polyphagia, polydipsia, gynecomastia, hirsutism, hand tremor.

Hematopoietic: abnormal bleeding, easy bruisability, adenopathy.

Psychiatric: anxiety, depression, insomnia, food phobias, or compulsions.

Self perception: body image, self image.

Value Belief: complementary health practices, advanced direction regarding sustenance, religious impact on food.

Source: Lisa A. Hark, PhD, RD and M. Elayne DeSimone, PhD, NP-C, FAANP, 2012. Used with permission.

disease states. Diagnoses that had not been anticipated may first become evident during a thorough review of systems. All positive and negative findings for each system are listed. All significant positive findings in the review of system warrant a comprehensive symptom analysis and possibly, diagnostic testing.

Nutrition-related questions can be found in several sections of the systems review and will vary according to the patient's age as shown in Table 2-3. Anorexia or loss of appetite is cause for concern and warrants further investigation, regardless of the patient's age. All patients should be asked to quantify the type of liquids typically consumed, as fluid intake may affect presenting symptoms such as headache, dehydration, constipation, or others.

Physical Examination
General Appearance

Immediately upon introduction, the Nurse Practitioner begins to collect data regarding nutritional status. Basic information regarding body habitus and development are readily obtained by initial observation and provide important clues to the differential diagnoses that begin to form. Through an informed and targeted approach to the physical examination, it is possible to validate nutrition data obtained through the history, and pick up clues to metabolic abnormalities and pathophysiologic changes. When terms such as obese, overweight, undernourished, thin, well nourished, well-developed, or cachectic are used, they should be supported by findings in the physical examination and noted in the problem list.

Vital Signs and Anthropometric Measures

Documents that report comprehensive encounters must contain the appropriate set of vital signs. In the adult, vital signs include blood pressure, heart rate, respiration rate, temperature, height, weight, and body mass index (BMI). It is also helpful to obtain a waist circumference. Additional documentation is often used in the pediatric setting to track height, weight, growth, and development.

Physical Findings

Nutrition-oriented aspects of the physical examination focus on the skin, head, hair, eyes, mouth, nails, extremities, abdomen, skeletal muscle, and fat stores. Areas to examine closely for muscle wasting include the temporal muscles and the interosseous muscles on the hands. The condition of skeletal muscles of the extremities may serve as an indicator of malnutrition. Subcutaneous fat stores should be examined for losses due to a sudden decrease in weight or for excess accumulation that commonly occurs in obesity. At the present time, the most commonly encountered nutritional problem seen in clinical practices in the US and many developed countries is obesity and its associated complications. Obesity complications are associated with distinct physical evidence and should be documented when noted. These include: elevated blood pressure (both arms, seated), pulse (rate, rhythm), xanthelasma (hyperlipidemia), retinopathy (diabetes and hypertension), acanthosis nigricans (insulin resistance), jaundice, petichiae, icterus, hepatomegaly (hepatic disease), loss of lateral eyebrows, thyroid enlargement or nodule, coarse hair and skin, delayed reflexes (hypothyroidism), abnormal heart sounds, pale conjunctivae and skin (cardiac disease).[10] Specific clinical signs that are attributable to nutrient deficiencies and significance on physical examination are shown in Table 2-4.

Body Mass Index

Body mass index (BMI) is a weight for height measurement which provides a more accurate reflection of total body fat than body weight alone (Figure 2-1).[8]

An international data bank, maintained by the World Health Organization (WHO) is available to classify a particular patient's body habitus as underweight, overweight, or obese (Table 2-5).[11] BMI values are age-independent and the same for both sexes (Figure 2-2). At present, the international classification is used for all ethnic groups despite some recent investigation into possible risk variation in Asian populations.[12,13] While a valuable and reliable indicator for most patients, there are several limitations

To calculate BMI using metric units:

$$BMI = weight\ (kg)\,/\,height\ (m^2)$$

To calculate BMI using Imperial units:

$$BMI = weight\ (lb) \times 703\ height\ (in^2)$$

Figure 2-1 Calculation of BMI
Source: NHLBI[10]

Table 2-4 Physical Examination Findings with Nutritional Implications

General Survey: overweight, obese, severely obese, cachectic, proximal or distal muscle wasting, muscle weakness, altered state of consciousness.

Vital Signs: temperature, blood pressure, pulse, respiratory rate, height, weight, BMI, waist circumference, percent weight change, loss of more than 1½ inches of adult height (osteoporosis).

Skin: decreased turgor (dehydration), hirsuitism (polycystic ovarian syndrome), jaundice (alcoholism, liver disease, substance use), acanthosis nigricans (obesity, metabolic syndrome, insulin resistance, diabetes), ecchymosis (vitamin K, C deficiency), dermatitis (marasmus, niacin, riboflavin, zinc, biotin, EFA deficiency), follicular hyperkeratosis (vitamin A deficiency), petechiae (vitamin A, C, K deficiency), pigmentation changes (niacin deficiency, marasmus), pressure ulcers/delayed wound healing (kwashiorkor, diabetes, vitamin C, zinc deficiency), psoriasiform rash, eczematous scaling (zinc deficiency), purpura (vitamin C, K deficiency), scrotal dermatosis (riboflavin deficiency), pallor (iron, folic acid, vitamin B_{12}, copper, vitamin E deficiency), thickening and dryness of skin (linoleic acid deficiency, hypothyroidism), smooth, silky skin (hyperthyroidism).

Hair: easy pluckability (protein deficiency), alopecia (zinc, biotin deficiency) change in thickness and texture (thyroid disease).

Head: temporal muscle wasting (marasmus and cachexia), delayed closure of fontanelle (pediatric malnutrition or growth retardation), lymphadenopathy (chronic illness, infection).

Eyes: night blindness, xerosis, Bitot spots, keratomalacia (vitamin A deficiency), photophobia, blurring, conjunctival inflammation, corneal vascularization (riboflavin deficiency), retinopathy (diabetes and hypertension), xanthelesma (hyperlipidemia), loss of lateral third of eyebrow (hypothyroidism), lid lag, exopthalmus (hyperthyroidism), icteric sclera (hepatic disease).

Mouth: angular stomatitis (riboflavin, iron deficiency), bleeding gums (vitamin C, K, riboflavin deficiency), cheilosis (riboflavin, niacin, vitamin B_6 deficiency), dental caries (fluoride deficiency, bone loss, poor hygiene, lack of access to care), hypogeusia (zinc, vitamin A deficiency), glossitis (riboflavin, niacin, folic acid, vitamin B_{12}, vitamin B_6 deficiency), nasolabial seborrhea (vitamin B_6 deficiency), papillary atrophy or smooth tongue (riboflavin, niacin, iron deficiency), fissuring, scarlet or raw tongue (niacin, folate, vitamin B_{12}, B_6 deficiency), halitosis (dental disease, renal disease), loss of enamel on rear front teeth surfaces (bulimia).

Neck: goiter (iodine deficiency), thyroid nodules, bruit (thyroid disease), parotid enlargement (marasmus), lymphadenopathy (chronic infection), bruits (cardiovascular disease).

Thorax: thoracic and rachitic rosary (vitamin D deficiency), kyphosis, scoliosis (osteoporosis, vertebral compression fractures, early satiety due to abdominal crowding).

Abdomen: abdominal obesity (metabolic syndrome, diabetes, heart disease), diarrhea (niacin, folate, vitamin B_{12} deficiency, marasmus), hepatomegaly/ascites (kwashiorkor, alcoholism), ascites (liver disease, cancer).

Cardiac: signs of heart failure S3, S4, gallops (thiamin, selenium deficiency, anemia, eating disorders, cardiac disease).

Genito/urinary: delayed puberty (marasmus, eating or exercise disorder), hypogonadism (zinc deficiency).

Back/Extremities: bone tenderness, kyphosis, edema (thiamin and protein deficiency), growth retardation, failure to thrive (energy deficiency), hyporeflexia (thiamin deficiency), kyphosis (osteoporosis), muscle wasting and weakness, bone pain (vitamin D, magnesium deficiency, marasmus), tenderness at end of long bones (vitamin D deficiency), squaring of shoulders-loss of deltoid muscles (kwashiorkor), diminished sensation to light touch (diabetes mellitus), kyphosis, scoliosis (osteoporosis).

Table 2-4 (*Continued*)

Nails: spooning (koilonychias) (iron deficiency), transverse lines (kwashiorkor)

Neurological: dementia (vitamin B deficiency, hypothyroidism), delirium (hypoglycemia, electrolyte imbalance), loss of reflexes, wrist drop, foot drop (thiamin deficiency), ophthalmoplegia (vitamin E, thiamin deficiency), peripheral neuropathy (thiamin, vitamin E, vitamin B_{12} deficiency, diabetes), tetany (vitamin D, calcium, magnesium deficiency), delayed reflexes in the relaxation phase (hypothyroidism), hyper-reflexia (hyperthyroidism), ataxia (vitamin B_{12} deficiency, vitamin B_6 toxicity) diminished vibratory sense @128 cps or diminished touch to filament (diabetes)

Source: Lisa A. Hark, PhD, RD and M. Elayne DeSimone, PhD, NP-C, FAANP Used with permission.

of its use. BMI may overestimate body fat in very muscular people and underestimate body fat in some underweight people, such as the elderly who have lost lean tissue. However, consistent, accurate trended measurements of BMI provide important data regarding nutritional health. As such, inclusion of this measurement should be seen as routine in both ambulatory and institutional settings. Nurse Practitioners who determine patient numeracy regarding BMI can more effectively use this number as an outcome measure when developing treatment plans with their patients. Sharing trends in BMI with patients gives them additional data to reinforce the treatment plan.

Table 2-5 WHO International Classification of Adult Underweight, Overweight, and Obesity According to BMI

	BMI (kg/m²)	
Classification	**Principal cut-off points**	**Additional cut-off points**
Underweight	<18.50	<18.50
Severe thinness	<16.00	<16.00
Moderate thinness	16.00–16.99	16.00–16.99
Mild thinness	17.00–18.49	17.00–18.49
Normal range	18.50–24.99	18.50–22.99
		23.00–24.99
Overweight	≥25.00	≥25.00
Pre-obese	25.00–29.99	25.00–27.49
		27.50–29.99
Obese	**≥30.00**	**≥30.00**
Obese class I	30.00–34.99	30.00–32.49
		32.50–34.99
Obese class II	35.00–39.99	35.00–37.49
		37.50–39.99
Obese class III	≥40.00	≥40.00

Source: WHO.[11,12]

Waist Circumference

Waist circumference is an independent measure of risk in normal weight patients, as well as in overweight and obese patients.[10,14,15] Excess visceral adipose tissue is associated with metabolic syndrome and is reflected by an increased waist circumference measurement.[14,16] Waist circumference is a predictor of morbidity and is considered

Figure 2-2 Body Mass Index Values and Classification.

	Normal						Overweight					Obesity Class I					Obesity Class II					Obesity Class III																
BMI	19	20	21	22	23	24	25	26	27	28	29	30	31	32	33	34	35	36	37	38	39	40	41	42	43	44	45	46	47	48	49	50	51	52	53	54
Height (inches)																					Body weight (pounds)															
58	91	96	100	105	110	115	119	124	129	134	138	143	148	153	158	162	167	172	177	181	186	191	196	201	205	210	215	220	224	229	234	239	244	248	253	258
59	94	99	104	109	114	119	124	128	133	138	143	148	153	158	163	168	173	178	183	188	193	198	203	208	212	217	222	227	232	237	242	247	252	257	262	267
60	97	102	107	112	118	123	128	133	138	143	148	153	158	163	168	174	179	184	189	194	199	204	209	215	220	225	230	235	240	245	250	255	261	266	271	276
61	100	106	111	116	122	127	132	137	143	148	153	158	164	169	174	180	185	190	195	201	206	211	217	222	227	232	238	243	248	254	259	264	269	275	280	285
62	104	109	115	120	126	131	136	142	147	153	158	164	169	175	180	186	191	196	202	207	213	218	224	229	235	240	246	251	256	262	267	273	278	284	289	295
63	107	113	118	124	130	135	141	146	152	158	163	169	175	180	186	191	197	203	208	214	220	225	231	237	242	248	254	259	265	270	278	282	287	293	299	304
64	110	116	122	128	134	140	145	151	157	163	169	174	180	186	192	197	204	209	215	221	227	232	238	244	250	256	262	267	273	279	285	291	296	302	308	314
65	114	120	126	132	138	144	150	156	162	168	174	180	186	192	198	204	210	216	222	228	234	240	246	252	258	264	270	276	282	288	294	300	306	312	318	324
66	118	124	130	136	142	148	155	161	167	173	179	186	192	198	204	210	216	223	229	235	241	247	253	260	266	272	278	284	291	297	303	309	315	322	328	334
67	121	127	134	140	146	153	159	166	172	178	185	191	198	204	211	217	223	230	236	242	249	255	261	268	274	280	287	293	299	306	312	319	325	331	338	344
68	125	131	138	144	151	158	164	171	177	184	190	197	203	210	216	223	230	236	243	249	256	262	269	276	282	289	295	302	308	315	322	328	335	341	348	354
69	128	135	142	149	155	162	169	176	182	189	196	203	209	216	223	230	236	243	250	257	263	270	277	284	291	297	304	311	318	324	331	338	345	351	358	365
70	132	139	146	153	160	167	174	181	188	195	202	209	216	222	229	236	243	250	257	264	271	278	285	292	299	306	313	320	327	334	341	348	355	362	369	376
71	136	143	150	157	165	172	179	186	193	200	208	215	222	229	236	243	250	257	265	272	279	286	293	301	308	315	322	329	338	343	351	358	365	372	379	386
72	140	147	154	162	169	177	184	191	199	206	213	221	228	235	242	250	258	265	272	279	287	294	302	309	316	324	331	338	346	353	361	368	375	383	390	397
73	144	151	159	166	174	182	189	197	204	212	219	227	235	242	250	257	265	272	280	288	295	302	310	318	325	333	340	348	355	363	371	378	386	393	401	408
74	148	155	163	171	179	186	194	202	210	218	225	233	241	249	256	264	272	280	287	295	303	311	319	326	334	342	350	358	365	373	381	389	396	404	412	420
75	152	160	168	176	184	192	200	208	216	224	232	240	248	256	264	272	279	287	295	303	311	319	327	335	343	351	359	367	375	383	391	399	407	415	423	431
76	156	164	172	180	189	197	205	213	221	230	238	246	254	263	271	279	287	295	304	312	320	328	336	344	353	361	369	377	385	394	402	410	418	426	435	443

Source: Adapted from [10].

an independent risk factor for diabetes, dyslipidemia, hypertension, and cardiovascular disease even when BMI is not markedly high (Chapter 8). In patients with a BMI greater than 35 kg/m², there is little additional risk from elevated waist circumference, as severe risk is already present.[10] Therefore, measuring waist circumference is only recommended in patients with a BMI less than 35 kg/m². The waist circumference measurement is particularly important to measure in patients with a family history of diabetes and those who may be borderline overweight.[17] Waist circumference may decrease as patients begin to exercise, even without significant weight loss.[18,19]

In order to obtain an accurate waist circumference measurement, the patient should be standing in only their underwear. A horizontal mark is drawn just above the uppermost lateral border of the right iliac crest, which should then be crossed with a vertical mark in the mid axillary line. The measuring tape is placed in a horizontal plane around the abdomen at the level of this mark on the right side of the trunk. The plane of the tape should be parallel to the floor and the tape should be snug but not tight. Patients should be advised to breathe normally when the measurement is taken.

Laboratory Data to Diagnose Nutritional and Medical Problems

No single blood test or group of tests accurately measures nutritional status. Therefore, clinical judgment is important when deciding what tests to order based on the patient's history and physical findings. Adherence to current national guidelines, such as the US Preventive Services Task Force, ensures that patients are screened at the appropriate age and intervals to achieve early detection of nutrition-related disease states such as diabetes, hyperlipidemia, hypertension, thyroid disease, cancer, kidney disease, and anemia. For adults who present with obesity it is prudent to measure fasting lipid and glucose levels, liver function tests, and hemoglobin A1C as baseline indicators of disease. The nutrition-related laboratory tests shown in Table 2-6 are grouped according to medical condition and can assist with diagnosis. Other diagnostic tests may be indicated, based on the patient's individual presentation.

Diagnosis of Malnutrition

Malnutrition is defined as a suboptimal or deficient supply of nutrients that interferes with an individual's growth, development, general health, or recovery from illness. A BMI of less than 18.5 kg/m² defines adults who are consistently underweight and at risk for malnutrition. The WHO defines mild (BMI 17–18.49), moderate (BMI 16–16.9) and severe thinness (BMI < 16) using BMI cut-off points (Table 2-5).[12] Infants and children who fall below the 5th percentile of weight-for-age or BMI-for-age on the pediatric growth charts should be refined to endocrinology (growth failure) and/or a GI/Nutrition Service. In acute malnutrition, a child's weight-for-age percentile on the growth chart falls first, followed by a decline in height growth. In extreme cases of malnutrition or starvation, a child's head circumference growth may also plateau. The importance of plotting pediatric growth parameters over time is paramount, as poor weight gain and/or weight loss are key to diagnosing malnutrition, failure to thrive, and other medical conditions associated with poor weight gain in the pediatric population, such as cystic fibrosis (Chapter 5).

Table 2-6 Nutrition-Related Laboratory Tests

Alcoholism: complete blood count (CBC), aspartate aminotransferase (AST), alanine aminotransferase (ALT), gamma-glutamyl transferane (GGT), thiamin, folate, and vitamin B_{12}.

Anemia: CBC with indices, iron, ferritin, total iron binding capacity (TIBC), transferrin saturation, red blood cell folate, serum vitamin B_{12}.

Diabetes: fasting glucose and lipids, hemoglobin A1C, insulin, C-reactive protein (CRP), serum and urinary ketone bodies, BUN, creatinine, creatinine clearance, urine microalbumin.

Thyroid disease: thyroid stimulating hormone, thyroid antibodies, lipid profile.

Eating disorders: CBC, potassium, albumin, serum amylase, thyroid studies, beta-carotene aspartate amino transferase (AST), alanine aminotransferase (ALT), anemia tests.

Fluid, Electrolyte, and Renal Function: sodium, potassium, chloride, calcium, phosphorus, magnesium, blood urea nitrogen (BUN), creatinine, urine urea nitrogen, urinary and serum, oxalic acid, uric acid.

Hyperlipidemia: cholesterol, fasting triglycerides, LDL-C, HDL-C, and thyroid stimulating hormone (TSH) (secondary cause).

Musculoskeletal pain, weakness: serum calcium, phosphate, 25(OH) vitamin D, PTH.

Malabsorption: 24-hour fecal fat, barium studies, electrolytes, albumin, fasting triglycerides, hydrogen breath test.

Metabolic Syndrome: fasting glucose and lipids, hemoglobin A1C, uric acid, FSH/LH, testosterone levels in women.

Refeeding Syndrome: albumin, calcium, phosphorous, magnesium, potassium.

Source: Lisa A. Hark, PhD, RD and Darwin Deen, MD, MS, 2012. Used with permission.

Marasmus results when the body's requirements for calories and protein are not met by dietary intake. Marasmus is characterized by severe tissue wasting, excessive loss of lean body mass and subcutaneous fat stores, dehydration, and weight loss. Decreased protein intake is usually associated with decreased calorie intake, but can occur independently.

Kwashiorkor describes a patient with protein deficiency and is characterized by lethargy, apathy, irritability, retarded growth, changes in skin (dermatitis) and hair pigmentation, edema, and low serum albumin. Both marasmus and kwashiorkor are associated with weakness, weight loss, decline in functional status (increased difficulties with activities of daily living), impaired immune function with increased susceptibility to infection, and increased risk of morbidity and mortality.

Malnutrition in Hospitalized Patients

Hospitalized patients are at significant risk for malnutrition and loss of lean body mass, particularly muscle.[20-22] Research shows that 30–50% of patients admitted to hospital are undernourished and up to 37% experience loss of lean body mass within a few days after admission.[23,24] Excess loss of lean body mass can lead to rapid decline in physical status and increased complications, such as decreased wound healing and increased rates of pressure ulcers.[20] It is therefore critical to assess patients' nutritional status early in their hospital stay as part of the admissions screenings and conduct early and continuous nutrition assessment throughout patient stays. Key conditions associated with accelerated loss of lean body mass and strength include advancing

Table 2-7 Common Causes of Malnutrition

Decreased Oral Intake: poverty, poor dentition, GI obstruction, abdominal pain, anorexia, dysphagia, depression, social isolation, and chronic pain.

Increased Nutrient Loss: glycosuria, GI bleeding, diarrhea, malabsorption, nephrosis, a draining fistula, or protein-losing enteropathy.

Increased Nutrient Requirements: hypermetabolic state or excessive catabolic processes (surgery, trauma, fever, burns, hyperthyroidism, severe infection, malabsorption syndromes, cancer, chronic obstructive pulmonary disease, cardiac cachexia, critical illness, and HIV/AIDS). Pregnant women and children are also at risk due to increased nutritional requirements during growth and development.

Source: Lisa A. Hark, PhD, RD, 2012. Used with permission.

age, diabetes, GI disease, pneumonia, pressure ulcers, and malnutrition. Table 2-7 outlines the most common causes of malnutrition.

Prevalence of Malnutrition

Children, older adults, and hospitalized and nursing home patients are particularly prone to malnutrition. According to the *Healthy People 2010*, 6% of low-income children under the age of 5 years were growth retarded due to malnutrition in 2006.[25] According to the WHO, 50% of deaths among children less than 5 years of age in developing countries are associated with malnutrition.[27] One in three people are affected by vitamin and mineral deficiencies and one out of four pre-school children suffer from malnutrition. One in six infants born in developing countries is of low birth weight.[27] Some degree of malnutrition occurs during most hospitalizations regardless of the type of injury or illness.[28] The prevalence of malnutrition in the outpatient population has not been determined.

Risk factors for malnutrition include chronic diseases, use of multiple prescription medications, poverty, inadequate nutritional knowledge, homebound and/or non-ambulatory status, poor social support structure, major psychiatric diagnosis, and alcoholism. Food insecurity is defined by the US Department of Agriculture (USDA) as lack of access to enough food to fully meet basic needs at all times due to lack of financial resources.[29] Households that are food insecure, even when hunger is not present, have such limited resources that they may run out of food and cannot afford balanced meals. Hungry households have been defined as those that lack adequate financial resources to the point where family members, especially children, are hungry on a regular basis and food intake is severely reduced.[30] Food insecurity and poor diet quality exist at unsettling levels throughout the US despite attempts to create a food and nutrition safety net.[31] Providing nutrition education to all food assistance program participants, including the benefits associated with the recommended intake of fruits and vegetables as well as the availability and affordability of fresh produce, is a priority.

Health Consequences of Malnutrition

According to the WHO malnutrition affects all age groups, from conception to older adults. Health consequences of underweight range from intrauterine brain damage and growth failure to reduced physical and mental capacity in childhood to an increased risk of developing diet-related chronic diseases later in life. Insufficient food intake results in loss of fat, muscle, and ultimately visceral tissue. This reduction in tissue mass is reflected in weight loss. The smaller tissue mass has reduced nutritional requirements, likely reflecting more efficient utilization of ingested food and reduction in work capacity at the cellular level. The combination of decreased tissue mass and reduction in work capacity impedes responses to illness or surgery. The stress of critical illness inhibits the body's natural conservation response to malnutrition. In addition, undernourished patients experience nutrient deficiencies and imbalances that exacerbate the natural reduction in cellular work capacity (Table 2-4). They also experience a decrease in the inflammatory response and immune function. These alterations result in increased morbidity and mortality; therefore, adequate nutrition is essential for reversing these physiological effects. Aggressive nutritional support, instituted early in critical illness, may reduce the adverse effects in critically ill patients (Chapter 13).

Assessing Protein Status

Clinically, visceral protein levels may be depleted due to increased protein losses in the stool and urine, as a result of wounds involving severe blood loss, or secondary to poor dietary protein intake. Following serum protein levels may prove useful in conjunction with other assessment parameters (Table 2-8). However, each of these tests has limitations because serum protein levels are affected not only by nutrition and hydration status, but by disease states, surgery, and liver dysfunction. The half-life ($t1/2$) of each protein is given because knowing its duration will allow Nurse Practitioners to use these tests to monitor changes in protein nutrition.

Table 2-8 Serum Protein Tests to Assess Nutritional Status

Serum Albumin

Serum albumin has a half-life of 18–20 days and reflects nutritional status over the previous 1–2 months. Levels may decrease irrespective of nutritional status with acute stress, overhydration, trauma, surgery, liver disease, and renal disease. False increases also occur with dehydration. This test is not a good indicator of recent dietary status or acute changes in nutritional status (less than 3 weeks) given its long half-life. Significantly reduced levels of serum albumin are associated with increased morbidity and mortality (<3.5 mg/dL).

Serum Transferrin

Serum transferrin has a half-life of 8–9 days. Changes in serum transferrin levels are influenced by iron status, as well as by protein and calorie intake. Results of this test reflect intake over the preceding several weeks.

Serum Prealbumin

With a half-life of 2–3 days, serum prealbumin reflects nutritional status as well as protein and calorie intake over the previous week. Prealbumin levels may be falsely elevated in renal disease and are reduced with severe liver disease.

Source: Hark 2009.[1]

Estimating Resting Energy Expenditure (REE)

The amount of energy required to maintain vital organ function in a resting state over 24 hours is referred to as the resting energy expenditure (REE). The basal metabolic rate (BMR) is the minimum caloric requirement at a neutral environmental temperature during a fasting state. BMR is generally impractical to measure. REE is approximately 10% above the BMR. Thus, the REE is used in clinical medicine for estimation of BMR. REE accounts for approximately 65% of total daily energy expenditure and varies considerably among individuals with different height, weight, age, body composition, and gender. REE significantly correlates with lean body mass. Regular physical activity, especially weight-bearing exercises, can increase lean muscle mass, and thus increase REE.

Energy is expressed in kilocalories (kcal) and is produced by the oxidation of dietary protein, fat, carbohydrate, and alcohol. A kilocalorie is the amount of heat required to raise the temperature of one kilogram of water by 1 degree Celsius. Due to the loss of lean body mass over time, regular exercise can play a significant role in maintaining REE, especially in older adults. The amount of energy produced by the oxidation of dietary macronutrients is shown in Table 2-9.

Table 2-9 Definition of Energy/Calorie

One gram of *protein* yields approximately 4 kcal
One gram of *carbohydrate* yields approximately 4 kcal
One gram of *fat* yields approximately 9 kcal
One gram of *alcohol* yields approximately 7 kcal

Energy and Protein Needs of Hospitalized or Critically Ill Patients

Equations to estimate energy requirements have been developed as part of the Dietary Reference Intake recommendations.[32] Activity factors are added to the REE as necessary to calculate total daily caloric needs, which vary for active and inactive patients. Total energy expenditure (TEE) is equal to the REE times the appropriate physical activity (PA) factor. Many hospitals still use the Harris-Benedict equations to estimate calorie requirements, which are shown in Table 2-10.[33] The physical activity factor for hospitalized patients or those confined to bed is 1.2; for non-hospitalized, sedentary patients, use 1.3. For healthy, active individuals a factor of 1.5 is used to estimate caloric needs for weight maintenance.

Protein requirements in a critically ill patient depend on the degree of catabolic stress the patient is experiencing. Protein calories should be calculated separately.

Some guidelines for protein needs are as follows:

- In unstressed well-nourished individuals: 0.8 to 1.0 g/kg/day.
- In post-surgical patients: 1.5 to 2.0 g/kg/day.
- In highly catabolic patients (burns, infection, fever): >2 g/kg/day.

Table 2-10 The Harris–Benedict Equation to Calculate Energy Requirements

The Harris-Benedict Equation estimates basal (resting) energy expenditure in adults, which varies with both body size and gender.

REE equation for males:

$66+[13.7 \times weight (kg)]+[5.0 \times height (cm)] - [6.8 \times (age)]=kcal/day$

REE equation for females:

$655+[9.7 \times weight (kg)]+[1.85 \times height (cm)] - [4.7 \times (age)]=kcal/day$

Total Energy Expenditure (TEE)

Multiply the REE by an activity factor to estimate the TEE: use 1.2 for those confined to bed, 1.3 for those with a sedentary lifestyle and low physical activity. For healthy, active individuals use a factor of 1.5 to estimate caloric needs for weight maintenance

The Harris–Benedict equation should be modified by using an adjusted body weight for patients who are obese because adipose tissue is not as metabolically active as lean body mass. The REE would be overestimated if this factor were not taken into account.

Adjusted body weight: $[(Current body weight - goal weight) \times 25\%]+goal weight$

Source: Japur 2009.[33]

Table 2-11 Key Nutrition Recommendations by Age and Disease

Infants: fluoride, iron, calories, protein, fat for growth and brain development.
Children: fluoride, iron, calcium, calories, protein, fat for growth and development.
Teenagers: iron, calcium, calories, protein for pubertal development (screen for eating disorders).
Pregnancy: folate, iron, calcium, protein, appropriate weight gain.

Alcoholism: folate, thiamin, vitamin B_{12}, calories
Anemia: iron, vitamin B_{12}, folate
Ascites: sodium, protein
Beriberi: thiamin
Cancer: adequate protein, calories, and fiber
Celiac Disease: avoid gluten, multi-vitamin and B-Complex supplement
Constipation: fiber, fluids
COPD, Asthma: vitamin D, calcium, weight loss, calories
Diabetes: carbohydrates, saturated fat, cholesterol, calories, fiber
Heart Disease: saturated fat, monounsaturated fat, cholesterol, fiber
Hyperlipidemia: saturated fat, monounsaturated fat, cholesterol, fiber
Heart Failure: sodium
Hypertension: sodium, calcium, potassium, alcohol, total calories
Kidney Stones: calcium, oxalate, uric acid, protein, sodium, fluid
Liver Disease: protein, sodium, fluid
Lactose Intolerance: vitamin D, calcium
Malabsorption: vitamins A, D, E, K
Obesity: total calories, portion sizes, saturated fat
Osteoporosis: vitamin D, calcium
Pellegra: niacin
Renal Failure: protein, sodium, potassium, phosphorous, fluid
Rickets: vitamin D, calcium
Scurvy: vitamin C
Vegetarian diet: protein, vitamin B_{12}, iron, calcium

Source: Lisa A. Hark, PhD, RD, 2012. Used with permission.

Determination of the Problem List

Nutrition-related problems are prioritized according to their severity and treatment urgency. Evidence of a nutrition disorder should be considered *primary* if it occurs in an individual with no other etiology that explains signs and symptoms of malnutrition. A primary nutrition problem is usually the result of imbalances, inadequacies, or excesses in the patient's nutrient intake. Manifestations may include obesity, weight loss, malnutrition, or poor intake of vitamins or minerals such as iron, calcium, folate, vitamin D, or vitamin B_{12}. Secondary nutrition problems occur when a primary pathologic process results in inadequate food intake, impaired absorption and utilization of nutrients, increased loss or excretion of nutrients, or increased nutrient requirements. Common causes of secondary nutritional disorders include thyroid disease, anorexia nervosa, malabsorption, diabetes, trauma, acute medical illness, cancer, and surgery. Undernutrition may occur as a result of a chronic condition or an acute episode complicating an underlying disease.

Patients of normal weight and no other risk factors should be encouraged to maintain their weight, evaluate the quality of their diet and make any necessary lifestyle alterations to preserve their health over time. Treatment plans for patients of abnormal weight should be devised in conjunction with the patient and family to reduce nutrition risk and effects of disease. Effective nutrition therapy contains both a diagnostic component and a treatment plan. Patient education is an essential part of nutrition therapy. Key dietary issues by age and disease are summarized in Table 2-11.

References

1. Hark LH, Deen DD, Pruzansky A. Overview of nutrition assessment in clinical care. In: Hark LH, Morrison G (Eds), *Medical Nutrition and Disease*. 4th edition. Wiley-Blackwell, Malden, MA, 2009.
2. Mini Nutrition Assessment (MNA). www.mna-elderly.com
3. Gans KM, Ross E, Barner CW, et al. REAP and WAVE: new tools to rapidly assess/discuss nutrition with patients. *J Nutrition* 2003;133:556S–562S.
4. Gans KM, Risica PM,Wylie-Rosett J, et al. Development and evaluation of the nutrition component of the Rapid Eating and Activity Assessment for Patients (REAP): a new tool for primary care providers. *J Nutr Educ Beh* 2006;38:286–292
5. Gans KM, Hixson ML, Eaton CE, et al. Rate Your Plate: an eating pattern assessment and educational tool for blood cholesterol control. *Nutr Clin Care* 2000;3:163–169, 177–178.
6. Soroudi N, Wylie-Rosett J, Mogul D. Quick WAVE Screener: a tool to address weight, activity, variety, and excess. *Diabetes Educ* 2004;30:616–628.
7. Vellas B, Villars H, Abellan G, et al. Overview of the MNA – its history and challenges. *J Nutr Health Aging* 2006;10:456–463.
8. Barner CW, Wylie-Rosett J, Gans KM. WAVE: a pocket guide for a brief nutrition dialogue in primary care. *Diabetes Educator* 2001;27:352–362.
9. Blackburn G, Bistrain B, Maini B, et al. Nutritional and metabolic assessment of the hospitalized patient. *J Parenter Enteral Nutr.* 1977;1:11–21.
10. National Institutes of Health, National Heart, Lung, and Blood Institute. Clinical guidelines on the identification, evaluation, and treatment of overweight and obesity in adults: the evidence report. *Obes Res* 1998;6S2:51S–210S.
11. World Health Organization. *Obesity and Overweight*. Fact sheet no. 311. Geneva: World Health Organization, 2006.

12. World Health Organization. Global Data Base on Body Mass Index. http://apps.who.int/bmi/index.jsp?introPage=intro3.html. Accessed 2012.

13. Asia Pacific Cohort Studies Collaboration. Central obesity and risk of cardiovascular disease in the Asia Pacific Region. *Asia Pac J Clin Nutr* 2006;15:287–292.

14. Welborn TA, Dhaliwal SS. Preferred clinical measures of central obesity for predicting mortality. *Eur J Clin Nutr* 2007;61:1373–1379.

15. Fox CS, Massaro JM, Hoffmann U, et al. Abdominal visceral and subcutaneous adipose tissue compartments: association with metabolic risk factors in the Framingham heart study. *Circulation* 2007;116:39–48.

16. Katzmaryzyk PT, Janssen I, Ross R, et al. The importance of waist circumference in the definition of metabolic syndrome. *Diabetes Care* 2006;29:404–409.

17. Price GM, Uauy R, Breeze E, et al. Weight, shape, and mortality risk in older persons – elevated waist-hip ration, not high body mass index, is associated with a greater risk of death. *Am J Clin Nutr* 2006;84:449–460.

18. Grundy SM, Hansen B, Smith SC Jr, et al. Clinical management of metabolic syndrome: a report of the American Heart Association/National Heart, Lung, and Blood Institute/American Diabetes Association conference on scientific issues related to management. *Circulation* 2004;109:551–556.

19. Grundy SM, Cleeman JI, Daniels SR, et al. Diagnosis and management of the metabolic syndrome: an American Heart Association/National Heart, Lung, and Blood Institute Scientific Statement. *Circulation* 2005;112:2735–2752.

20. Demling RH. Nutrition, anabolism and the wound healing process: an overview. *Eplasty* 2009;9:65–94.

21. Paddon-Jones D, Sheffield-Moore M, Cree MG, et al. Atrophy and impaired muscle protein synthesis during prolonged inactivity and stress. *J Clin Endocrinol Metab* 2006;91:4836–4841.

22. Evans WJ, Morley JE, Argilés J, et al. Cachexia: a new definition. *Clin Nutr* 2008;27:793–799.

23. Pichard C, Kyle UG, Morabia A, et al. Nutritional assessment: lean body mass depletion at hospital admission is associated with an increased length of stay. *Am J Clin Nutr* 2004;79:613–618.

24. Schiesser M, Kirchhoff P, Müller MK, et al. The correlation of nutrition risk index, nutrition risk score, and bioimpedance analysis with postoperative complications in patients undergoing gastrointestinal surgery. *Surgery* 2009;145:519–526.

25. US Department of Health and Human Services. *Healthy People 2010*. US Government Printing Office, Washington, DC. 2010. http://www.healthypeople.gov.

26. Rice AL, Sacco L, Hyder A, et al. Malnutrition as an underlying cause of childhood deaths associated with infectious diseases in developing countries. *Bulletin of the World Health Organization* 2000;78:1207–1221.

27. Carlo W, Goudar SS, Jehan I, et al. High mortality rates for very low birth weight infants in developing countries despite training. *Pediatrics* 2010;126:1072–1080.

28. Joosten K, Hulst J. Malnutrition in pediatric hospital patients: current issues. *Nutrition* 2011;133–137.

29. United States Department of Agriculture. Economic Research Services. http://www.ers.usda.gov/Briefing/FoodSecurity/. Accessed 2012.

30. USDA. Economics research service. *Household Food Security in the US*, 2007.

31. Nord M, Andrews M, Carlson S. Household food security in the United States, 2008. *Economic Research Report No. (ERR-83)*, 2009: 66.

32. Otten JJ, Pitzi Hellwig J, Meyers LD. *Dietary Reference Intakes: Essential Guide to Nutrient Requirements*. Institute of Medicine, National Academies Press, Washington DC, 2006.

33. Japur CC, Penaforte FR, Chiarello PG, et al. Harris-Benedict equation for critically ill patients: are there differences with indirect calorimetry? *J Crit Care* 2009;24:628.

3 Nutrition Counseling for Effective Behavior Change

Darwin Deen, MD, MS
Virginia Biddle, PhD, RN, PMHNP-BC, CPNP
Dara Dirhan, MPH, RD, LDN

OBJECTIVES

- Outline the Health Belief Model and explain what motivates a patient to change health behaviors.

- Explain the Transtheoretical Model, outline the stages of change, and evaluate the patient's stage of change.

- Describe the goals of Motivational Interviewing and present examples of probing questions.

- Recognize the importance of self-efficacy and describe activities that influence self-efficacy.

Introduction

Although Nurse Practitioners counsel patients on a daily basis, training in the area of lifestyle behavior change counseling can be strengthened. This chapter aims to increase the effectiveness of nutrition and physical activity lifestyle counseling for Nurse Practitioners and provides an overview for the content covered in each of the clinical chapters. This chapter focuses on the Stages of Change Theoretical Model and Motivational Interviewing. Modules to help Nurse Practitioners assess patients' readiness to change, set goals, and provide effective counseling in a variety of clinical settings are provided. One of the many challenges in providing nutrition counseling to patients is that simply providing accurate information regarding the relationship between their diagnosis and their diet is only the beginning of the process to help change behavior. As described in Chapter 2, assessing diet and lifestyle is a key component of the patient's medical and social history and should be ascertained during non-acute visits. Given the large number and variety of diseases encountered in primary care by Nurse Practitioners, diet and lifestyle advice is an important part of routine care.[1] Many patients are open to behavioral counseling and would benefit and be satisfied if this counseling were integrated into traditional procedures, such as during a routine checkup or when discussing their medical history.[2] Through

---

The Nurse Practitioner's Guide to Nutrition, Second Edition. Edited by Lisa Hark, Kathleen Ashton and Darwin Deen.
© 2012 John Wiley & Sons, Inc. Published 2012 by John Wiley & Sons, Inc.

Table 3-1 Counseling Strategies for Effective Behavior Change

- Set realistic goals.
- Celebrate small successes.
- Expect setbacks.
- Be lavish with praise.
- Use group visits for support.
- Refer to a dietitian when indicated.

Source: Darwin Deen, MD, MS, 2012. Used with permission.

Table 3-2 The Health Belief Model

The Health Belief Model (HBM) seeks to explain what motivates patients to change health behaviors. Patients vary greatly in their interest in health and in their willingness to change personal habits in the pursuit of improved health.

Perceived Susceptibility: Does the patient consider himself or herself to be at-risk from their current behavior? For example, help the patient understand that saturated fat contributes to increasing serum low-density lipoprotein (LDL) levels.

Perceived Severity: Does the patient believe that the potential outcome is bad enough that it needs to be changed? For example, if an overweight patient understands that he or she may become diabetic, they may be more likely to make dietary and lifestyle changes to control weight and decrease risk.

Outcome Efficacy: Does the patient appreciate the impact of making dietary and lifestyle changes? Explain that patients who exercise regularly are more likely to lose weight and keep it off.[5,6]

Cost vs Benefit: Does the patient consider that the outcome is worth the effort expended? This may be the hardest challenge to address for any given individual. Any change is difficult and some changes are more difficult than others.

Source: Adopted from Becker 1974.[7]

assessments of body mass index (BMI), waist circumference, co-morbidities of overweight and obesity, as well as ongoing counseling, goal setting, encouragement, and monitoring, Nurse Practitioners play a very important role in educating patients about the importance of maintaining a healthy weight.[3] Counseling strategies for effective behavior change are shown in Table 3-1.

The cornerstone of treatment for overweight and obesity is lifestyle intervention, which requires counseling patients about their diet and physical activity.[4] The appropriate place to begin a discussion of a recommended lifestyle behavior change is with the patient's understanding of the health implications of their current behavior. Just because patients are aware of their diagnosis does not mean that they understand the implications that their diagnosis has on their health and risk for disease. Using the Health Belief Model (see Table 3-2), a discussion of potential outcomes based on specific behavior changes is essential to help motivate patients to make changes. This process involves eliciting information from the patient about their expectations, not merely providing information. This will provide the Nurse Practitioner and the patient with a common language to use in determining what changes to make and how to go about the process of making those changes.

Understanding Patients' Stage of Change

An assessment of the patient's readiness to change will guide Nurse Practitioners in determining how best to proceed and will provide an atmosphere of patient-centeredness. Since nutrition interventions requires active involvement of the patient, formulating a joint agenda and setting weekly and monthly goals will make it possible to include effective advice and guidance for the patient.[1]

The Transtheoretical Model was developed by Prochaska and DiClemente in an effort to identify a unifying theory of how people with addictions change their behavior.[8,9] Prochaska describes a sequence of attitudes and intentions and behavioral steps people take to change behavior. The model focuses on specific strategies found effective at various points in the change process and suggests outcome measures, including decision balance and self-efficacy.[9]

The stages that individuals go through in the Transtheoretical Model begin with pre-contemplation (not considering making a change in the target behavior – see Case 1), and advance through contemplation (considering the pros and cons of making a behavioral change – see Case 2), preparation (planning steps to make changes), action (actually changing the targeted behavior – see Case 3), maintenance (making the changed behavioral habitual – see Case 4), and relapse (when a formerly altered behavior pattern returns – see Case 5). The use of the Transtheoretical Model in dietary assessment is shown in Table 3-3.

Table 3-3 Using the Transtheoretical Model in Dietary Assessment

Behavioral Stage	Key Assessment Focus	Nurse Practitioner's Goal
Pre-contemplation	Patient is not yet considering dietary or lifestyle changes to reduce health risks or prevent disease. "I can't" or "I won't ..."	Determine patient's knowledge and understanding of behaviors associated with health risk.
Contemplation	Patient is considering making some lifestyle changes. "I may..."	Identify short- and long-term goals and select one change to try first.
Preparation	Patient is planning to make lifestyle changes and attitudes reflect their commitment. "I will..."	Support patient's decision, help with the process, and review potential obstacles to success.
Action	Patient initiates new behavior change Statements reflect affirmation. "I tried...," I can..., " "I do"	Ensure follow-up for problem-solving and reinforce commitment.
Maintenance	Patient becomes comfortable with making dietary or lifestyle changes habitual. Focus on how to continue lifestyle changes. "I usually ..."	Congratulate and support patients' commitment and recognize potential for relapse. Begin to identify new behaviors to modify.
Relapse	Patient has abandoned new behavior or returned to previous behaviors. "I failed..." or "I'm so mad at myself..."	Discuss patient's emotional state and frame relapse as a learning opportunity.

Source: Darwin Deen, MD, MS, 2012. Used with permission.

Case 1

Dave is a 14-year-old teen who comes in with his mother for a school physical. He is 5'6" and weighs 200 lb (BMI: 32.3). He loves junk food and hates vegetables. Mom says he watches a lot of television and when questioned, he admits to playing video games for at least 3 hours every day. He does not exercise. He is an honor roll student in school, but doesn't have many friends. He states he is not interested in talking about these issues.

STAGE OF CHANGE: Pre-contemplation.

APPROACH: Ask Dave how he thinks things would be different for him if he weighed 180 lb instead of 200 lb. He responds that he would feel better about his body and would be more motivated to play the sports he enjoys. Ask Dave to keep a food journal and think about what changes he could make that would help him lose 20 lb. Schedule him for a follow-up appointment in 2 weeks.

Case 2

Rich is a 30-year-old consultant who comes in for a check-up, admitting that his cholesterol is high (LDL 160 mg/dL). He travels a lot for work and eats most meals out. He tries to exercise but admits he is too busy. He does not smoke cigarettes. He is 5'10" and weighs 210 lb (BMI: 30.2). He played football in college and his weight has remained stable since that time.

STAGE OF CHANGE: Contemplation.

APPROACH: Rich is interested in his health, but questions the reality of changing his lifestyle to reduce his cholesterol. However, he leads a busy life and is not able to prepare healthy meals and increase his exercise. Therefore, focus on healthy selections when eating out. Strategies at lunch and dinner include skipping bread, limiting alcohol; eating red meat no more than once a week; ordering broiled, grilled, and baked fish and chicken; eating smaller portions; and sharing dessert. He may be able to eat oatmeal for breakfast. In addition, brainstorm with him about ways to increase exercise, e.g., using gyms at hotels, or walking instead of taxis (see Chapter 7).

It is important to recognize that behavior change is not necessarily a linear process where patients move smoothly from one stage to the next. As patients move through the behavioral stages, attitudes shift from an inability or unwillingness to consider dietary recommendations to a "can do" attitude in which counseling focuses on how to make behavioral changes. Sometimes patients will relapse and be unable to move forward again until they are able to successfully address whatever barriers interfered with their continued progress.

Table 3-4 Determining Stages of Change: Questions to Discuss

An assessment of readiness to change can be obtained with a self-administered questionnaire or by interview.

- Have you *ever* (tried to) change the way you eat to lose weight or improve your health? (no = pre-contemplation)
- Are you currently following a dietary plan for any reason?
- How long have you been following this plan and why? (less than 6 months = *action stage*, longer than 6 months = *maintenance stage*)
- During the past month, have you thought about dietary changes you could make to lose weight or improve your health? (yes = contemplation)

Source: Darwin Deen, MD, MS, 2012. Used with permission.

The Transtheoretical Model of Behavioral Change has been used to assess patients' motivation and readiness to make lifestyle changes to address obesity, diabetes, and cardiovascular related risks.[10-13] Nutrition-related questions to discuss with patients to determine their stage of change is shown in Table 3-4.

Discussing past experiences with weight loss or previous attempts to make other dietary changes can be helpful in opening the dialogue. As eating is a social and cultural activity, effective dietary change is facilitated when the entire family makes changes together. It may therefore be necessary to address concerns about the health effects of a given dietary intervention on other family members.

The stage of behavioral readiness is fluid; life stressors can easily move a person from maintenance to pre-contemplation. The risk of relapse is greater for the "veteran" dieter, who may be quite knowledgeable, than for the novice who may be ready for change and seeking information. Making dietary changes is often fraught with ambivalence and conflict over the commitment to behave differently in eating situations and to change food choices. While readiness to lose weight may be fairly global, the stage of readiness for specific food items or behaviors may vary. For different individuals who want to lose weight, some may be ready to substitute low fat or skim milk for whole milk, while others may be reluctant to make this substitution. These individuals may switch roles related to another food behavior such as reducing portion sizes. Thus, assessing why a change may be difficult can facilitate discovery of a potential solution. At a pre-contemplation or contemplation stage, open-ended questions provide valuable information about how the patient views dietary changes. This technique may uncover some of the emotional or cultural components of eating behaviors. Thus, the interviewer asks "why" questions about eating habits, rather than "what" questions used to quantify food intake. Much of the dialogue will focus on the ambivalence elicited regarding the perceived pros and cons of making dietary changes. At the preparation or action stage, "what" questions can identify food items that can be targeted for behavioral change. At the maintenance stage, "when" questions can be used to identify situations producing risk of relapse.

Case 3

Leslie is a 40-year-old woman with fatigue. She works full-time and is a single mother. She often skips breakfast, but cooks dinner most nights for her family. She is 5'8" and weighs 200 lb (BMI: 30.5). She doesn't have any time to exercise and is under a lot of stress. She asks for help with a weight loss program.

STAGE OF CHANGE: Action.

APPROACH: Leslie is stressed from work and financial issues and is asking for help to lose weight. She is in the action stage and ready to follow advice. Explain the importance of eating breakfast, as this will help regulate her appetite throughout the day. In a supportive, non-judgmental manner, emphasize that she needs to set a good example and provide a healthy diet for both her and her children. There is so much going on in her life, it would be useful to address one thing at a time (see Chapter 6).

Motivational Interviewing

Motivational Interviewing is an approach that has been shown to be effective at helping patients modify addictive behaviors and is increasingly being applied to lifestyle problems no matter what stage of change the patient is in.[14] Habitual behavior patterns, such as unhealthy eating and a sedentary lifestyle, share aspects of addictive behaviors. The goal of Motivational Interviewing is to understand the motivational state of the patient at the time and to act appropriately. For example, in the pre-contemplation stage, a person needs information and feedback to better understand the problem and to begin to imagine that change is possible. Giving advice about how or what to change at this point is not effective.

Motivational Interviewing is designed to elicit motivation from the patient, and avoids trying to impose it from the outside. It is defined as a patient-centered counseling style for eliciting behavior change by helping patients to explore and resolve ambivalence.[15] Resolving ambivalence is a key to Motivational Interviewing and can be done in conjunction with the Stages of Change Model. When people move into the contemplation stage – when they are thinking about changing versus not changing, balancing out the pros and cons – they are more susceptible to real change. However, a helping professional who starts pushing behavior change on the patient at this stage may meet resistance. Examples of Motivational Interviewing techniques are shown in Table 3-5.

Examples of probing nutrition-related questions to ask during motivational interviewing are shown in Table 3-6.

Table 3-5 Motivational Interviewing Techniques

- Express empathy.
- Roll with resistance.
- Develop discrepancy.
- Avoid argumentation.
- Support self-efficacy.
- Listen actively.
- Show warmth.
- Exhibit genuineness.

Table 3-6 Examples of Probing Questions During Motivational Interviewing

---

- What do you like about the way you eat now? (*Convenience, flavor, feelings.*)
- What changes do you feel are necessary in the way you currently eat? (*Assess which behavior the patient is most ready to change at the present time.*)
- What benefits do you gain from the way you eat? (*Visualize eating situations and feelings after eating.*)
- How does your eating relate to bad feelings? (*Anger, frustration, anxiety, stress.*)
- How does your eating relate to your method of coping? (*Examine coping style for various stressors and how that relates to eating.*)
- What would your life be like if you changed the way you eat? (*Visualize lifestyle changes and explore potential feeling of loss, concern about being hungry.*)
- What foods that you like do you think you would have to give up or be "told" to eat less of? (*Favorite foods, foods at social events, snacking pattern.*)
- What foods do you dislike that you think you "should" or will be "told to" eat? (*"Diet food" perceptions, food groups not currently eaten, e.g., vegetables, etc.*)

Source: Darwin Deen, MD, MS, 2012. Used with permission.

It is the patient's task, not the Nurse Practitioner's, to identify and resolve his or her ambivalence. Direct persuasion is not an effective method to resolve ambivalence. The patient needs help listing pros and cons as well as a health professional who really listens. The patient determines whether their current behavior is consistent with their goals and values and then makes choices to move toward a decision to act. Presenting arguments for the need to change will leave the patient in the role of defending arguments against change; the counselor must leave room for the patient to provide both the pros and cons. The counseling style is generally an empathetic and eliciting one. Readiness to change is not a patient trait but a fluctuating product of interpersonal interaction. Within this model, the therapeutic relationship is more like a partnership than one of expert and novice. Successful patient motivation begins with establishing a therapeutic relationship from which motivation can grow. In this setting, similar to effective patient education, there is more listening than talking.

Motivation as a Behavioral Probability

The Nurse Practitioner can never really know what the patient is thinking and feeling. We infer these things from what patients say, the emotions they show, and how they act. If patients adhere well to a prescribed plan, we expect they are more likely to have positive outcomes. We can turn this around and say, "motivation can be defined as *the probability that a person will enter into, continue, and adhere to a specific change strategy*".[16] This shifts the emphasis from "motivated" as a passive adjective to the active "motivate", which is the counselor's job to perform. The counselor does not just give advice, but motivates, and increases the likelihood that the patient will understand and perform all the parts of action required to change. The patient cannot be blamed for being unmotivated: it is the counselor's job to provide the appropriate input at each stage of the process. Motivation is a part of the helping professional's job.

The goals of a Motivational Interviewing session will be achieved when the Nurse Practitioner has used active listening, when the patient's self-esteem has been maintained or enhanced, when the interview focuses on specific behaviors that are steps to an overall goal, and when incidental goals are set that will create progress toward an overall outcome. For example, if the patient usually drinks several cups of coffee with half-and-half each day and one of his/her goals is to cut down on the saturated fat content of his/her diet, then he/she should:

1. Recognize that half-and-half cream is an important source of saturated fat.
2. Refine that overall statement to recognize how much of an impact changing to whole or low-fat milk could have on his/her saturated fat intake.
3. Consider how best to institute a change, e.g. he/she might decide to use whole milk when getting coffee at a restaurant but buy 1% low-fat milk to use at home. This would be a good step toward changing their taste preference for half-and-half cream. Alternatively, he/she might prefer to continue using half-and-half cream but use less or drink fewer cups of coffee each day.

Using Motivational Interviewing to Identify Ambivalence

Developing and maintaining motivation is crucial to making lifestyle changes. The assessment should be focused on identifying and addressing the internal ambivalence about giving up "unhealthy" habits that are associated with increased risk, e.g., smoking or unhealthy eating habits.[17] The goal of Motivational Interviewing is to have the patient, rather than the provider, present the reasons for change. People persuade themselves better than any other person can.[18] In discussion, point out discrepancies between what the patient says he or she wants and the consequences of their current behavior. Discrepancies between their current behavior and their own goals are a starting point for change. It is also important to avoid direct

---

Case 4

Gary is a 50-year-old man who comes in for a blood pressure check. He is on thiazide diuretic and an ACE inhibitor and his blood pressure is 145/90 mmHg. He works as a supervisor and his shifts are 12 hours long. He is married and he often does the cooking. He and his wife both use salt. He is 5'11" and weighs 200 lb. He states he doesn't have any time to exercise. You identify the following issues: (1) BMI: 27.9 kg/m² (diagnostic of overweight), (2) stage 1 hypertension on medication, (3) salt ingestion, (4) sedentary lifestyle.

STAGE OF CHANGE: Maintenance.

APPROACH: His blood pressure today is 140/90. He is on medication and he is following the DASH diet, adds no salt to his food (except occasionally) and drinks only one to two glasses of wine on weekends. Your plan today is to discuss exercise with him. Ask Gary if it is okay to talk a little about his exercise habits. Congratulate him on all the dietary changes he has made, and ask him what he thinks about today's blood pressure reading.
1. If he expresses dissatisfaction, ask if he has thought about things he can do to lower his blood pressure further.
2. If he is not interested in exercise, tell him you respect his decision and let it go.
3. On the other hand, if he feels that exercise might be possible, highlight the importance of daily physical activity to control blood pressure.
4. See what he thinks about these suggestions and what he thinks he could do to try to be more active.

Table 3-7 Eliciting Benefits of Changing Lifestyle and Eating Patterns

- What benefits do you think you might gain from changing the way you eat? (*Brainstorm the range of potential benefits, e.g., fit into clothes, feel better, keep family from nagging.*)
- How does your eating (and lifestyle) pattern relate to "chronic" health problems (e.g., diabetes, hypertension)? (*Explore how nutrition therapy may affect control of cardiovascular disease risk factors, and medication dosage/side effects, e.g., sexual function, etc.*)
- How could changing your lifestyle improve your long-term health and ability to function? (*Explore important personal events.*)
- How could lifestyle changes improve your every day functioning now? (*Explore fatigue, energy, ability to concentrate, stamina, etc.*)
- What food or lifestyle changes do you think you may like? (*Explore potential misperceptions of restrictions, or how some of the dislikes may be addressed, e.g., feeling hungry.*)
- How do you think you could change your lifestyle to get the potential benefits without feeling deprived? (*List some of the reasons given for not changing your intake.*)

Source: Darwin Deen, MD, MS, 2012. Used with permission.

confrontational messages. Eliciting benefits of changing lifestyle and eating behaviors are shown in Table 3-7.

The Importance of Self-Efficacy

Self-efficacy is a person's belief that they can carry out a change or a task.[19] The Nurse Practitioner must convey messages that he/she has confidence in the patient's ability to carry out tasks leading to change. Telling the patient what you think they should do is often counterproductive. If the patient has made some changes, build on these early successes. If the patient has experienced setbacks, emphasize that there are many paths to the goal and the best approach still needs to be uncovered. Self-efficacy predicts when knowledge will influence behavior.[20] Self-efficacy is the patient's perception of their ability to exert control. Once knowledge gaps have been identified, addressing self-efficacy may be the most effective method of promoting behavior change. Self-efficacy can be assessed by inquiring about who the patient feels is most in control of their diet, who they feel was responsible for any past failures, and how the patient has responded to obstacles in the past.

If the patient does not feel in control of his/her behavior, helping them to identify those areas where they can gain control will make behavior change more likely. If the patient blames themselves for past failures (low self-efficacy), they need a plan to address how to make this time different. If the patient feels that external factors were responsible for past failures, ask them to describe what has changed in the environment that will prevent this from happening again. To influence self-efficacy, patients must be asked to make a realistic appraisal of their abilities (Table 3-8). For example, rather than concentrating on the health benefits of a new dietary regimen, which are long term, advise the patient to think instead about how good they will feel about accomplishing a short term goal that they set for themselves. Examples include fitting into an old suit that used to fit or buying a new item in a smaller size.

Table 3-8 Sources of Self-Efficacy

- Verbal persuasion (including self-talk).
- Performance accomplishment.
- Vicarious performance.
- Physiologic arousal.

Activities That Have Been Shown to Influence Self-Efficacy
- Modeling behavior (such as cooking classes).
- Reflection on past accomplishments (positive reinforcement).
- Role plays (practising potential difficult situations).
- Placing emphasis on effective benefit (short-term benefits).

Source: Darwin Deen, MD, MS, 2012. Used with permission.

Practice What You Preach

Nurse Practitioners can enhance credibility and ability to relate to patients by practicing healthy lifestyles. Become an expert on exercise options in your community (advertise fundraising and lunchtime walks in your office, join them when you can, let your patients see you out there). Participate in physical activity yourself, make sure your children are involved in local team sports, etc., get involved in your local school district, and be a voice for more physical activity and healthier cafeteria foods. Encourage your office staff to eat healthy and to exercise regularly (if we don't promote work-site health, who will?). If you maintain a library for your patients make sure that it has useful nutrition information resources and send out heath-promoting mailings, e-mail, etc. When your patients see how important this is to you, they will be more inclined to seek out your advice when they need help. Become a resource in your community, speak out whenever and wherever you can

---

Case 5

Julie is a 63-year-old woman who comes in with type 2 diabetes (hemoglobin A1C: 7.5%). Her cholesterol is 220 mg/dL, she has an LDL-C of 120 mg/dL and her HDL-C is 45 mg/dL. She is taking a statin and an oral hypoglycemic agent. She had been seeing a dietitian for several years but recently lost her job and no longer has health insurance. Julie says she is under a lot of stress and gained back 20 of the 40 lb she has lost. She is 5'9" and weighs 180 lb (BMI: 27 kg/m²).

STAGE OF CHANGE: Relapse.

APPROACH: Julie has been successful at losing weight, lowering her cholesterol, and controlling her blood sugar but now she has gained weight and her lab values are slowly worsening. She should be congratulated for her previous success and encouraged to continue with her healthy eating and exercise program. Explore her unemployment status and discuss options for support, such as Weight Watchers, to provide weight loss counseling at lower cost. She would probably benefit from a group class for patients with diabetes as well (see Chapters 6 and 8).

(block parties, town hall meetings, church suppers), and help your neighbors to identify ways to eat healthier and become more physically active. The more experience you have with these lifestyle challenges, the more of a resource you will be for your patients.

Summary: Role of Nurse Practitioners

Nutrition counseling provided by Nurse Practitioners can produce beneficial changes in diet, risk factors (BMI, blood pressure), waist circumference, and lab values (glucose, hemoglobin A1C, lipids). Research demonstrates that the combination of primary care-based programs providing nutrition counseling and a low-cost office support system has beneficial effects on patients' dietary fat intake, weight, and blood lipid levels.[21] Models for multidisciplinary care vary depending on whether they are designed for an individual medical practice or as part of the health care services of a larger facility. For example, lifestyle changes for healthy weight management must be permanently incorporated into a patient's daily lifestyle to reduce obesity and its associated risks.

Within the current organization of primary care, it could be argued that there is limited time to give detailed dietary advice. To be effective, acceptable, and useful, dietary interventions need to be individualized and applied in the context of family life.[22] Patients who are seen frequently and on a continuous basis benefit from the effectiveness of individual lifestyle interventions.[23] Working closely with registered dietitians using multidisciplinary approaches to patient education and chronic disease prevention and management will help improve patient outcomes.[24] Examples of when to refer to a dietitian are shown in Table 3-9.

A well-motivated, informed, and educated team can play a major role in facilitating dietary change in patients, translating nutritional guidelines into meaningful and practical terms, and offering advice that reflects the social and cultural mix of the local community. Group practices could connect with local community agencies/advocates to help address specific local issues and increase the relevance to community members who may or may not be patients.[22] "In these times of changing health care priorities there are great opportunities to maximize the health gain possible with diet. The potential contribution that diet could make to the nation's health is significant and it therefore needs to be put firmly on the health care agenda".[22]

Table 3-9 When to Refer to a Dietitian

- Unable to lose weight.
- Loss of appetite and appetite changes.
- Chronic diseases (e.g. cancer, diabetes, renal disease, heart disease).
- Pregnancy.
- Restricted eating (vegetarianism, macrobiotic, raw food, vegan).
- Nutrition support (enteral nutrition, parenteral nutrition).
- Food allergies or intolerances.
- Social factors that may limit appropriate intake (e.g., religion, poverty).
- Eating disorders.

Source: Lisa Hark, PhD, RD and Darwin Deen, MD, MS, 2012. Used with permission.

References

1. Van Weel C. Dietary advice in family medicine. *Am J Clin Nutr* 2003;77(4 Suppl):1008S–1010S.
2. Wolff LS, Massett HA, Weber D, et al. Opportunities and barriers to disease prevention counseling in the primary care setting: a multisite qualitative study with US health consumers. *Health Promot Int* 2010;25:265–276.
3. Rippe JM, McInnis KJ, Melanson KJ. Physician involvement in the management of obesity as a primary medical condition. *Obesity Res* 2001;(Suppl 4):302S–311S.
4. Kushner RF, Kushner N. Weight management counseling using a targeted lifestyle patterns approach. *Diabetes Spectrum* 2009;22:26–28.
5. Catenacci VA, Ogden LG, Stuht J, et al. Physical activity patterns in the National Weight Control Registry. *Obesity* 2008;16:153–161.
6. Catenacci VA, Wyatt HR. The role of physical activity in producing and maintaining weight loss. *Nat Clin Prac Endocrin Metab* 2007;3:518–529.
7. Becker MH. *The Health Beliefs Model and Personal Health Behavior CB Slack*, Inc., Thorofare, NJ. 1974.
8. Prochaska JO, DiClemente CC, Norcross JC. In search of how people change: applications to addictive behaviors. *Am Psychol* 1992;47:1102.
9. Prochaska JO, Norcross JC, DiClemente CC. *Changing for Good*. William Morrow, New York, NY. 1994.
10. Prochaska, JO, DiClemente, CC. Transtheoretical therapy toward a more integrative model of change. *Psychother Theor Res Pract* 1982;19:276–287.
11. Sutton K, Logue E, Jarhoura D, et al. Assessing dietary and exercise stage of change to optimize weight loss interventions. *Obesity Res* 2003;22:641–652.
12. Vallis M, Ruggiero L, Greene G, et al. Stages of change for healthy eating in diabetes: relation to demographic, eating-related, health care utilization, and psychosocial factors. *Diabetes Care* 2003;26:1468–1474.
13. Molaison EF. Stages of change in clinical nutrition. *Nutr Clin Care* 2002;5:251–257.
14. Miller WR, Rollnick S. *Motivational Interviewing: Preparing People for Change*, 2nd edition. Guilford Publishing, New York, NY. 2002.
15. Miller WR, Rollnick S. *What is MI?* www.motivationalinterview.org
16. Miller WR. Motivation for treatment: a review with special emphasis on alcoholism. *Psych Bull* 1985;98:84–107.
17. Rollnick S, Miler WR, Butler CC. *Motivational Interviewing in Health Care*. Guilford Publishers, New York, NY. 2008.
18. Rose GS. Towards a theory of motivational interviewing. *Am Psychol* 2009;64:527–537.
19. Zimmerman GL, Olsen CG, Bosworth MF. A 'Stages of Change' approach to helping patients change behavior. *Am Fam Physician* 2000;61:1409–1416.
20. Rimal RN. Closing the knowledge-behavior gap in health promotion: the mediating role of self-efficacy. *Health Comm* 2000;12:219–237.
21. Woolf SH, Glasgow RE, Krist A, et al. Putting it together: finding success in behavior change through inegration of services. *Am Fam Med* 2005;3(Suppl 12)s20–s27.
22. Van Weel C. Morbidity in family medicine: the potential for individual nutritional counseling, an analysis from the Nijmegen Continuous Morbidity Registration. *Am J Clin Nutr* 1997;65(6 Suppl):1928S–1932S.
23. Moore, H, Adamson AJ, Gill T, et al. Nutrition and the health care agenda: a primary care perspective. *Family Practice* 2000;17:197–202.
24. Ockene IS, Hebert JR, Ockene JK, et al. Effect of physician-delivered nutrition counseling training and an office-support program on saturated fat intake, weight, and serum lipid measurements in a hyperlipidemic population: Worcester Area Trial for Counseling in Hyperlipidemia (WATCH). *Arch Intern Med* 1999;159:725–731.

Section 2
Nutrition During the Lifespan

4 Nutrition from Pre-conception Through Lactation

Amy McKeever, PhD, CRNP
Patricia Digiacomo, MSN, RNC
Lisa Hark, PhD, RD
Kathleen Larkins, MSN, CNS, RNC-OB

OBJECTIVES

- Review the physiological changes during pregnancy.
- Identify the current nutritional recommendations for pregnancy appropriate to the antepartum and post-partum mother.
- Recognize the medical and psychosocial issues that affect the nutritional status of the antepartum and lactating mother.
- Develop a plan of care for the appropriate antepartum and the lactating mother and incorporate the current American Dietetic Association recommendations.

Introduction

Adequate nutrition during pregnancy and lactation involves balancing the increased demands of the growing fetus and the energy requirements of the pregnant woman. The antenatal period is a critical time when maternal nutrition and dietary intake can influence fetal outcomes. Studies have linked maternal dietary deficiencies to premature birth, low birth weight, neural tube defects, maternal pre-eclampsia, obesity, and diabetes.[1] Additionally, research has indicated that higher maternal body mass index (BMI) in pregnancy and greater gestational weight gain are predictors of obesity risk for the offspring.[2] Since the goal of adequate nutrition during pregnancy and lactation is positive maternal and neonatal outcomes, the prenatal period provides an opportunity for Nurse Practitioners to assess adequate nutrition, evaluate healthy eating, and educate the antenatal patient regarding appropriate nutritional plans to meet the demands of pregnancy.[1,3,4]

This chapter reviews nutritional requirements before, during, and after pregnancy. Nurse Practitioners caring for pregnant women must recognize the risk factors for altered nutrition and nutritional deficiencies that may develop during pregnancy and lactation as well as the medical and psychosocial conditions that may impair the mother's nutritional status throughout the antepartum period.[1-5] In addition, poor antenatal nutrition has long-term health sequela for the mother and fetus.[6]

The Nurse Practitioner's Guide to Nutrition, Second Edition. Edited by Lisa Hark, Kathleen Ashton and Darwin Deen.

Obesity Rates in Pregnancy

Over the past 50 years, the number of women of reproductive age who are overweight (BMI > 25.0–29.9 kg/m²) has remained stable at approximately 30%.[7,8] Over the same time period, there has been an almost threefold increase in obesity rates (BMI > 30 kg/m²) from 13 to 35% in the same population.[9] This increase in obesity is disproportionately reflected in three minority populations; Hispanic, African American, and Native American women.[8] In 2009, the Institute of Medicine (IOM) published revised recommendations for weight gain in pregnancy that stressed the importance of: (1) achieving appropriate pre-gravid weight, (2) beginning pregnancy at a healthy weight, (3) all women having individualized pre-conception, prenatal and post-partum care to assist in attaining a healthy weight gain, within the guidelines, and (4) returning to a healthy pre-gravid weight after delivery.[5] All women should also have a nutrition assessment during their pre-conception phase with the goal of optimizing maternal, fetal, and infant health. Dietary changes should begin pre-conceptually with appropriate modifications throughout the antenatal period and then continuing into post-partum and lactation.[10] Antenatal patients who are identified as having dietary deficiencies pre-conceptually or during the antenatal period require a referral to a registered dietitian for nutrition counseling and management. Issues that warrant nutrition assessment and counseling before and during pregnancy are shown in Table 4-1.

Components of the Prenatal Evaluation

Conducting a comprehensive obstetric history, including a nutrition assessment, is essential at the first prenatal visit. This typically takes place at approximately 10 weeks gestation. This visit should include a comprehensive health history and physical examination.[11,12] A comprehensive nutrition history includes previous weight-gain patterns during pregnancy, prior history of nausea, vomiting, or hyperemesis during pregnancy, gestational diabetes, pre-eclampsia, anemia, pica (eating non-food items, e.g. ice, detergent, starch, chalk, clay, or rocks, etc.), and weight status (BMI).[13–15] Nurse Practitioners conducting a thorough evaluation of a woman's nutritional status

Table 4-1 Issues that Warrant Nutrition Assessment and Counseling

- Pregnancy involving multiple gestations (twins, triplets).
- Frequent gestations (less than a 3 month inter-pregnancy interval).
- Use of tobacco, alcohol, or chronic medicinal or illicit drugs.
- Severe nausea and vomiting (hyperemesis gravidarum).
- Eating disorders, including anorexia, bulimia, and compulsive eating.
- Inadequate weight gain during pregnancy.
- Adolescence.
- Restricted eating (vegetarianism, macrobiotic, raw food, vegan).
- Food allergies or food intolerances.
- Gestational diabetes mellitus (GDM) or history of GDM.
- Prior history of low-birth-weight babies or other obstetric complications.
- Social factors that may limit appropriate intake (e.g. religion, poverty).
- Obesity.

Source: Lisa Hark, PhD, RD and Darwin Deen, MD, MS, 2012. Used with permission.

prior to, and during pregnancy, will elicit dietary information including appetite status, meal patterns, dieting regimens, cultural or religious dietary practices, vegetarianism, food allergies, cravings and/or aversions. Questions about abnormal eating practices, such as following food fads, bingeing, purging, laxative or diuretic use, or pica should also be included.[14,16]

Other relevant information includes the habitual use of caffeine-containing beverages, tobacco, alcohol, recreational drug consumption, and any vitamin or herbal supplementation or alternative pharmacological therapies the woman may be consuming.[17] Information about dietary supplements may not be readily volunteered but their use may be inappropriate or dangerous during pregnancy, such as high intake of vitamin A. Nurse Practitioners should review their patient's current dietary intake by asking her to describe everything she ate and drank the day before, or have her complete a diet history questionnaire (Chapter 2).

The medical history should identify maternal risk factors for nutritional deficiencies (fad diets or eating disorders) or chronic diseases with nutritional implications (e.g. absorption disorders, eating disorders, metabolic disorders, infections, diabetes mellitus, PKU [phenylketonuria], sickle cell trait, or renal disease). Women who have had closely spaced pregnancies (i.e. less than a year between pregnancies) are at increased risk of having depleted nutrient reserves.[14] Maternal nutrient depletion may also be associated with an increased incidence of pre-term birth, intrauterine growth restriction (IUGR), and maternal mortality/morbidity.[18,19].

Once the medical history is completed, questions regarding professional, social, economic, and emotional stresses and specific religious practices may be included in the assessment (including dietary restrictions and fasting) since these factors may impact a woman's nutritional status. Some work environments adversely impact dietary intake, as they may provide inadequate time during the day to eat proper meals or allow access to nutritionally marginal food. For this reason, it is important to ask pregnant women about the conditions of their employment and identify limitations and potential solutions. Women with lower socio-economic status often need support to obtain nutritious food and referral to food assistance programs may be appropriate (e.g. Women, Infants, and Children Program [WIC]).

Assessing Nutrition Prior to Pregnancy

Nurse Practitioners may choose to institute nutrition counseling during pre-conceptual counseling sessions since many women are receptive to nutrition counseling just prior to or during pregnancy. Therefore, this is an opportune time to encourage the development of good nutrition and physical activity practices aimed at preventing future medical problems such as obesity, diabetes, hypertension, and osteoporosis. Elements of the nutrition assessment prior to pregnancy are listed in Table 4-2 and pre-conception nutrition counseling recommendations are shown in Table 4-3.

Nutritional Recommendations During Pregnancy

Adequate nutrition is important before conception as well as during the pregnancy. Inadequate nutrient intake during the first 2 months of pregnancy may lead to

Table 4-2 Assessing Nutrition Prior to Pregnancy

- Gravidity and parity.
- Obstetrical history (extensive pregnancy history, dates, length of pregnancy complications, outcomes).
- Obstetrical complication summary (infections in pregnancy, anemia, medical conditions, low-birth-weight babies, large for gestational age babies, spontaneous abortions, neonatal deaths, weight patterns in pregnancies, nausea/vomiting, hyperemesis, PICA).
- Post-partum infections.
- Lactation history.
- Medical conditions affection absorption (PKU, eating disorders, metabolic disorders, diabetes mellitus, renal disease, sickle cell trait).
- Pre-term deliveries.
- Nicotine use.
- Substance use.
- Caffeine intake.
- Herbal supplement use.
- Chronic medicinal use.
- Work environment.
- Cultural/religious practices.

Source: ACOG[20], Viswanathan et al.[21]

Table 4-3 Preconception Nutrition Counseling Recommendations

- Obtain an optimal pre-pregnancy weight.
- Increase folic acid supplementation (1 mg/day).
- Include a daily prenatal vitamin at time of conception.
- Limit caffeine intake (<200 mg/day).
- Eliminate vitamin A supplementation.
- Eliminate nicotine use.
- Eliminate alcohol and recreational drug use.
- Eliminate mega-doses of vitamin and mineral supplements.
- Eliminate herbs and natural substances.

Source: ACOG[20], AAOP[22], Lee.[23]

teratogenic effects or to spontaneous abortion.[5,18] After the second month, inadequate nutrition can inhibit fetal growth causing small for gestational age (SGA) or intrauterine growth retardation (IUGR). After 24 weeks gestation, inadequate nutrition can increase the chance of premature birth and decrease fetal stores of essential nutrients, mostly iron, magnesium, and calcium.[24,25] Generally, folic acid and iron supplementation are the only recommended supplements during pregnancy.

Maternal Nutrient Needs: Current Recommendations (RDA Shown in Appendices S and T)

Energy

Daily caloric requirements have been estimated by dividing the gross energy cost (80 000 kcal) by the approximate duration of pregnancy (250 days after the first month), producing an average additional 300 kcal/day for the entire pregnancy. During the first trimester, total energy expenditure does not change greatly and weight gain is minimal assuming the woman began her pregnancy without depleted body reserves. Therefore, additional energy intake is recommended primarily in the second and third trimesters. Current recommendations are an additional 340 kcal/day above the non-pregnant energy requirements during the second trimester and 452 kcal/day during the third trimester.[26]

Protein

Additional protein is required during pregnancy for fetal, placental, and maternal tissue development. Maternal protein synthesis increases in order to support expansion of the blood volume, uterus, and breasts.[26] Protein retention increases fivefold from the first to the second trimester and about 80% from the second to the third trimester with a total of approximately 925 g of protein retained during pregnancy.[26] Protein recommendations are therefore increased from 46 g/day for an adult, non-pregnant woman to 71 g/day during pregnancy.[26] This represents a change in protein recommendation from 0.8 g/kg/day for non-pregnant women to 1.1 g/kg/day during pregnancy.[5]

Polyunsaturated Fatty Acids

Humans cannot synthesize polyunsaturated fatty acids with double bonds (omega-3 and omega-6), therefore they must be obtained from the diet as either linoleic (omega-6) or alpha linolenic (omega-3) which are converted to eicosapentaenoic (EPA) and docosahexaenoic acid (DHA). There are numerous studies reporting the beneficial effects of omega-3 fatty acids on lipid levels, cardiovascular and immune function (Chapter 8). During pregnancy omega-3 fatty acids support pregnancy and healthy baby development. Adequate intake of omega-3 fatty acids during pregnancy and the post-natal period has been shown to reduce the incidence of premature birth and miscarriages.[27,28] Women who have been supplemented also have reduced incidence of pre-term labor and intrauterine infection rates, which have been linked to the reduction in the inflammatory marker interleukin-10 and interleukin-13 in the fetus.[29,30] Infants born to women who continue to consume DHA and EPA supplements while breastfeeding, have shown improvements in cognitive function, visual acuity, attention span, and sleep patterns.[31] The availability of the DHA and EPA to the fetus depends on maternal dietary intake as well as placental function.[32,33]

Although the US expert panel recommends that pregnant women consume at least 300 mg/day of DHA, the mean intake of DHA for pregnant and lactating women was only 52 mg/day and 20 mg/day for EPA.[34,35] This may in part be explained by the decrease in fish consumption after the Food and Drug Administration (FDA) issued an advisory aimed at pregnant women to avoid consuming fish due to high levels of mercury and raw fish which may contain food-borne illness.[36,37] High levels of mercury can affect the developing nervous system in a fetus and young child.[37] Advise pregnant and lactating mothers to consume less than 12 ounces of a variety of fish per week.[38] Five of the most commonly eaten fish low in mercury are shrimp, canned light tuna, salmon, pollock, and catfish. Fish high in mercury are shark, swordfish, king mackerel, and tile fish.[38] Flaxseed is a source of omega-3 fatty acids and some medical experts recommend that women avoid flaxseed and flaxseed oils during pregnancy or while breastfeeding since it is a plant source of phytoestrogens.[39,40] It is therefore important for the Nurse Practitioner to assess dietary consumption of DHA and EPA products during pregnancy and post-partum while breastfeeding. Once the assessment is complete the Nurse Practitioner can provide patient education regarding the types of foods that contain DHA and EPA, and develop a plan to increase omega-3 fatty acids during pregnancy. Food sources of omega-3 fatty acids are shown in Appendix M.

Vitamin A

Vitamin A is a fat-soluble vitamin and refers to compounds or mixtures of compounds having vitamin A activity. Severe vitamin A deficiency is rare in the US and an adequate intake of vitamin A is readily available in a healthy diet. Vitamin A deficiency during pregnancy weakens the immune system, increases risk of infections and has been linked with night blindness.[19] However, increasing dietary intake of vitamin A, rather than using supplements, is advised since excess retinol intake is a known human teratogen.[19,41] Critical periods for damage from birth defects appear during the first trimester and are related to abnormalities in the cranial neural crest cells.[42] Over-the-counter multivitamin supplements may contain excessive doses of vitamin A and thus should be discontinued during pregnancy. Additionally, topical creams that contain retinol derivatives, commonly used to treat acne, should be avoided during pregnancy and in women trying to get pregnant. Doses exceeding 15 000 µg/day are associated with an increased risk of birth defects and should not be used in pregnancy.[42] Monthly pregnancy tests are a standard of care for women receiving these medications.

Folate

Folate and its metabolically active form tetrahydrofolate function as coenzymes involved in one-carbon transfer reactions that include the synthesis of nucleic acids and several amino acids.[43] Therefore, adequate levels of dietary folate are important during pregnancy to support rapid cell growth, replication, cell division, and nucleotide synthesis for fetal and placental development.[44] The increased demand for folate during pregnancy is also related to maternal erythropoesis, mainly during the second and third trimesters. However, since embryonic neural tube closure is complete by 18–26 days after conception, it is especially crucial that pregnant women consume adequate folate before and during the first 4 weeks of pregnancy.[44] Unfortunately, folate deficiency is the most prevalent vitamin deficiency during pregnancy, with well-known associations with birth defects.[45,46]

Spina bifida and anencephaly, the two most common types of neural tube defects (NTD), occur in approximately 3000 pregnancies (0.76/1000 births) each year in the US.[47] Women who have had a previous pregnancy affected by a NTD or who are personally affected by a NTD are at a higher risk (2–3%) in a current pregnancy.[43] Supplementation with 4000 µg/day (4 mg/day) of folate, initiated one month prior to attempting to conceive and continued throughout the first trimester of pregnancy, has been shown to reduce the risk of a repeat NTD by 72%.[44,48] Several controlled and observational trials have shown that periconceptional and early pregnancy consumption of folate supplements can reduce a woman's risk for having an infant with an NTD by as much as 50–70%.[45] Food sources of folate are shown in Appendix F.

Case 1

Patty is a 32-year-old married woman who has missed her period and discovers that she is pregnant. This was an unplanned pregnancy and her first prenatal visit is scheduled at 5 weeks gestation (normal gestation period is 40 weeks). Patty's previous delivery was by cesarean section and she had a normal delivery. Her infant weighed 7.5 lb (3.4 kg) at birth. She is not hypertensive and has no history of pregnancy-induced hypertension during her previous gestation. Her 1-hour glucose tolerance test at 28 weeks was normal in her prior pregnancy. She currently takes no medications, vitamins, minerals, or herbal supplements. She denies any allergies or sensitivities to medications or foods. Patty stays at home to care for her 2-year-old daughter. She reports having little free time to exercise. She does not smoke or drink alcohol. She is 5'6" (168 cm) and her current weight is 145 lb (66 kg). BMI: 23.5.

PROBLEM: On most days, Patty's diet consists of a bagel with cream cheese and coffee for breakfast, a turkey breast sandwich and diet coke with pretzels for lunch and fish or chicken for dinner with either corn or pasta. She snacks on frozen yogurt before bed. Patty has a significant family history of neural tube defects and her diet only contains 238 μg of folate, well below her recommended intake. Patty's sister-in-law (her husband's sister) had a miscarriage at 24-weeks gestation and the baby was found to have anencephaly, a type of neural tube defect. She does not usually eat vegetables and fruits and does not drink juice.

ADVICE: By following the *My Plate* suggestions to eat three to five servings of vegetables, two to four servings of fruits, and six to 11 servings of grain daily, Patty would be able to increase her folate intake. Recommended dietary modifications could include either adding orange juice or a fresh orange or grapefruit to breakfast, carrots sticks to lunch, and a green vegetable, such as broccoli or asparagus to dinner. In addition to these naturally occurring sources of folate, a ready-to-eat fortified breakfast cereal could contribute significantly to Patty's folate intake. Folate is also contained in whole grains such as oatmeal or oat bran cereals, wheat germ, whole grain breads, and brown rice that could easily be incorporated into Patty's diet. She should also be prescribed a prenatal vitamin supplement containing 1 mg of folic acid.

Vitamin D

Vitamin D intake is essential for proper absorption of calcium and normal bone health. During pregnancy, vitamin D is also critically important for fetal growth and development as well as for the regulation of genes associated with normal implantation and angiogenesis.[49-52] Low maternal vitamin D status has been associated with reduced intrauterine long bone growth, shorter gestation, reduced childhood bone-mineral accrual, and decreased birth weight.[52-54] Low maternal vitamin D status may also have consequences for fetal "imprinting" that may affect neurodevelopment, immune function, and chronic disease susceptibility later in life as well as soon after birth.[51,55] Maternal vitamin D status may also be an independent risk factor for pre-eclampsia and supplementation may be helpful in promoting neonatal well-being and preventing pre-eclampsia.[56] To evaluate vitamin D levels prior to and during pregnancy, check serum 25(OH)D levels and aim for vitamin D levels greater than 30 nmol/l and prescribe 1000–5000 mg/day of vitamin D_3 depending on the level of deficiency.[25,51,57] Food sources of vitamin D are shown in Appendix B.

Calcium

Large quantities of calcium are essential for the development of the fetal skeleton, fetal tissues, and hormonal adaptations during pregnancy. These include changes in calcium regulatory hormones affecting intestinal absorption, renal reabsorption of calcium, and bone turnover of calcium.[58] The presence of $1,25(OH)_2D_3$ stimulates increased intestinal absorption of calcium during the second and third trimesters, protecting maternal bone, while meeting fetal calcium requirements. Fetal calcium needs are highest during the third trimester, when the fetus absorbs an average of 300 mg/day in response to the increased maternal $1,25(OH)_2D_3$.[58] Studies suggest that inadequate calcium during pregnancy is associated with gestational hypertension, pre-term delivery, and pre-eclampsia.[59,60]

Consuming at least three servings of dairy foods every day, including calcium fortified juices and soy beverages, can help meet these requirements.[14] Women who limit their intake of dairy foods because of lactose intolerance seem to be able to tolerate yogurt and cheese on a daily basis, but may also require a supplement. The standard prenatal vitamin typically contains 150–300 mg/serving. Calcium carbonate, gluconate, lactate, or citrate may provide 500–600 mg/day of calcium to account for the difference between the amount of calcium required and that consumed. Food sources of calcium are shown in Appendices G and H.

Iron

Iron is an essential component of hemoglobin production and requirements increase significantly during pregnancy. Additional iron is needed to expand maternal red cell mass by 20–30% as well as for fetal and placental tissue production. Throughout pregnancy, an additional 450 mg of iron is delivered to the maternal marrow and 250 mg is lost in blood during delivery. Therefore, approximately 1000 mg is required during pregnancy and the RDA has been established at 27 g/day compared with 18 mg/day for non-pregnant women. Food sources of iron are shown in Appendix L.

According to the CDC, screening for anemia should take place prior to pregnancy, as well as during the first, second, and third trimester in high-risk individuals as shown in Table 4-4. Iron deficiency anemia increases the risk of maternal and infant death, pre-term delivery, low neonatal birth weight, and has negative consequences

Table 4-4 Diagnosis of Anemia in Pregnancy

Lab test	1st Trimester	2nd Trimester	3rd Trimester
Hemoglobin (g/dL)	<11	10.5	<11
Hematocrit (%)	<33	32	<33

Source: Centers for Disease Control and Prevention: Iron Deficiency (www.cdc.gov).[65]

for normal infant brain development and function.[61,62] The prevalence of iron deficiency in pregnancy is higher in African-American women, low-income women, teenagers, women with less than a high school education, and women with multiple parity.[63] *Healthy People 2020* goals include reducing anemia among pregnant females in their third trimester from 29 to 20% and reducing ethnic and income disparities.[3] Hemoglobin <11 g/dL or hematocrit below 33% in the first or third trimester indicate anemia. Hemoglobin <10.5 g/dL or hematocrit below 32% in the second trimester also indicates anemia.[65] As the significant increase in maternal blood volume during pregnancy typically reduces hemoglobin levels, serum ferritin and mean corpuscular volume should be used as diagnostic criteria as these measures are not affected by the increased blood volume. Serum ferritin is also useful in assessing the post-gastric bypass pregnant patient. A serum ferritin level of <15 ng/mL warrants aggressive treatment and may require intramuscular injection rather than oral supplementation.

Nutrition and Substance Abuse During Pregnancy
Alcohol
Each year in the US, at least 500 000 fetuses are exposed to alcohol, a known teratogen.[66] Alcohol consumption varies widely during pregnancy, but approximately 10 of every 1000 live births are negatively affected by alcohol.[67] Excessive alcohol consumption can result in fetal alcohol syndrome (FAS), manifesting as microcephaly, cleft palate, and micrognathia. Maternal alcoholism contributes to fetal nutritional deficiencies by inhibiting maternal absorption of nutrients and providing a toxic environment for the developing fetus. According to the ACOG, there is no known safe level of alcohol consumption during pregnancy. Therefore, it is currently recommended that alcohol intake be avoided by pregnant women and women attempting to become pregnant (www.acog.org). In addition, the Council on Science and Public Health of the American Medical Association recommends abstinence from alcohol throughout pregnancy.[68]

Cigarette Smoking
There are over 4000 chemicals produced from a cigarette, with some chemicals being known carcinogens. Nicotine is primarily metabolized in the liver, eliminated by the kidneys, and can easily cross the placenta with fetal concentrations that are generally 15% higher than maternal levels.[69] Nicotine consumption during pregnancy has been consistently associated with low neonatal birth weight, pre-term delivery, and spontaneous abortion.[15] Smokers have a 40% higher risk of pre-term births than non-smokers.[70] Recent research has shown a correlation between smoking during pregnancy and childhood asthma, obesity, and sudden infant death syndrome (SIDS).[71] These risks are associated with maternal smoking in late pregnancy.[72] If women who smoke become pregnant, they should be advised to discontinue cigarette smoking.

Caffeine
Caffeine is metabolized more slowly in pregnancy and passes readily through the placenta to the fetus.[69,73] Women who consume 200 mg of caffeine daily are twice as likely as women who consume no caffeine to have a miscarriage.[17] According to the March of Dimes, women who are pregnant or trying to become pregnant should limit

Table 4-5 Nutrition Counseling Recommendations During Pregnancy

- Eat a healthy diet with at least five servings of fruits and vegetables daily.
- Eat three meals per day and avoid skipping meals.
- Consume three servings of dairy foods daily.
- Increase omega-3 fat intake.
- Increase folic acid supplementation (1 mg/day).
- Take a daily prenatal vitamin.
- Limit caffeine intake (<200 mg/day).
- Avoid vitamin A supplementation.
- Avoid nicotine use.
- Avoid alcohol and recreational drug use.
- Avoid mega-doses of vitamin and mineral supplements.
- Avoid herbs and natural substances.
- Avoid consuming flax seed.

Source: ACOG[20], AAOP.[22]

their caffeine intake to no more than 200 mg/day (www.marchofdimes.com). This is equivalent to about one 12-ounce cup of coffee. The FDA recommends pregnant women reduce their caffeine intake from all sources, including teas, hot cocoa, chocolate, energy drinks, coffee ice cream, and soda (FDA). Therefore, it is best to advise decaffeinated beverage consumption for women who are pregnant or trying to become pregnant. Nutrition counseling recommendations during pregnancy are shown in Table 4-5.

Maternal Weight-Gain Recommendations

Maternal weight gain is attributable both to increases in the mother's tissue (increased circulating blood volume, breast mass, uterine size) and feto-placental growth within the uterus (increased size of the fetus, placenta, and amniotic fluid volume).[74] During the first half of gestation, weight gain primarily reflects changes in maternal stores and fluid status. In the second half of gestation, weight gain is the result of a continued increase in maternal stores and fluid, as well as fetal growth.[14] Rapid weight gain near the end of gestation, after approximately 32 weeks, often represents the accumulation of tissue edema. The rate of weight gain during pregnancy is important because maternal weight gain and infant birth weight are correlated. Most weight gain should occur in the second and early third trimesters (18–30 weeks). Adequate weight gain in the second trimester of pregnancy appears to be predictive of fetal and neonatal weight, even if weight gain is inadequate during the remainder of the pregnancy.[15,75] However, 60% of pregnant women fail to gain the recommended amount of weight during pregnancy. Excess weight gain increases post-partum obesity and obesity during pregnancy increases the risk of overweight newborns.[76] Weight gain recommendations are shown in Table 4-6.

Low Pre-Conception BMI (Underweight)

Women with low pre-conception BMI (<18.5 kg/m²) are at risk for delivering low-birth-weight infants and/or developing toxemia. The IOM recommends that women

Table 4-6 Recommendations for Gestational Weight Gain With Single Pregnancies Based on Pre-Pregnancy Body Mass Index

Pre-pregnancy Body Mass Index (kg/m²)	Total Gestational Weight Gain (lb)
Underweight (<18.5)	28–40
Normal weight (18.5–24.9)	25–35
Overweight (25.0–29.9)	15–25
Obese (≥30.0)	11–20

Source: Sheih, 2011[4], IOM, 2009.[5]

with low pre-pregnancy body mass indices (BMI < 18.5 kg/m²) should increase their caloric intake substantially to attain a weight gain between 28 and 40 lb during the course of pregnancy.[5] However, this may be unrealistic in many cases. A woman with a BMI of less than 18.5 kg/m² who is considering pregnancy should be encouraged to gain weight before conceiving. Protein-calorie supplementation may assist in correcting pre-conception nutritional deficits and provide adequate nutrients for fetal development. Inadequate weight gain (<2 lb/month during the second and third trimesters) is associated with low-birth-weight infants, IUGR, and fetal complications. Inhibited fetal growth usually correlates with inadequate weight gain. Women with inadequate weight gain or weight loss should have repeated and thorough nutritional evaluations. Careful diet histories should be taken to determine the adequacy of dietary intake and supplementation prescribed as necessary.[77]

Overweight and Obesity

In pregnancy, obesity increases the risk of less than optimal reproductive outcomes and increases the risk of maternal complications and the chance of spontaneous abortions.[78,79] Pre-pregnancy obesity increases the chance of congenital problems, such as neural tube defects, macrosomia, stillbirth, childhood obesity, and metabolic syndrome as an adult.[13,77,80,81] Obesity in pregnancy places the mother at risk for gestational diabetes, hypertensive disorders, shoulder dystocia, cesarean birth, and post-partum complications of hemorrhage, infection, and depression.[13,80,82,83]

Women with high pre-conception BMI (>25 kg/m²) are at risk for developing diabetes, hypertension, and thromboembolic events, and for delivering macrosomic infants (> 4000 g or 8 lb, 13 oz). Although there is considerable controversy regarding the management of pregnancy in obese women, the current guidelines call for limited maternal weight gain of up to 15 lb in obese women. To avoid inadequate intake of crucial nutritional components, which can adversely impact both mother and fetus, pregnant women with BMI > 30 kg/m² should limit their weight gain during the course of their pregnancies.[20] However, they should not severely restrict their caloric intake such that the nutrients required to sustain a healthy pregnancy are insufficient. Even in severe obesity carbohydrate recommendations are 175 g/day.

Adequate consumption of omega-3 fatty acids, calcium, iron, folate, B vitamins, and protein are particularly crucial during pregnancy, regardless of maternal weight. If caloric intake is inadequate, ingested proteins are catabolized for energy needs and are therefore unavailable for maternal and fetal protein synthesis. An estimated 32 kcal/kg/day is necessary for optimal use of ingested protein. Severe restriction of caloric intake, or severe restriction of and/or carbohydrate intake, can result in ketosis, which is detrimental for the developing fetus. Studies have also suggested an association between ketosis and reduced uterine blood flow. Ketone bodies are concentrated in amniotic fluid and absorbed by the developing fetus. The mental development of children whose mothers have had ketonuria during pregnancy has been shown to be stunted, although the direct causal link between fetal ketosis and inhibited mental development has yet to be definitively established.[84]

Rapid and excessive weight accumulation is usually the result of fluid retention, which is associated with, but does not cause, toxemia. Fluid retention in the absence of hypertension or proteinuria is not an indication for salt restriction or diuretic therapy, but women who retain fluid should be monitored for other signs of toxemia. Edema in the lower extremities is caused by the accumulation of interstitial fluid secondary to obstruction of the pelvic veins and commonly occurs during the later stages of pregnancy.[85] Nurse Practitioners should instruct the mother with edema in the lower extremities to elevate the legs and wear support hose.

Excessive weight gain during pregnancy may also be caused by fat deposition. As excessive weight gain is associated with both maternal and fetal morbidities, weight gain that exceeds the recommendations appropriate for pre-conception BMI should be monitored. A careful dietary history should be taken to determine the source of excess weight gain, and recommendations for dietary changes should be offered accordingly.[14] Preliminary evidence supports the case of a low glycemic index diet for weight control during pregnancy rather than a low fat diet.

Conditions Affecting Nutritional Status of Pregnant Women

The Adolescent Patient

It is very important to obtain detailed risk assessments for adolescent pregnant patients due to their complex emotional, social, and economic concerns. Important factors to assess in pregnant adolescents include: excessive pre-pregnancy weight, anemia, unhealthy lifestyles (smoking, drugs, alcohol), history of eating disorders, and young age at menarche. Both the pattern of weight gain and the total weight gain are especially significant among pregnant adolescents. Inadequate weight gain before 24 weeks gestation, regardless of total pregnancy weight gain, has been associated with low-birth-weight among infants born to adolescent mothers. Due to an adolescent's anatomic and physiologic immaturity, if an adolescent becomes pregnant less than 4 years after menarche, she will be at increased nutritional risk.[29] Younger adolescents may need to gain additional weight (above the amount recommended for their pre-conception BMIs) in order to support their own normal growth during the course of their pregnancies. Iron and calcium supplements should be prescribed for adolescent pregnant patients (see Appendix T for RDA for pregnant and lactating adolescents). Pregnant adolescents who consume diets that consist of large amounts of carbohydrates and limited amounts of protein and fat seem to have a reduced risk of delivering low-birth-weight infants or pre-term infants as compared with pregnant adolescents who consume diets lower in carbohydrates.[86,87]

Multiple Gestations

Evidence supports a link between optimal maternal nutrition and weight gain and improved outcomes in multiple gestations including reduced risk of low-birth-weight infants.[5,88] Early weight gain during the first trimester is important to build maternal nutrient stores for later placental growth. Optimal outcomes (birth weight ≥ 2500 g) have been associated with a maternal weight gain of 24 lb by 24 weeks gestation.[89,90] With multiple fetuses, there is an increased depletion of the woman's nutritional reserves. These include increased plasma volume, increased basal metabolic rate, and increased insulin resistance.[91] The Institute of Medicine recommendations for gestational weight gain with twin pregnancies are based on pre-pregnancy BMI.[5,88] No guidelines are available for women with a BMI less than 18.5.

Recommendations are as follows:

- Normal weight (BMI: 18.5–24.9): gain: 37–54 lb.
- Overweight (BMI: 25.0–29.9): gain: 31–50 lb.
- Obese (BMI: ≥30.0): gain: 25–42 lb.

There is an increase in maternal resting expenditure by 10% in twin pregnancies and, therefore, a 40% increase in caloric requirements is necessary to meet the nutritional demands. The larger placenta results in an increase in placental hormone and steroid production which leads to greater maternal carbohydrate use and depletion of maternal hepatic glycogen stores. This may lead to maternal ketonemia. A low glycemic index diet with 40% carbohydrates, 40% fat, and 20% protein with a caloric intake of 3000–4000/day (based on pre-pregnancy BMI) has been recommended.[89] This dietary intake should be divided into three meals and three snacks to decrease the chance of hypoglycemia and ketosis. The importance of nutrition continues after the delivery of twin gestation to support breastfeeding.[92,93] Nutritional recommendations during a twin pregnancy are shown in Table 4-7.

Twins are at risk for decreased fetal growth and premature labor in which case micronutrient supplementation may have significant benefits. There is little research on twin micronutrient supplementation; however, based on the expectations of

Table 4-7 Twin Pregnancy Nutritional Recommendations

	Underweight	Normal Weight	Overweight	Obese
Calories (kcal/day)	4000	3000–3500	3250	2700–3000
Protein (g/day)	200	175	163	150
Carbohydrate (g/day)	400	350	325	300
Fat (g/day)	178	156	144	133

Source: Goodnight, 2009.[91]

Table 4-8 Twin Pregnancy Micronutrient Supplementation Requirements

	First Trimester	Second Trimester	Third Trimester
MV with iron (30 mg/day elemental tablets)	1	2	2
Calcium (mg/day)	1500	2500	2500
Vitamin D (IU/day)	1000	1000	1000
Magnesium (mg/day)	400	800	800
Zinc (mg/day)	15	30	30
DHA/EPA (mg/day)	300–500	300–500	300–500
Folic acid (mg/day)	1	1	1
Vitamin C (mg/day)	500–1000	500–1000	500–1000
Vitamin E (IU/day)	400	400	400

Source: Goodnight, 2009.[91]

similar or higher requirements for twin versus singleton pregnancies, additional supplements are recommended.[91] Table 4-8 lists supplementation needs.

Hypertension During Pregnancy

It is important that Nurse Practitioners provide the hypertensive pregnant patient with additional nutritional guidance on a well-balanced diet including increasing the amount of protein, limiting sodium, and encouraging the proper amount of vitamin D supplementation.

The pregnant hypertensive patient needs to have a well-balanced diet high in protein to promote cellular growth and to replace any protein lost in the urine. Sodium intake should not exceed 1.5 g/day.[5] Current research supports the importance of vitamin D in lowering the risk of pre-eclampsia. In the US, a 20 ng/mL or lower 25(OH)D concentration of vitamin D doubled the risk of pre-eclampsia.[94] In Norway, a vitamin D intake of 600–800 IU/day, compared with an intake of <200 IU/day, lowered the risk of pre-eclampsia in pregnant women.[95] The IOM Committee (2009) has increased their recommendation of vitamin D intake from 200 IU/day to 600 IU/day.[5]

Pregnancy Following Gastric Bypass Surgery (Chapter 7)

Pregnant women who have had gastric bypass surgery should be monitored closely for nutrient malabsorption and malnutrition.[96] Although their risk of complications is less than an obese patient, women who are post-bariatric surgery are at risk for anemia, gestational diabetes, pre-eclampsia, and cesarean birth.[97] The most common risk factors for the fetus include premature birth, low-birth-weight, macrosomia, and perinatal mortality.[98,99] There is one case report in the literature of maternal and fetal death post-gastric bypass due to an intestinal infarction.[100] Most clinicians recommend that women of childbearing age avoid pregnancy for at least one year after gastric bypass. Adjustable gastric banding (AGB) for women planning conception is often the recommended procedure because of the importance of vitamin and mineral requirements during pregnancy.[101] Following bariatric surgery, the pregnant woman is at increased risk of vitamin B$_{12}$, folate, iron, vitamin D, and calcium deficiencies.[13]

For patients who have had a Roux-en-Y procedure, laboratory values such as vitamin B_{12}, CBC, and comprehensive metabolic panels should be checked monthly. To reduce the risk of dumping syndrome, screening for gestational diabetes is done using 2-hour post-prandial blood glucose measure rather than a one hour glucola or 3-hour oral glucose tolerance tests. Many patients require folate in doses of up to 2 g/day, and vitamin B_{12} supplementation when levels consistently fall below 80 pg/mL.[102] More research is needed to develop guidelines for pregnancy after bariatric surgery (Chapter 7).

Diabetes During Pregnancy

Women with type 1 diabetes mellitus (DM) must be diligent to avoid both hypoglycemia and hyperglycemia with ketosis during pregnancy.[103] Fetal glucose utilization may also cause maternal fasting hypoglycemia. Therefore, it is especially important that women who enter pregnancy with type 1 DM understand the importance of frequently monitoring their blood sugar.[87,104,105] Women with pre-diabetes or type 2 diabetes who become pregnant may develop increased insulin resistance and may require additional insulin to control their diabetes (Chapter 9).

Nurse Practitioners need to include pre-conception nutrition counseling for pregnant women with diabetes. Strict blood glucose control prior to conception (minimum of 2 months) and during the first 3 months of pregnancy has been shown to reduce the risk of significant infant anomalies.[106] The incidence of infants born with congenital anomalies from mothers who have diabetes is 5–10% and usually includes cardiac, central nervous system, and skeletal system defects.[107] The American College of Obstetrics and Gynecology (ACOG) recommends maintaining a fasting blood glucose less than 95 mg/dL and a 2-hour post-prandial glucose less than 120 mg/dL to decrease the risk of perinatal mortality and congenital anomalies.[5]

Pregnant women with diabetes are also at increased risk of having a miscarriage or spontaneous abortion secondary to inadequate glycemic control during the embryonic phase.[108,109] When maternal insulin secretion cannot accommodate normal pregnancy induced glucose intolerance, gestational diabetes mellitus (GDM) results. GDM is usually diagnosed during the second or third trimester of pregnancy, at which time insulin-antagonist hormone levels increase, usually resulting in insulin resistance. After delivery, approximately 90% of all women with GDM become normoglycemic.[87] Research indicates that 35–75% of these patients will have GDM during their subsequent pregnancy and 50% of these patients will likely develop type 2 diabetes over the 15–20 years following pregnancy.[110] Reducing BMI after pregnancy decreases a women's risk of becoming diabetic by 25%.[108]

Risk factors for GDM include obesity, family history of diabetes, prior history of gestational diabetes, and the presence glycosuria.[111] The diagnosis of GDM is crucial in preventing perinatal morbidity and mortality.[112] The current practice is to screen all pregnant patients for GDM between 24 and 28 weeks gestation.[113] Risk factors alone may fail to identify up to 50% of patients with GDM.[87] According to the American Diabetes Association women with low-risk status do not require glucose testing.[114] There is limited research to support screening for GDM prior to 24 weeks gestation.[115]

Table 4-9 Nutrition Counseling Recommendations for Gestational Diabetes

---

- Maintain consistent carbohydrate intake at each meal and snack:
  - 130 g/day of carbohydrates during pre-conception and the first trimester of pregnancy
  - 175 g/day of carbohydrates during the second and third trimesters
- High fiber, 28 g/day, from whole grains, fruits, and vegetables.
- Limit simple sugars to less than 10% of total calories.
- Maintain reasonable body weight:
  - Add 300 calories/day during second and trimesters
  - Obese patients should subtract 500 calories/day.
- Eat at similar times each day.
- Control portion sizes.
- ACOG recommends the following calorie distribution: 10–20% at breakfast, 5–10% at mid-morning snack, 20–30% at lunch, 5–10% at mid-afternoon snack, 30–40% at dinner, and 5–10% at bedtime snack.
- The bedtime snack is most important and should include complex carbohydrates and protein to prevent night-time hypoglycemia.
- Include initiating insulin therapy in patients who fail to maintain a fasting plasma glucose ≤105 mg/dL, or 1-hour post-prandial plasma glucose ≤155 mg/dL, or 2-hour post-prandial plasma glucose ≤130 mg/dL.

Source: Adapted from the ADA.[116]

There is a two-step approach for the glucose challenge test. The first measure is performed 1-hour after a 50 g oral glucose load. A threshold level greater than or equal to 130 mg/dL for the 1-hour screen should be used. Roughly 20% of patients will test positive, and these patients will require a second screening during a 3-hour, 100 g glucose load. The diagnosis of GDM is made when two or more serum glucose values are outside the normal range proposed by the American Diabetes Association; less than 95 mg/dl for fasting glucose, less than 180 mg/dl 1-hour post-100 g glucose, less than 155 mg/dl 2-hour post-100 g glucose, and less than 140 mg/dl 4-hours post-100 g glucose.

Key points for education of pregnant women with GDM are shown in Table 4-9. Consulting a nutritionist to work with the diabetic patient to develop meal plans based on the patient's lifestyle, cultural, and ethnic food preferences is essential for a low-risk pregnancy.[116] HbA1C levels should be monitored during a woman's pre-conception, first prenatal visit, and every 2–3 months throughout the pregnancy.[103,117] HbA1C values above 10% are associated with an increased chance of congenital anomaly at rates of 20–25%. Nutritional goals in caring for pregnant women who are diabetic include strict blood glucose control, maintaining or obtaining an appropriate BMI during pregnancy, proper nutrition, and absence of ketone bodies.[108]

Patients with serum glucose levels consistently above recommendations require insulin therapy to achieve normoglycemia. Recommendations include initiating insulin therapy in patients that fail to maintain a fasting glucose ≤ 105 mg/dL, or 1-hour post-prandial plasma glucose ≤ 155 mg/dL, or 2-hour post-prandial plasma glucose ≤ 130 mg/dL.[114] Recent data evaluating the use of second-generation sufonylureas (e.g. glyburide) are encouraging but they are not FDA approved for the treatment of GDM.[112,114]

The US Preventive Services Task Force found fair to good evidence that screening, combined with diet and insulin therapy can reduce the rate of fetal macrosomia in women with GDM.[118] Whether or not insulin therapy is implemented, the management goal should be to prevent the maternal and fetal complications associated with GDM. All women with GDM should receive nutrition counseling as standard of care.[103] Maternal complications include fetal macrosomia and resultant delivery complications (e.g. increased risk of cesarean section, operative vaginal delivery, shoulder dystocia). Fetal complications include possible increased incidence of fetal demise and ketonemia, which have been associated with lower IQ scores in children 2–5 years of age. The data remain inconclusive as to whether the complications are entirely preventable using the currently accepted therapies.

Promotion of breastfeeding is especially important as recent research shows it may provide protection from diabetes for both mothers and babies.[105,119] Breastfeeding increases HDL-cholesterol levels and decreases fasting and 2-hour post-prandial blood glucose levels.[120] Therefore, insulin requirements are less and carbohydrate and protein snacks may be necessary. Calories need to be increased to 500–800/day. Oral hypoglycemic medications are contraindicated during breastfeeding. Nurse Practitioners must assess risk for mastitis and nipple infections because the diabetic patient is at increased risk.[121]

Psychosocial Issues Affecting Nutritional Status

The US continues to have relatively high perinatal morbidity and mortality, compared with other developed countries. Thus, societal factors have an impact on pregnancy outcomes.[122] ACOG defines psychosocial issues as non-biomedical factors that affect mental and physical well-being. Maternal psychosocial and nutritional status in the early weeks of pregnancy can affect placental development (Table 4-10).[123] These factors can contribute to attitudes towards food, appetite, and knowledge deficit regarding the importance of food and nutrition. Nurse Practitioners should screen and assess for the following psychosocial factors each trimester and offer resources that the mother could access for support if indicated. In addition,

Table 4-10 Psychosocial Factors Affecting Pregnancy

- Age.
- Occupation/economic status.
- Educational level/access to information.
- Intimate partner violence.
- Stress.
- Depression/anxiety.
- Trauma.
- Unintended pregnancy.
- Marital status.
- Religious practices.
- Smoking.
- Alcohol.
- Chemical dependency.
- Homelessness.
- Exercise.
- Obesity.

Source: Sokol.[122]

Table 4-11 Social Factors Thought to Influence Diet

- Social support.
- Societal and cultural norms.
- Food and agricultural policies.
- Food assistance programs.
- Economic price systems.
- Knowledge and attitudes.
- Skills.

Source: *Healthy People*, 2020.[3]

Healthy People 2020 objectives include social factors thought to influence diet (Table 4-11).

Strategies for Managing Nausea, Vomiting, Heartburn, and Constipation

Nausea and vomiting during pregnancy are associated with increased levels of the pregnancy hormone human chorionic gonadotropin (hCG). HCG doubles every 48 hours in early pregnancy, peaking at about 12 weeks of gestation. Women are more likely to have nausea or vomiting during pregnancy if they have the following:[14,81,124]

- Pregnant with twins or higher multiples.
- History of nausea and vomiting in a previous pregnancy.
- History of nausea or vomiting as a side effect of taking birth control pills.
- History of motion sickness.
- Relative (mother or sister) who had morning sickness during pregnancy.
- History of migraine headaches.

Nausea affects about 70% of pregnant women and can impact quality of life. Of those women who experience nausea during early pregnancy, 2% require hospitalization for severe hyperemesis gravidarum.[125] In severe cases of hyperemesis gravidarum, total parental nutrition should be considered. According to ACOG, increasing consumption of protein and pyridoxine (vitamin B_6)-25 mg every 8 hours with or without doxylamine may provide effective treatments for mild cases.[126] It is important for Nurse Practitioners to provide patient education regarding how to manage morning sickness as shown in Table 4-12. This information may assist in improving the quality of life during the first trimester. Reflux esophagitis is also a common complaint during pregnancy and is caused by the increased abdominal pressure secondary to the enlarging uterus. Hormonal changes may relax the cardiac sphincter, permitting chyme to be redirected into the esophagus.

Recommendations for alleviating the symptoms of heartburn in pregnancy include: (1) elevating the head of the bed four inches, (2) avoiding meals or snacks 2–3 hours before reclining, (3) avoiding alcohol entirely, (4) avoiding acidic fruits, caffeine, carbonation and peppermint, (5) eating small, frequent meals, and (6) taking antacids as needed.

Table 4-12 Managing Morning Sickness

- Ingest ginger tea. Peel dime sized piece of ginger and place it in a cup of boiling water. Allow to boil for 5–8 minutes. Note: 2 g of dried ginger or 1 g of ginger syrup is the daily dosage allowed in the first trimester of pregnancy.[127]
- Drink warm ginger ale (sugar only, not artificial sweetener).
- Increase dietary consumption of foods rich in potassium and magnesium. (Appendix J and K).
- Try an acupressure wristband which stimulates the P6 acupuncture site. This site is located three finger widths above the wrist on the anterior side.[128]
- Eat foods high in carbohydrates such as dry crackers or toast in the morning.
- Eat frequent, small amounts of food throughout the day.
- Eat small, frequent, low fat meals and snacks (e.g., fruit, pretzels, yogurt, crackers).
- Avoid foods that may cause stomach irritation such as spearmint, peppermint, caffeine, citrus fruits, spicy foods, high-fat foods, or tomato products.
- Avoid eating or drinking for 1–2 hours before lying down.
- Take a walk after meals.
- Wear loose fitting clothes.
- Avoid fragrances, such as perfume, household cleaners, and air fresheners.
- Increase fluid intake to 2 or 3 quarts per day, including water, juice, milk, and soup.
- Increase daily dietary fiber intake through ingestion of high-fiber cereals, whole grains, legumes, fruits, and vegetables.
- Brush teeth after eating to prevent symptoms.

Source: Lisa Hark, PhD, RD, 2012. Used with permission.

Antacids do inhibit iron absorption, however, and should be used sparingly and only when all other management strategies have proven ineffective. The amount of calcium from antacids should be taken into consideration when assessing total calcium intake.[87] Nurse Practitioners should inform patients that antacids may contain aluminum and cause constipation, or magnesium which may cause diarrhea. Education should also include avoiding baking soda and Alka Seltzer because these may cause electrolyte disturbances.[29]

Constipation is common during pregnancy as a result of abdominal pressure from the enlarging uterus, hormonal changes, and iron supplementation. Smooth muscle relaxation and increased water reabsorption in the large intestine during pregnancy result in decreased gastrointestinal motility, compounding the problem of constipation. Constipation during pregnancy can cause marked discomfort, including bloating and aggravation of hemorrhoids. Strategies for managing constipation include increased fluid intake of two or three quarts daily, increased low-impact physical activity (e.g. walking, swimming, yoga), increased dietary fiber intake through food (e.g. in the form of high-fiber cereals, whole grains, legumes, fruits or vegetables), use of supplemental psyllium (Metamucil), and use of a stool softener in conjunction with iron supplements.[14]

Nurse Practitioners can also teach the antepartum patient to take special care regarding food safety as shown in Table 4-13. During pregnancy, the immune system is weakened, which makes it harder for the body to fight off harmful food-borne microorganisms that cause food-borne illness (Table 4-14). Unborn babies are at risk because bacteria can cross the placenta and infect the fetus.

Table 4-13 Key Points to Improve Food Safety

Clean
- Wash hands thoroughly with warm water and soap.
- Wash hands before and after handling food, and after using the bathroom, changing diapers, or handling pets.
- Wash cutting boards, dishes, and countertops with hot water and soap.
- Rinse raw fruits and vegetables thoroughly under running water.

Separate
- Separate raw meat, poultry, and seafood from ready-to-eat foods.
- If possible, use one cutting board for raw meat, poultry, and seafood and another one for fresh fruits and vegetables.
- Place cooked food on clean plate.

Cook
- Cook foods thoroughly.
- Use a food thermometer to check temperature.
- Keep foods out of the Danger Zone: the range of temperatures at which bacteria can grow (usually between 40 °F and 140 °F).
- 2-hour Rule: discard foods left out at room temperature for more than 2 hours.

Chill
- Your refrigerator should register at 40 °F or below and the freezer at 0 °F. Place an appliance thermometer in the refrigerator and check the temperature periodically.
- Refrigerate or freeze perishables.
- Use ready to eat perishable food (dairy, meat, poultry, seafood) as soon as possible.

Source: FDA[129], (CDC www.cdc.gov).[130]

Lactation

Breast milk is the optimal food source for infants. Nurse Practitioners have a responsibility to promote, protect, and support breastfeeding. Nurse Practitioners should understand the physiology of lactation, the process of lactogenesis, and the benefits of breastfeeding to the mother/baby dyad in order to optimally encourage and support pregnant women to breastfeed their babies when they are born. Position papers published by the American Academy of Pediatrics (AAP), American Dietetic Association (ADA), and the International Lactation Consultants Association (ILCA) provide guidance for clinicians in supporting breastfeeding efforts. The American Academy of Family Physicians (AAFP) also has very helpful guidelines on the clinical management of breastfeeding. The only contraindications for breastfeeding are shown in Table 4-15.

Composition of Breast Milk

Breast milk is species-specific (made for human infants) and offers many advantages over infant formula. The nutrients in breast milk are proportioned appropriately for the neonate and vary to meet the newborn's changing needs. Breast milk changes composition according to gestational age at birth and continues transformation throughout the stages of development in the infant's life (Table 4-16). Breast milk provides protection against infection and is easily digested.[135]

Table 4-14 Food-Borne Illnesses

Food-Borne Illness	Sources	Fetal Effects	Maternal Effects	Recommendation
Listeriosis: a harmful bacterium that can grow at refrigerator temperatures	Soil Groundwater Plants Animals Refrigerated, ready to eat foods and unpasteurized milk and milk products	Chorioamnionitis Premature labor Spontaneous abortion Fetal demise	Fever Chills Headache Muscle and backaches GI symptoms	Avoid: hot dogs, luncheon meats, bologna, or other deli meats unless they are reheated until steaming hot. Refrigerated pate, meat spreads from a meat counter, or smoked seafood in the refrigerated section of the store. Raw milk or food
Toxoplasmosis: *T. gondii* is harmful parasite	Cat feces Litter boxes Gardens and outdoor places where there may be cat feces (sandboxes) Raw and undercooked meats Unwashed fruits and vegetables Contaminated water	Infected babies can suffer hearing loss, mental retardation, and blindness Stillbirth and early prenatal death	A pregnant woman may have no symptoms but can pass the parasite on to the fetus if exposed during the first few months of pregnancy	Avoid changing litter boxes Wear gloves for gardening or handling sand from sand boxes Cover sand boxes Do not get a new cat while pregnant Cook meat thoroughly

(Continued)

Table 4-14 Food-Borne Illnesses (*Continued*)

Food-Borne Illness	Sources	Fetal Effects	Maternal Effects	Recommendation
Salmonella and Campylobacter	Raw unpasteurized milk Raw and undercooked meat Poultry Eggs Salads Cream desserts Filling Contaminated water	Abortion Stillbirth Premature labor	Headache Diarrhea Abdominal pain Nausea Chills Fever Vomiting	Wash hands often, especially after handling pets or working in the garden
Heavy Metals	Methyl mercury Lead Cadmium Nickel Selenium	Miscarriage Stillbirth Premature Neurotoxicity Teratogenicity Embryotoxicity	No effects	Avoid: highly carnivorous fish, e.g. tuna, shark, tilefish, swordfish Mackerel Mercury can be removed from vegetables by washing well with soap and water All dairy foods and juices should be pasteurized

Source: March of Dimes[131], Jacobson[132], Delgado[133], USDHHS.[134]

Table 4-15 Contraindications to Breastfeeding

- Human immunodeficiency virus (HIV) type I & II infection.
- Use of antiretroviral medications.
- Use of or dependency upon illicit drugs or alcohol.
- Human T-cell leukemia virus type I & II.
- Prescribed cancer chemotherapy agents.
- Radiation therapies (can require weaning).

Source: CDC (www.cdc.gov).[130]

Table 4-16 Types of Breast Milk

Colostrum/First Milk: Produced during the later stages of pregnancy and is present in highest concentration during the first few days of lactation. It is a thick yellow substance that is high in protein, fat-soluble vitamins (A, E, and K) and minerals. Colostrum also contains large amounts of antibodies and immunoglobins, especially IGA, which helps protect the infant's gastrointestinal tract from infection. First milk helps establish the normal flora in the intestines and has a laxative effect which speeds the passage of meconium.

Transitional Milk: Serves as a bridge between first milk and mature milk. The amounts of immunoglobulins and proteins decrease, and lactose, fat content, and calories increase. The vitamin content is approximately the same as that of mature milk.

Mature Milk: Replaces transitional milk after approximately 2 weeks of lactation. It has a bluish color and is not as thick as colostrum. Mature milk contains approximately 20 kcal/oz and nutrients sufficient to meet the infant's needs.

Foremilk: Breast milk that is delivered in the first 5–10 minutes of a feeding. It is lower in calories than hindmilk.

Hindmilk: Breast milk that is delivered at the end of a feeding session. It is higher in fat and energy and probably controls infant satiety.

Source: Lawrence.[135]

Breast milk is rich in most nutrients required to sustain the newborn's appropriate growth during the first 6 months of life. The total amount of fat in breast milk is constant, but its composition varies with the duration of the feeding. Initially, breast milk has a relatively low fat content. Following the first let-down reflex, breast milk becomes higher in fat and calories. The fat content of breast milk provides 50% of the infant's total energy requirements in readily absorbable form. Therefore, it is essential that the infant be allowed to nurse on each breast until he or she is satisfied to derive the appropriate fat calories from the feeding. Encouraging the infant to suckle on each breast for 10 minutes or more ensures adequate calorie consumption.[14] Nurse Practitioners should evaluate maternal vitamin D levels to determine if the mother or baby needs a vitamin D supplement. Breast feeding has many advantages for the mother as shown in Table 4-17.

Research regarding protection against the development of allergies and autoimmune diseases continues to confirm that early nutrition is a factor in immune system development. Although the immune system continues to develop throughout the lifespan,

Table 4-17 Breastfeeding Benefits for Women and Children

	Mechanism
Benefits for the Mother	
Post-partum Recovery	Oxytocin release reduces bleeding after delivery and uterus contraction and causes return to its normal size more quickly.
Psychological Benefits	Faster rate of weight loss after pregnancy in some patients. Empowerment decreases risk of post-partum depression. Creates a special bond (less chance of child abuse and neglect).
Reduced Health Risks	Can reduce risk of breast and ovarian cancer, osteoporosis, cardiovascular disease, hyperlipidemia, and diabetes.
Benefits for the Infant	Decrease in otitis media. Decrease in gastrointestinal infections. Reduction in upper respiratory infections. Reduction in asthma. Decreased risk for obesity, cardiovascular disease, diabetes, childhood leukemias, Crohn's disease, SIDS.

Source: Lawrence[135], CDC.[136]

Case 2

Jennifer is a 15-year-old adolescent female who presents to the obstetric clinic due to missing her period for 4 months. She is found to be 20 weeks pregnant and is a late presenter for prenatal care. On exam the patient has only gained 2 lb and admits that she rarely eats breakfast due to nausea, she eats a pretzel and iced tea for lunch, and then her family orders out for dinner or she makes herself a sandwich or cereal for dinner since her mother often does not cook.

PROBLEM: Since this was an unplanned pregnancy the patient has not received appropriate prenatal testing, has not gained the recommended gestational weight, failed to take prenatal vitamins, and failed to follow the nutritional recommendations for a pregnant adolescent.

ADVICE: Jennifer needs to increase her caloric intake by 500 calories/day. Recommendations include daily prenatal vitamins with 1 mg/day of folic acid and calcium supplementation of 1000 mg/day. To enhance her nutrient intake we encouraged her to follow the *My Plate Guide* and to increase her intake of whole grain or enriched breads and cereals, fruit and vegetables, 2% milk or yogurt, and include an iron-rich snack, such as raisins, or dried fruit, or orange juice in the morning. She should increase her fluid intake (up to 2 liters/day) with skim milk, 100% juices, and water.

Adolescents should be encouraged to not skip meals and to eat regularly throughout the day, three meals with two snacks or five small meals. The pregnant female should also be encouraged to eat foods high in iron: dried fruit, orange juice, and broccoli. Additionally, she should increase her calcium intake with the use of milk and ice cream, aiming for three cups per day. Lastly, the adolescent female should remember to avoid alcohol intake, be as active as possible, and take her prenatal vitamins.

the neonate's conditioned response forms by exposure to certain bioactive components of breast milk. Evidence suggests that upon exposure to antigens, breast milk educates the neonatal immune system in the decision-making process underlying the immune response.[137] Additional research supports the formation of the immune system response patterns at the beginning of life which continue throughout the lifespan.[138]

Nurse Practitioners may advise the mother about the duel benefits of breastfeeding and guide the mother through the prevention and early recognition and treatment of breastfeeding problems (Table 4-18). Initial assessment of the breasts to determine if

Table 4-18 Breastfeeding Complications

Mastitis: Inflammatory condition of the breast caused by clogged milk duct.
- Treated with heat, frequent nursing, ibuprofen.
- Assess the mother for evidence of fever of 101 °F, (38.4 °C), increased pulse rate, flu-like aching, nausea, chills, pain or swelling over the area of blockage.
- If an infection is present, treatment should consist of a 10–14 day course of antibiotics against *Staphylococcus aureus* as well as heat, massage, alternate feeding positions, and frequent nursing.

Sore Nipples
- Avoid soaps and ointments.
- Demonstrate proper latch-on and positioning of the infant.
- Warm water compresses, hydrogel dressing, lanolin.
- Temporary use of a breast shield to protect blisters or cracks.
- Initiate infant feeding on the least sore breast to avoid the strong sucking required for the "letdown response".

Breast Engorgement
- Engorgement can be prevented by frequent feeding (every 2–3 hours day and night is recommended). Giving a bottle at night and skipping a feeding can cause engorgement.
- If the breasts are hard and tender, hand expression or pumping; mild heat and gentle massage may soften the areolar mound before feeding.
- Pain medication can be used before feeding.
- Cold is best treatment after a feed. A rice sock or bag of ice or frozen vegetables may be used as a compress.
- Chilled cabbage leaves applied to exposed nipples for 20 minutes after a feeding.

Inverted Nipples
Prior to feeding evert nipple by:
- Applying cold compresses.
- Rolling and gently pulling out on the nipple.
- Using a breast pump to draw the nipple out before feeding.
- Using a device fashioned from a 10 or 20 mL disposable plastic syringe.
- The syringe can be modified by removing the plunger, cutting off the end of the syringe 0.25 inches above where a needle would attach, and inserting the plunger through the end that was cut. The mother places the smooth end over her nipple, gently pulling back for 30–60 seconds before each feeding.

Abscess: Infrequent complication of mastitis which can be caused by untreated mastitis, or delayed or ineffective treatment, failure to drain the mastic breast, or acute weaning during mastitis.
- Confirm the presence of an abscess by ultrasound, needle aspiration incision.
- Drainage should be considered.
- Advise patients to continue breastfeeding since weaning or inhibiting lactation during treatment may hinder the rapid resolution of the abscess.

Source: Lawrence[135], Walker[139], Joanna Briggs Institute.[140]

the nipples are erect, flat, or inverted may assist with the preparation for breastfeeding. Teaching should be initiated regarding proper positioning of the infant at the breast and proper latch-on. Instruction designed to teach the correct breastfeeding mechanics is the best prevention for nipple pain. The primary cause of sore nipples is thought to originate from faulty breastfeeding mechanics, that is, poor positioning, disorganized or dysfunctional sucking, improper latch-on, or failure to form a teat (the ability of the infant to draw the nipple and part of the areola deep into the mouth). Nurse Practitioners can readily manage most of the common problems associated with breastfeeding; however, referral to a mother-to-mother support group or a certified lactation consultant may be indicated.[14,139]

Nutritional Recommendations for Lactating Women
Energy and Protein
Approximately 85 calories are required to produce 100 mL of breast milk. Stored energy from maternal fat reserves provides 100–150 kcal/day, but this may not be sufficient. Therefore, current recommendations advise that the daily caloric intake of lactating women be increased by 500 kcal/day for the first 6 months and 400 kcal/day for the remaining 7–9 months. Post-partum women should avoid diets and medications that promise rapid weight loss. Weight loss should always be gradual, particularly for lactating women, who require more calories than non-lactating women to support breast milk production. No more than 1–2 lb/month is considered a safe loss while breastfeeding.[135] Protein requirements for lactating women are recommended at 71 g/day.

Calcium
Normally 2–8% of total body calcium is mobilized for breast milk production during lactation which will be restored following the onset of menses. Diets of adults of low socio-economic status are often low in calcium. In the US, studies of lactating women consuming 2700 kcal/day suggest that they frequently don't meet the RDAs for calcium and zinc. Diets that contain less than 2700 kcal/day may also be low in magnesium, vitamin B_6, and folate.

Iron
Iron requirements are lower during lactation (9 mg/day) than during pregnancy (27 mg/day) until menstruation resumes (18 mg/day). Adolescent mothers' diets may be particularly low in iron and supplements may be advised.

Vitamin Supplements
Prenatal vitamin supplements are routinely prescribed to lactating women to ensure adequate intake. However, lactating women should be encouraged to obtain their nutrients from a well-balanced, varied diet. Also, they should continue to drink to thirst, or about 2 to 3 quarts of fluids per day to prevent dehydration. New

---

Case 3

Suzie is a 26-year-old woman who delivered a healthy 8 lb, 2 ounce baby boy who is now 6 weeks old. This was her first pregnancy. She has lost 20 lb (9 kg) since giving birth and currently weighs 140 lb (63.5 kg). She is 5'7". BMI: 22.

PROBLEM: Suzie is very busy with her baby and finds it hard to sit down for a meal. Yesterday she ate a bowl of corn flakes with skim milk for breakfast, a peanut butter and jelly sandwich and orange juice for lunch, and a half of a baked chicken breast for dinner with a baked potato, apple sauce, and a diet cola. She likes ice cream at night if she has time between feedings. Suzie says she is even hungrier than she was during her pregnancy, but cannot find time to eat and knows she is not drinking enough because her mouth is dry. She is afraid that she is not producing enough milk because the baby always appears hungry and is not as chubby as her friend's formula-fed baby. Her mother told her she should avoid eating vegetables and chocolate because they will upset the baby's stomach and produce gas. Suzie is also concerned about how to feed the baby when she returns to work in 2 months.

ADVICE: Suzie is not consuming enough calories to maintain her weight and simultaneously produce adequate amounts of breast milk to feed her baby. Her calorie requirements when she is breastfeeding are estimated to be 2700 kcal/day, calculated on the basis of 30 kcal/kg/day plus an additional 500 kcal/day for lactation. Her diet does not provide enough iron, calcium, vitamin A, vitamin B$_{12}$, folate, or zinc. To enhance her nutrient intake encourage her to follow the *My Plate for Moms*, which she can access online to assist her to plan her meals ahead of time. Using this guide will help her dietary plan to increase her intake of whole grain or enriched breads and cereals, fruit and vegetables, 1% low-fat milk or yogurt, and include an iron-rich snack, such as raisins or dried fruit in the morning. Advise her to continue to take her prenatal vitamin. In addition, her fluid intake is low and she should be encouraged to drink more nutritious fluids (up to 2 liters/day), such as skim milk, 100% juices, and water. Suzie should also be given the information to contact a local lactation consultant for assistance in planning her return to work.

---

guidelines from the American Academy of Pediatrics advise supplementation with 400 IU of vitamin D that should be initiated within days of birth for all breast-fed infants.

Alcohol Consumption

The use of alcohol by breastfeeding mothers is widespread and even considered "usually compatible" with breastfeeding by the AAP. However, data suggest that when used excessively, the infant may suffer various complications, including developmental delay. Whether or not to use alcohol is a choice that all breastfeeding mothers must make for themselves. Nurse Practitioners should assist mothers to adjust alcohol consumption appropriately in both timing and volume.[135]

References

1. Gennaro S, Biesecker B, Fantasia HC, et al. Nutrition profiles of American women in the third trimester. *Am J Clin Nutr* 2011;36:120–126.

2. Reynolds RM, Osmond C, Phillips DIW, et al. Maternal BMI, parity, and pregnancy weight gain: influences on offspring adiposity in young adulthood. *J Clin Endocrinol Metab* 2010;95:5365–5369.

3. *Healthy People 2020.* Department of Health and Human Services, Washington, DC. www.healthypeople.gov

4. Sheih C, Carter A. Online prenatal nutrition education. *Nursing for Women's Health* 2011; 15:26–33.

5. Institute of Medicine. *Weight Gain During Pregnancy: Reexamining the Guidelines.* National Academies Press, Washington DC, 2009.

6. Sewell MF, Huston-Presley L, Super DM, et al. Increased neonatal fat mass not lean body mass, is associated with maternal obesity. *Am J Obstet Gynecol* 2006;195:1100–1103.

7. Flegal KM, Carroll MD, Ogden CL, et al. Prevalence and trends in obesity among US adults, 1999-2-000. *JAMA* 2002;288:1723–1727.

8. Ogden CL, Carroll MD, Curtin LR, et al. Prevalence of overweight and obesity in the US1999–2004. *JAMA* 2006;295:1549–1555.

9. Flegal KM, Carroll MD, Ogden CL, et al. Prevalence and trends in obesity among US adults, 1999–2008. *JAMA* 2010;303:235–241.

10. Goldstein JG, Funai EF, Roque H. Nutrition in pregnancy. *Up To Date.* www.uptodate.com/contents/nutrition-in-pregnancy. Accessed 2012.

11. Deen DD, Hark LA. Feeding the mother-to-be. In *The Complete Guide to Nutrition in Primary Care.* Wiley-Blackwell Publishing, Malden, MA, 2007.

12. Fejzo MS, Ingles SA, Wilson M, et al. High prevalence of severe nausea and vomiting of pregnancy and hyperemesis gravidarum among relatives of affected individuals. *Eur J Obst Gyn Repr Biology* 2008;141:13–17.

13. Cox JT, Phelan ST. Nutrition during pregnancy. *Obstet Gynecol Clin North Am* 2008;35:369–383.

14. Hark LA, Deen DD. Nutrition in pregnancy and lactation. In *Medical Nutrition and Disease.* 4th edition. Wiley-Blackwell Publishing, Malden, MA, 2009.

15. Armstrong E, Harris LH, Kukla R, et al. Maternal caffeine consumption during pregnancy and the risk of miscarriage. *Am J Obstet Gynecol* 2008;198: 279.

16. Beyan C, Kaptan K, Infran A, et al. Pica: a frequent symptom in iron deficiency anemia. *Arch Med Sci* 2009;5:471–474.

17. Weng X, Odouli R, Li DK. Maternal caffeine consumption during pregnancy and the risk of miscarriage: a prospective cohort study. *Am J Obstet Gynecol* 2008;198:279.

18. Institute of Medicine. *Nutrition During Pregnancy: Weight Gain, Nutrient Supplements.* Committee on Nutritional Status During Pregnancy and Lactation. National Academies Press, Washington, DC, 1990.

19. Shils ME, Shike M, Ross AC, et al. *Modern Nutrition in Health and Disease.* 10th edition. Lippincott, Williams and Wilkins. Philadelphia, PA, 2006.

20. American Congress of Obstetricians and Gynecologists. *Your Pregnancy and Birth.* 4th edition. ACOG, Washington, DC, 2005.

21. Viswanathan M, Siega-Riz AM, Moos M-K, et al. Outcomes of maternal weight gain, evidence report/technology assessment No. 168 AHRQ Publication No. 08-E-0-09. Agency for Healthcare Research and Quality, Rockville, MD, 2008.

22. American Academy of Pediatrics (AAOP) and The American College of Obstetricians and Gynecologists (ACOG). *Guidelines for Perinatal Care.* AAOP and ACOG, Washington DC, 2007.

23. Lee JM, Smith JR, Philipp BL, et al. Vitamin D deficiency in a healthy group of mothers and newborn infants. *Clin Pediatr* 2007;46:42–44.

24. Kretchmer N, Zimmermann M. *Developmental Nutrition*. Allyn and Bacon, Boston,1997.

25. McCullough ML. Vitamin D deficiency in pregnancy: bringing the issues to light. *J Nutr* 2007;137:305–306.

26. Food and Nutrition Board, Institute of Medicine. *Dietary Reference Intakes for Energy, Carbohydrate, Fiber, Fat, Fatty Acids, Cholesterol, Protein, and Amino Acids*. National Academies Press, Washington, DC, 2002.

27. Elias SL, Innes SM. Infant plasma trans, n-6 and n-3 fatty acids and conjugated linoleic acids are related to maternal plasma fatty acids, length of gestation and birth weight and length. *Am J Clin Nutr* 2001;73:807–14.

28. Groh-Wargo S, Jacobs J, Auestad N, et al. Body composition in preterm infants who are fed long-chain polyunsaturated fatty acids: a prospective, randomized, controlled trial. *Pediatr Res* 2005;57:712–718.

29. London M, Ladewig P, Ball J, et al. *Maternal and Child Nursing Care*. 3rd Edition. Pearson, New York, 2011.

30. Dunstan JA, Mon TA, Barden A, et al. Maternal fish oil supplementation in pregnancy reduces interleukin-13 levels in cord blood of infants at high risk of atopy. *Clin Exp Allergy* 2003;33:442–448.

31. Harper M, Thom E, Klebanoff MA, et al. Omega-3 fatty acid supplementation to prevent recurrent preterm birth: a randomized controlled trial. *Obstet Gynecol* 2010;115:234–242.

32. Innes SM, Elias SL. Intakes of essential n-6 and n- polyunsaturated fatty acids among pregnant Canadian women. *Am J Clin Nutr* 2003;77:473–478.

33. Haggarty P. Effect of placental function on fatty acid requirements during pregnancy. *Eur J Clin Nutr* 2004;58:1559–1570.

34. Simopoulos AD, Leaf A, Salem N. US Expert Panel: essentiality of an recommended diet intakes for omega-6 and omega-3 fatty acids. *Ann Nutr Metab* 1999;43:127–130.

35. Peyron-Caso E, Quignard-Boulange A, Laromiguiere M, et al. Dietary fish oil increases lipid mobilization but does not decrease lipid storage-related enzyme activities in adipose tissue of insulin-resistant, sucrose-fed rats. *J Nutr* 2003;133:2239–2243.

36. Oken E, Kleinman KP, Berland WE, et al. Decline in fish consumption among pregnant women after a national mercury advisory. *Obstet Gynecol* 2003;102:346–351.

37. American Medical Association Council on Science and Public Health. Mercury and Fish Consumption: Medical and Public Health Issues. AMA-ASSN.org. 2004. Accessed 2012.

38. US Department of Health and Human Services and US Environmental Protection Agency. What you need to know about mercury in fish and shellfish. 2005. www.epa.gov. Accessed 2012.

39. March of Dimes Foundation. www.marchofdimes.com. Accessed 2012.

40. Brooks JD, Ward WE, Lewis JE, et al. Supplementation with flaxseed alters estrogen metabolism in postmenopausal women to a greater extent than does supplementation with an equal amount of soy. *Am J Clin Nutr* 2004;79:318–325.

41. Rothman KJ, Moore LL, Singer MR, et al. Teratogenicity of high vitamin a intake. *NEJM* 1995;333:1369–1373.

42. The Teratogen Information System (TERIS). Vitamin A. depts.washington.edu/terisweb. Accessed 2012.

43. Laanpere M, Altmäe S, Stavreus-Evers A, et al. Folate-mediated one-carbon metabolism and its effect on female fertility and pregnancy viability. *Nutr Rev* 2010;68:99–113.

44. Molloy AM, Kirke PN, Brody LC, et al. Effects of folate and vitamin B_{12} deficiencies during pregnancy on fetal, infant, and child development. *Food Nutr Bull* 2008;29:S101–S111.

45. Blencowe H, Cousens S, Modell B, Lawn J. Folic acid to reduce neonatal mortality from neural tube disorders. *Intern J Epid* 2010;39:110.

46. Black M. Effects of vitamin B_{12} and folate deficiency on brain development in children. *Food Nutr Bull* 2008;29:126–131.

47. US Preventive Services Task Force. Agency for Healthcare Research and Quality. Folic acid for the prevention of neural tube defects: US Preventive Services Task Force recommendation statement. *Ann Intern Med* 2009;150:626–631.

48. Goh YI, Bollano E, Einarson TR, et al. Prenatal multivitamin supplementation and rates of congenital anomalies: a meta-analysis. *J Obstet Gynecol Can* 2006;28:680–689.

49. Hollis BW, Wagner CL. Vitamin D deficiency during pregnancy: an ongoing epidemic. *Am J Clin Nutr* 2006;84:273.

50. Hollis BW, Wagner CL. Nutritional vitamin D status during pregnancy: reasons for concern. *CMAJ* 2006;174:1287–1290.

51. Hollis, BW. Vitamin D requirement during pregnancy and lactation. *J Bone Min Res* 2007;22(S2):V39–V44.

52. Ainy E, Ghazi AA, Azizi F. Changes in calcium, 25(OH) vitamin D_3 and other biochemical factors during pregnancy. *J Endocrinol Invest* 2006;29:303–307.

53. Scholl TO, Chen X. Vitamin D intake during pregnancy: association with maternal characteristics and infant birth weight. *Early Human Devel* 2009;85:231–234.

54. Lapillonne A. Vitamin D deficiency during pregnancy may impair maternal and fetal outcomes. *Med Hypotheses* 2010;74:71–75.

55. McGrath J. Does 'imprinting' with low prenatal vitamin D contribute to the risk of various adult disorders? *Med Hypotheses* 2001;56:367–371.

56. Bodnar LM, Catov JM, Simhan HN, et al. Maternal vitamin D deficiency increases the risk of preeclampsia. *J Clin Endocr Metab* 2007;92:3517–3522.

57. Ginde AA, Sullivan AF, Mansbach JM, et al. Vitamin D insufficiency in pregnant and nonpregnant women of childbearing age in the US. *Am J Obstet Gynecol* 2010; 202:436.

58. Food and Nutrition Board, Institute of Medicine. *Dietary Reference Intakes for Calcium, Phosphorous, Magnesium, Vitamin D, and Fluoride*. National Academy Press, Washington, DC, 1997.

59. Atallah AN, Hofmeyer GJ, Duley L. Calcium supplementation during pregnancy for preventing hypertensive disorders and related problems. Cochrane Database of Systemic Reviews 2006;(1).

60. Solomon CG, Seely EW. Hypertension in pregnancy. *Endoc Metab Clin N Am* 2006;35: 157–171.

61. Georgieff MK. The role of iron in neurodevelopment: fetal iron deficiency and the developing hippocampus. *Biochem Soc Trans* 2008;36:1267–1272.

62. American Congress of Obstetrics and Gynecology Practice Bulletin. *Anemia in Pregnancy*, No. 95, 2008.

63. Belfort M, Rifas-Shiman SL, Rich-Edwards JW, et al. Maternal iron intake and iron status during pregnancy and child blood pressure at age 3 years. *Int J Epidemiol* 2008;37:301–308.

64. Shah PS, Ohlsson A. Effects of prenatal multimicronutrient supplementation on pregnancy outcomes: a meta-analysis. *Can Med Assoc J* 2009;180:E99.

65. Centers for Disease Control and Prevention. Recommendations to prevent and control iron deficiency in the United States. www.cdc.gov. Accessed 2012.

66. Bookstein FL, Connor PD, Huggins JE, et al. Many infants prenatally exposed to high levels of alcohol show one particular anomaly of the corpus callosum. *Alcoholism: Clin Exp Res* 2007;31:868–879.

67. Streissguth AP, Barr HM, Martin DC, et al. Effects of maternal alcohol, nicotine, and caffeine use during pregnancy on infant mental and motor development at eight months. *Alcoholism: Clin Exp Res* 2008; 4:152–164.

68. American Medical Association Council on Science and Public Health. Alcoholism and Alcohol Abuse Among Women. AMA-ASSN.org. 1997. Accessed 2012.

69. Einarson A, Riordan S. Smoking in pregnancy and lactation: a review of risks and cessation strategies. *Eur J Clin Pharm* 2009;65:325–330.
70. Wisborg K, Henriksen TB, Hedegaard M, et al. Smoking during pregnancy and preterm birth. *BJOG* 2005;103:800–805.
71. Aliyu M. Preventive Medicine 2010: the Annual Meeting of the American College of Preventive Medicine: Abstract 212669. Presented February 19, 2010.
72. Jaddoe V, Troe EW, Hofman A, et al. Active and passive maternal smoking during pregnancy and the risks of low birthweight and preterm birth: the Generation R Study. *Pediatr Perinatal Epid* 2008;22:162–171.
73. Browne ML, Burns TL, Drusschel CM, et al. Maternal caffeine consumption and risk of neural tube defects. *Birth Defects Part A: Clin Mol Teratol* 2009;85:879–889.
74. *Weight Gain During Pregnancy: Reexamining the Guidelines.* Rasmussin KM, Yaktin AL (Eds). Institute of Medicine. National Academies Press, Washington DC, 2009.
75. Stotland NE, Chang YW, Hopkins LM, et al. Gestational weight gain and adverse neonatal outcomes among term infants. *Obstet Gynecol* 2006;108:635–643.
76. Nohr EA, Vaeth M, Baker JL, et al. Combined associations of prepregnancy body mass index and gestational weight gain with the outcome of pregnancy. *Am J Clin Nutr* 2008;87:1750–1759.
77. Gale C, Javaid M, Robinson S, et al. Maternal size in pregnancy and body composition in children. *J Clin Endocrinol Metab* 2007;92:3904–3911.
78. Lashen H, Fear K, Sturde D. Obesity is associated with increased risk of first trimester and recurrent miscarriage: matched case control study. *Hum Reprod* 2004;19:1644–1646.
79. Kiel DW, Dodson EA, Artal R, et al. Gestational weight gain and pregnancy outcomes in obese women: how much is enough? *Obstet Gynecol* 2007;110;752–758.
80. Gardiner P, Nelson L, Shellhaas C, et al. The clinical content of pre-conception care: nutrition and dietary supplements. *AJOG* 2008;199(6B):S310–S327.
81. King T, Murphy PA. Evidence-based approaches to managing nausea and vomiting in early pregnancy. *J Midwifery Woman's Health* 2009;54:430–444.
82. Chu S, Bachman D, Callaghan W, et al. Association between obesity during pregnancy and increased use of health care. *N Engl J Med* 2008;358:1444–1453.
83. Rasmussen KM, Catalano PM, Yaktin AL. New guidelines for weight gain during pregnancy: what obstetrician/gynecologists should know. *Curr Opin Obstet Gynecol* 2009;21: 521–526.
84. Burstein E, Levy A, Mazor M, et al. Pregnancy outcome among obese women: a prospective study. *Am J Perinatol* 2008;195:S220–S220.
85. Butte NF, King JU. Energy requirements during pregnancy and lactation. *Public Health Nutr* 2005;8:1010–1027.
86. Chen XK, Wen SW, Fleming N, et al. Teen-age pregnancy and adverse birth outcomes: a large population-based retrospective cohort study. *Intern J Epid* 2007;35:368–373.
87. Nicholson J, Sullivan C, Holt M. Feeding the mother-to-be. In: Deen D, Hark L. (Eds), *The Complete Guide to Nutrition in Primary Care.* Wiley-Blackwell, Malden, MA, 2007.
88. Fox NS, Rebarber A, Roman AS, et al. Weight gain in twin pregnancies and adverse outcomes: examining the 2009 Institute of Medicine Guidelines. *Obstet Gynecol* 2010; 116:100–106.
89. Luke, B. Improving multiple pregnancy outcomes with nutritional interventions. *Clin Obstet Gynecol* 2004;134:1820–1826.
90. Luke, B. Nutrition and multiple gestation. *Semin Perinatol* 2005;29:349–354.
91. Goodnight W, Newman R. Optimal nutrition for improved twin pregnancy outcome. *Obstet Gynecol* 2009;114:1121–1134.
92. Luke B, Hediger ML, Nugent C, et al. Body mass index – specific weight gains associated with optimal birth weights in twin pregnancies. *J Reprod Med* 2003;48:217–224.

93. Luke B, Leurgans S. Maternal weight gains in ideal twin outcomes. *J Am Diet Assoc* 1996;96:178–181.

94. Bodnar LM, Simhan HN, Powers RW, et al. High prevalence of vitamin D insufficiency in black and white pregnant women residing in the northern United States and their neonates. *J Nutr* 2007;137:447–452.

95. Haugen M, Brantsaeter AL, Trogstad L, et al. Vitamin D supplementation and reduced risk of preeclampsia in nulliparous women. *Epidemiology* 2009;20:720–726.

96. Hark L, Catalano P. Nutritional Management During Pregnancy. In: Gabbe SG, Simpson JL, Niebyl JR, Driscoll DD (Eds), *Obstetrics: Normal and Problem Pregnancies*. Churchill Livingston, London, 2012.

97. Dixon JB, Dixon ME, O'Brien PE. Birth outcomes in obese women after laparoscopic adjustable gastric banding. *Obstet Gynecol* 2005;106:965–972.

98. Maggard M, Li Z, Yermilov I, et al. Bariatric surgery in women of reproductive age: special concerns for pregnancy. Evidence Report/Technology Assessment No. 169. (Prepared by the Southern California Evidence-based Practice Center under Contract No. 290-02-003). Rockville, MD: Agency for Healthcare Research and Quality. November 2008.

99. Chu SY, Callaghan WM, Bisch CC, et al. Gestational weight gain by body mass index among US women delivering live births, 2004–2005: fueling future obesity. *Am J Obstet Gynecol* 2009;200:271–277.

100. Moore K, Ouyang D, Whang E. Maternal and fetal deaths after gastric bypass surgery for morbid obesity. *N Engl J Med* 2004;351:721–722.

101. Skull AJ, Slater GH, Duncombe JE, et al. Laparoscopic adjustable banding in pregnancy: safety, patient tolerance and effect on obesity-related pregnancy outcomes. *Obes Surg* 2007;14:230–235.

102. Ducarme G, Revaux A, Rodrigues A, et al. Obstetric outcome following laparoscopic adjustable gastric banding. *Int J Gynecol Obstet* 2007;98:244–247.

103. American Congress of Obstetricians and Gynecologists. Pregestational diabetes mellitus (ACOG Practice Bulletin No. 60). Washington, DC, 2005.

104. Reese EA, Homko CJ. Diabetes mellitus and pregnancy. In: Gibbs RS, Karlan BY, Haney AF, Nygaard IE (Eds), *Danforth's Obstetrics and Gynecology*. 10th Edition. WoltersKluwer/ Lippincott Williams & Wilkins, Philadelphia, PA, 2008.

105. Steube AM, Rich-Edwards JW, Willett WC, et al. Duration of lactation and incidence of type 2 diabetes. *JAMA* 2005;294:2601–2610.

106. Slocum JM. Preconception counseling and type 2 diabetes. *Diabetes Spectrum* 2007;20: 117–123.

107. Wyatt JW, Frias JL, Hoyme HE, et al. Congenital anomaly rate in offspring of mothers with diabetes treated with insulin lispro during pregnancy. *Diabetic Medicine* 2005;22:803–807.

108. Kitzmiller J, Dang-Kilduff L, Taslimi M. Gestational diabetes after delivery. *Diabetes Care* 2007;30:S225.

109. Dudley D. Diabetic-associated stillbirth: incidence, pathophysiology, and prevention. *Obstet Gynecol Clin North Am* 2007;34:293–307.

110. Bottalico JN. Recurrent gestation diabetes: risk factors, diagnosis, management, and implications. *Semin Perinatol* 2007;31:176–184.

111. American Diabetes Association (ADA). Position statement: nutrition recommendations and interventions for diabetes. *Diabetes Care* 2007;30:S61.

112. Perkins JM, Dunn JP, Jagasia S. Perspectives in gestational diabetes mellitus: a review of screening, diagnosis, and treatment. *Clinical Diabetes* 2007;25:57–62.

113. Rodbard HW, Jellinger PS, Davidson J, et al. American Association of Clinical Endocrinologists/ American College of Endocrinology consensus panel on type 2 diabetes mellitus: An algorithm for glycemic control. *Endocrine Practice* 2009;15:540–559.

114. American Diabetes Association (ADA). Position statement: gestational diabetes mellitus. *Diabetes Care* 2004;27:S88.

115. Agency for Healthcare Research and Quality (AHRQ) and US Department of Health and Human Services (USDHHS): *Outcomes of maternal weight gain, Publication No. 08-E009, Rockville, MD, 2008, AHRQ*. www.ahrq.gov/clinic/tp/admattp.htm. Accessed 2012.

116. American Diabetes Association. Position statement: diagnosis and classification of diabetes mellitus *Diabetes Care* 2008;31(Suppl 1):S62.

117. US Preventive Services Task Force (USPSTF): Screening for gestational diabetes mellitus: Recommendation statement, AHRQ. 2008.

118. US Preventive Services Task Force. *The Guide to Clinical Preventive Services 2005*. Department of Health and Human Services. Oxford University. New York, 2005.

119. Chen A, Rogan WJ. Breastfeeding and the risk of post-neonatal death in the United States. *Pediatrics* 2004;113:e435–9.

120. Agency for Healthcare Research and Quality (AHRQ): Therapeutic management, delivery, and post-partum risk assessment and screening in gestational diabetes, Evidence Report/ Technology Assessment No. 162. 2008.

121. Gilbert, E. *Manual of High Risk Pregnancy and Delivery*. 5th Edition. Mosby, Inc., St Louis, MO, 2011.

122. Sokol RJ, Miller SI, Reed G. Alcohol abuse during pregnancy: an epidemiologic study. *Alcoholism: Clin Exper Res* 2008;4:135–145.

123. Fowles E, Murphy C, Ruiz R. Exploring relationships among psychosocial status, dietary quality and measures of placental development during the first trimester in low-income women. *Biol Res Nurs* 2011;13:70–79.

124. Bradley CS, Kennedy CM, Turcea AM, et al. Constipation in pregnancy: prevalence, symptoms, and risk factors. *Obstet Gynecol* 2007;110:1351–1357.

125. American Congress of Obstetrics and Gynecology (ACOG). *Nausea and vomiting of pregnancy*. Practice Bulletin No. 52, Washington, DC, 2004.

126. Jewell D, Young G. Interventions for nausea and vomiting in early pregnancy. *Cochrane Database Syst Rev*. 2003;4:CD000145.

127. Born D, Barron, ML. Herb use in pregnancy. *Am J Mater Child Nurs* 2005;30:201–206.

128. National Institute for Health and Clinical Excellence (NICE). *Quick Reference Guide: Antenatal Care for the Healthy Pregnant Woman*. 2nd Edition. RCOG Press, London, 2008.

129. Food and Drug Administration. Food safety for moms-to-be. 2009. www.fda.gov. Accessed 2012.

130. Centers for Disease Control and Prevention. Disease listing food-borne illness, general information. www.cdc.gov. Accessed 2012.

131. March of Dimes. Food-borne risks in pregnancy. 2008. www.marchofdimes.com. Accessed 2012.

132. Jacobson L, Serwint J. Listeriosis. *Ped Rev* 2008;29:410–411.

133. Delgado, Ana. Listeriosis in pregnancy. *J Midwifery Women's Health* 2008;53:255–259.

134. US Department of Health and Human Services and US Environmental Protection Agency. What you need to know about mercury in fish and shellfish. 2005. www.epa.gov. Accessed 2012.

135. Lawrence RA, Lawrence, RM. *Breastfeeding: A Guide for the Medical Profession*. 7th edition. Mosby, USA, 2011.

136. Centers for Disease Control and Prevention. Guide to Breast Feeding. www.cdc.gov. Accessed 2012.

137. Vidal K, Donnet-Huges A. Bioactive components of milk. *Advances Experimental Med Biol* 2008;606:195–216.

138. Enke U, Seyfarth L, Schleussner E, et al. Impact of PUFA on early immune and fetal development. *Br J Nutr* 2008;100:1158–1168.
139. Walker M. Conquering common breastfeeding problems. *J Perinatal Neonatal Nurs* 2008; 22: 267–274.
140. The Joanna Briggs Institute. The management of nipple pain and/or trauma associated with breastfeeding. Best Practice: evidence-based information sheets for health professionals. 2009;13:17–20.

5 Nutrition from Infancy Through Adolescence

Susan Breakell Gresko, MSN, CRNP, PNP-BC
Bridget S. Sullivan, MSN, MS, CRNP, RD

OBJECTIVES

- Identify age appropriate rates of growth and nutritional intake in pediatric patients.
- Identify markers of nutritional risk in pediatric patients.
- Identify and manage common nutritional problems and utilize preventative measures to decrease risk of acute and chronic diseases.
- Manage common variations in nutritional status in pediatric patients.

Introduction

Adequate and appropriate nutrition from infancy through adolescence is critical for the developing human being. Proper nutrition supplies the immediate energy needs for physical activity, the protein to develop and grow, and the micronutrients that support these processes. Dietary intake and physical activity, along with genetic predisposition, set the stage for adult health. The incidence of overweight and obesity across all age groups of the US population has increased at an alarming rate in recent years. Nurse Practitioners need to identify families with children at risk and provide age-appropriate anticipatory guidance to prevent obesity and other chronic diseases. To be effective in nutrition counseling, Nurse Practitioners must be aware of the cultural, economic, and social implications of food. It can be challenging for families to identify foods and implement lifestyle changes surrounding nutrition and physical activity. Primary care Nurse Practitioners can serve as significant resources for nutrition information and provide guidance on appropriate eating behaviors.

Growth

Evaluation of growth is the cornerstone of pediatric nutrition assessment.[1] The Centers for Disease Control and Prevention (CDC) recommends that health care providers:

- Use the WHO growth standards to monitor growth for infants and children from birth to 2 years
- Use the CDC growth charts for children ages 2 years and older

---

The Nurse Practitioner's Guide to Nutrition, Second Edition. Edited by Lisa Hark, Kathleen Ashton and Darwin Deen.
© 2012 John Wiley & Sons, Inc. Published 2012 by John Wiley & Sons, Inc.

Plotting a child's growth is a sensitive, non-invasive method to identify relatively normal physiologic function.[2] The early detection of abnormal growth patterns by the Nurse Practitioner in well-child visits allows for effective preventive and therapeutic interventions. The importance of plotting children's growth cannot be overstated.[2] Therefore, it is critical to accurately measure and plot children's weight, height, and head circumference using current growth chart measurements. Inaccurate measurements may result in misdiagnosis of growth failure, or a child with a normal growth pattern being referred for unnecessary evaluation. Gilluly et al.[2] reviewed data from 878 children measured in 55 pediatric or family primary care practices in seven US cities. Baseline results indicate only 30% of children were measured accurately. It is strongly recommended that a recumbent length-board be used to measure infants and young children from birth to 36 months. A stadiometer should be used to measure height in standing 2–18 year olds. Body mass index (BMI) is not calculated until a standing height can be measured.

Growth charts are not intended for use as a sole diagnostic instrument. Instead, growth charts are tools that contribute to forming an overall clinical impression of the child being measured.[3] Inadequate nutritional intake impacts growth and ultimately may interfere with children achieving their developmental potential. Children undergo two rapid periods of growth (reflected in growth velocity charts): the first during infancy and early childhood, the second during adolescence. Between these periods slow, steady growth occurs. Growth is documented by serial measurements of weight and length (or height) from birth to 18 years, and head circumference from birth to 36 months, plotted on growth curves derived from observations of large numbers of normal, healthy children. These curves, first developed by the National Center for Health Statistics (NCHS) in 1977, have been revised by the CDC Growth Charts.[3] Most of the data used to construct these growth charts comes from the National Health and Nutrition Examination Surveys (NHANES), collected from 1971 to 1994, which include all ethnic and racial groups, and both breast-fed and formula-fed infants (CDC Growth Charts). A recent innovation in the current growth charts was the inclusion of BMI values for age and gender for children aged 2–20 years. BMI provides an objective measure of weight in relationship to height to assess the degree of adiposity.

Interpretation of growth chart plots is an important function of Nurse Practitioners in primary care. Children require evaluation for underweight if their weight- and/or height-for-age plots below the 5th percentile. Crossing over 2% lines with weight loss or, when weight or linear growth plateaus on the growth chart, further medical and nutritional evaluation is required. Remaining between the 5th and the 85th percentile (within ±2 percentile lines) represents a normal growth pattern. Children plotting between the 85th percentile and the 95th percentile should be considered overweight.[3,4] Children plotting above the 95th percentile are considered obese.[3,4] Growth charts for premature infants are available on the CDC website and should be used when appropriate. Initially, during acute malnutrition the child's weight decreases or the rate of weight gain slows or plateaus. After 4–6 months the condition is considered chronic, resulting in slowing of linear growth (height). Chronic malnutrition harms brain growth in children under 3 years of age, and may result in reduced head circumference growth.

Overweight and Obesity

The epidemic of childhood overweight and obesity represents a dramatic setback in the progress toward assuring the future health of the US population. This epidemic is occurring nationwide, in young children as well as in adolescents, across all socio-economic and ethnic groups. Specific subgroups, particularly those of lower socio-economic status (SES), African Americans, Hispanic and Native Americans, are disproportionately affected.[4] Over the past three decades, the rate of obesity has more than doubled for preschool children aged 2–5 years and adolescents aged 12–19 years, and more than tripled for children aged 6–11 years.[4,5] The medical complications associated with obesity in children include sleep apnea, hypertension, hyperlipidemia, insulin resistance, type 2 diabetes, orthopedic problems (such as slipped capital femoral epiphysis), pseudo tumor cerebri, and psychosocial problems.[6,7,8]

Etiology of Obesity: Genetics and Environment

A strong genetic component has been found in studies comparing the BMI of children with that of their biologic or adoptive parents.[9] According to current estimates, a child with two obese biological parents has an 80% chance of becoming obese. The proportion drops to 40% of children with only one obese parent.[7] Acknowledging the strong genetic predisposition to obesity, environmental influences determine its expression. Environmental and lifestyle change correlate with the epidemic of childhood obesity over the last 30 years. These changes include both parents working outside the home, increased food marketing aimed at children, changes in the school environment (more high-fat foods and sugary beverages, as well as decreased physical activity), and more meals eaten outside the home, particularly fast food. Increased television viewing, as well as time devoted to sedentary activities, such as computer and video games, are also major contributing factors. Direct marketing to children through television commercials has influenced the foods they desire and eat, including fast food and sodas, often in "super-sized" portions.

Prevention and Treatment of the Overweight and Obese Child

Comprehensive treatment programs that include behavior modification have been shown to be moderately effective in the treatment of childhood obesity.[7,10] The best outcome of weight loss programs is achieved when the entire family works together to improve their diet and physical activity level. While weight loss may be indicated for obese children, weight maintenance in overweight pre-pubertal children is a more reasonable approach until linear growth is complete. Clearly, the most effective way to address the epidemic of obesity in children is through prevention.

Preventing children from becoming overweight involves providing adequate calories to support growth and development, while ensuring enough physical activity to prevent inappropriate weight gain.[4,11] Nurse Practitioners should be able to identify those at risk for the development of obesity using growth charts and family history.[12] At-risk groups include those who have one or both parents who are overweight or low socio-economic status, or are from at-risk ethnic groups. Mexican Americans have the highest incidence of obesity followed by African Americans. Maternal factors that increase a child's risk of obesity include formula-feeding instead of breastfeeding, excessive maternal weight gain during pregnancy (>15.9 kg), gestational diabetes, and large-for-gestational-age infants.[8] It is extremely difficult to overfeed a breast-fed child; a good reason to promote breastfeeding as an important part of obesity prevention. Nurse Practitioners can identify high risk children by reviewing family history of overweight and obesity, assessing maternal weight gain during pregnancy, monitoring growth over time, including BMI, and tracking growth percentiles. Nurse Practitioners have unique opportunities to guide families in their efforts to raise healthy, normal weight children. They can guide parents with knowledge and tools to provide nutritious foods at mealtimes while avoiding over-restriction. Limiting exposure to foods and providing adequate opportunities for physical activity is critical. Children have the responsibility to decide which of these foods and what quantities they will consume. Establishing this practice starting from infancy will support self-regulation, a key to life-long weight control.[13]

Laboratory Assessment

As part of a regular nutritional evaluation, broad screening using laboratory tests is generally not recommended. General assessments can include a complete blood count (CBC), serum electrolytes, creatinine, and albumin. Serum albumin is commonly used as an assessment of general nutritional and protein status. Evaluation of the CBC, including white blood cell morphology and red blood cell size, can provide evidence of deficiencies in iron, folate, and vitamin B_{12}. Blood chemistries can indicate electrolyte and mineral imbalances, though blood levels are not always good indicators of whole body balance.

Fasting Glucose

Data from a nationally representative sample indicate that approximately 0.5% of US adolescents have diabetes (American Diabetes Association). Seventy percent of these youth have type 1 diabetes and 30% have type 2 diabetes. An estimated 39 000 US adolescents have type 2 diabetes and nearly 2.8 million have impaired fasting glucose (>100 mg/dL; 5.6 mmol/L). In selected high-risk groups, glucose intolerance and type 2 diabetes occur more frequently. In a predominantly Hispanic and African American cohort of over 1700 eighth grade students in which 29% had BMIs ≥ 95th percentile for age and sex, elevated fasting glucose (≥100 mg/dL) was present in 40% of the cohort.[14] Impaired glucose tolerance (glucose ≥140 mg/dL 2-hour post-glucose challenge) occurred in 2.3%. The frequency of impaired glucose tolerance was nearly twice as high (4.1%) in the heaviest subset, those with BMI ≥95th percentile. Rates of impaired glucose tolerance were also higher in Hispanic (3.2%) and Native American (7.3%) youth than in the overall cohort. Among children in a weight management clinic, impaired glucose tolerance was reported in 14 of 55 (25%) severely obese children (4–10 years of age) and in 23 of 112 (21%) of severely obese adolescents (11–18 years of age). In severely obese youth, the progression from impaired glucose tolerance to type 2 diabetes may be rapid, particularly in those with continuing weight gain. Adolescence is a period of particularly high risk for the onset of type 2 diabetes. Overweight children and adolescents, particularly those with a family history of type 2 diabetes, are at increased risk of developing glucose intolerance and eventually type

Table 5-1 Testing for Type 2 Diabetes in Asymptomatic Children and Adolescents

---

- Overweight (BMI > 85th percentile for age and sex, weight for height > 85th percentile, or weight 120% of ideal for height).

Plus any two of the following risk factors:
- Family history of type 2 diabetes in first- or second-degree relative.
- Race/ethnicity (American Indian, African-American, Hispanic, Asian American, Pacific Islander).
- Signs of insulin resistance or conditions associated with insulin resistance (acanthosis nigricans, hypertension, dyslipidemia, PCOS, or small-for-gestational-age birth weight).

Age of Initiation: Age 10 years or at onset of puberty, if puberty occurs at a younger age.

Frequency: Every 3 years.

Test: Fasting plasma glucose (FPG) preferred.
- Clinical judgment should be used to test for diabetes in high-risk patients who do not meet these criteria.

Source: American Diabetes Association.[15]

2 diabetes. The recommended screening test is fasting plasma glucose. The American Diabetes Association criteria for type 2 diabetes screening in children and adolescents are shown Table 5-1.[15] In the evolution of type 2 diabetes, post-prandial glucose increases earlier than fasting glucose; some experts therefore recommend determining plasma glucose two hours after a standard glucose load or two hours after a meal.

Lipids

Screening for hypercholesterolemia should start at the age of 2 years for children with a positive family history of dyslipidemia or premature cardiovascular disease (CVD). It is also recommended that pediatric patients for whom family history is not known or those with other CVD risk factors, such as overweight (BMI ≥ 85th percentile, < 95th percentile), obesity (BMI ≥ 95th percentile), hypertension (blood pressure ≥ 95th percentile), cigarette smoking, or diabetes mellitus, be screened with a fasting lipid profile.[16] A positive family history of early atherosclerotic vascular disease (AVD) or hypercholesterolemia is defined as a parent or grandparent with a heart attack, sudden death thought to be related to AVD, angina, angioplasty, peripheral vascular disease, or cerebrovascular disease before age 55 for men and before age 65 for women. Children or adolescents with high cholesterol levels tend to become adults with high cholesterol levels. However, as tracking of lipid levels over time is not perfect, not all hypercholesterolemic children will become hypercholesterolemic adults. Also, there are concerns that with universal screening, more children may be placed on inappropriately restrictive, nutritionally inadequate diets. Current recommendations focus on screening children and adolescents at high risk for hypercholesterolemia, in order to identify those who should receive aggressive intervention. According to the *US Dietary Guidelines for Americans*[17], fat intake should be between 30 and 35% of total calories for children 2–3 years of age and between 25 and 35% of calories for children and adolescents 4–18 years of age, with most fats coming from sources of polyunsaturated and monounsaturated fatty acids, such as fish, nuts, and vegetable oils.

Iron Status

Iron deficiency, a relatively common problem, is usually due to inadequate dietary intake of iron and occurs most commonly during times of rapid growth or due to increased blood loss, toddlerhood, and adolescence (for girls). Iron deficiency is associated with cognitive and developmental abnormalities in children. Hematocrit, hemoglobin, and red blood cell indices are the laboratory parameters most commonly used to evaluate children and teens for iron deficiency. While more specific measures of iron stores are available (e.g. serum ferritin, transferrin, iron binding capacity, free erythrocyte protoporphyrin) they are costly and not widely utilized. *Healthy People 2020*[18] reports that 9% of children aged 1–2 years and 40% of children aged 3–4 are iron deficient. In addition, these analyses identified a substantially increased risk of iron deficiency with and without anemia in overweight and obese children compared with normal weight children, with iron deficiency prevalent in 15% of obese adolescent girls.[19]

A later examination of data from toddlers (ages 1–3) surveyed during NHANES IV (1999–2002) revealed an iron deficiency prevalence of 20% among obese toddlers compared with a prevalence of 7–8% among overweight and normal weight toddlers. A study of children (mean age 11.3±3.6 years) referred to a university-affiliated endocrinology clinic showed a significant inverse relationship between BMI and serum iron levels; iron deficiency was noted in 39%, 12%, and 4% of obese, overweight, and normal weight children, respectively.[19] Data from NHANES 2002 indicate that the overall prevalence of iron deficiency in US children under 5 years still exceeds the *Healthy People 2020* target of 1–5%.[18] Of 4.5 million low-income children under 5 years old participating in federally funded maternal and child health programs in 2006, 14% had anemia. Even in the absence of anemia, iron deficiency is associated with poor growth and neuro-cognitive development in infants and behavioral and learning problems in older children and adolescents. Iron deficiency and iron-deficiency anemia are also associated with decreased exercise capacity and physical endurance and therefore may contribute to the diminished exercise capacity observed in obese children and adolescents. Thus, it is important to evaluate overweight and obese children regardless of age for the presence of iron deficiency and/or iron-deficiency anemia. Iron-rich food sources are shown in Appendix L.

Energy and Protein Requirements

Energy requirements vary throughout childhood and correspond to the variations in rate of weight gain seen from birth through adolescence. The energy and nutrient requirements of children are proportional to their resting energy expenditure plus the energy needs of activity and normal growth. According to the Food and Nutrition Board, Institute of Medicine, National Academy of Science Dietary Reference Intake (DRI) values for energy requirements range from 520 kcal/day in girls aged 0–6 months up to 3152 kcal/day in boys aged 14–18 years (Table 5-2).[20]

For more details on estimating individual energy requirements (EER) in children from birth to 18 years, see the National Academy of Science, National

Table 5-2 Energy and Protein Requirements

Age	Energy (kcal/day)		Protein (g/day)	
	Males	Females	Males	Females
0–6 months	570	520	9.1	9.1
7–12 months	743	676	11.0	11.0
1–2 years	1046	992	13.0	13.0
3–8 years	1742	1642	19.0	19.0
9–13 years	2279	2071	34.0	34.0
14–18 years	3152	2368	52.0	46.0

Source: IOM: Food, and Nutrition Board. Dietary Reference Intakes for Energy and Protein, 2005.

Academies Press website (www.NAP.edu). Calculation of calories and protein consumed by an individual child, best performed by a nutrition professional, can be of use when weight gain falls below or exceeds average rates for individual ages. An emphasis on calorie levels in guiding families toward good nutrition and adequate intake should be avoided. It is better to help families understand nutritional requirements for children of various ages and the importance of age-appropriate portions and a balanced diet based on My Plate Guide,[21] in addition to the assessment of a child's growth curve to determine if growth and weight gain are within normal ranges.

Deviations from Normal Growth
Failure to Thrive

Failure to thrive describes the child who is not gaining weight appropriately due to inadequate calorie intake, malabsorption, and/or increased nutrient needs.[22] Commonly used criteria include children with weight (or weight-for-height) less than two standard deviations below the mean (5th percentile) for sex and age; and/or their weight curve has crossed more than two percentile lines (channels) on the National Center for Health Statistics/CDC growth charts after having achieved a previously stable pattern.[4] Evaluation of a child with growth failure should begin with a thorough history and physical exam, including a nutritional assessment. In the majority of cases, a history and physical will provide sufficient information to determine the etiology of failure to thrive (Table 5-3). Non-organic growth failure is the most common cause presenting in the US; therefore simple, non-invasive screening for medical problems should be undertaken.[24] Many children with poor growth suffer from behavioral and developmental problems, as well as social and economic disadvantages. When further medical evaluation is warranted, laboratory assessment should include complete blood count, comprehensive metabolic panel, thyroid function tests, and celiac panel. Other tests such as sweat testing, growth hormone, and inborn errors of metabolism should be performed as indicated by the history and physical findings.

Table 5-3 Differential Diagnosis of Failure to Thrive

Inadequate caloric intake
Incorrect preparation of formula (too diluted, too concentrated)
Unsuitable feeding habits (food fads, excessive juice)
Behavior problems affecting eating
Poverty and food shortages
Neglect
Disturbed parent–child relationship
Mechanical feeding difficulties (oromotor dysfunction, congenital anomalies, central nervous system damage, severe reflux)

Inadequate absorption
Celiac disease
Cystic fibrosis
Cow's milk protein allergy
Vitamin or mineral deficiencies (acrodermatitis enteropathica, scurvy)
Biliary atresia or liver disease
Necrotizing enterocolitis or short-gut syndrome

Increased metabolism
Hyperthyroidism
Chronic infection (human immunodeficiency virus or other immunodeficiency, malignancy, renal disease)
Hypoxemia (congenital heart defects, chronic lung disease)

Defective utilization
Genetic abnormalities (trisomies 21, 18, and 13)
Congenital infections
Metabolic disorders (storage diseases, amino acid disorders)

Source: Niedbala 2005.[23]

The Importance of Breakfast

Nurse Practitioners can promote important family time before the start of the day by encouraging eating breakfast together. Parents can model desired behavior and eat a healthy breakfast daily, regardless of how busy they are. A review of recent research suggests that eating breakfast may help children do better in school by improving memory, test grades, school attendance, psycho-social function, and mood.[25] The body and brain need glucose to function and to replenish glycogen stores after 8–12 hours of fasting. Eating breakfast helps improve mental alertness and physical performance and is positively associated with improvements in short-term memory. Breakfast should provide approximately 20% of a child's daily energy intake and nutrient needs. In children and adolescents, it is estimated that 12–34% regularly skip breakfast and these percentages increase with age.[26] Girls are more likely to skip breakfast while boys are more likely to eat breakfast daily.[26] Skipping breakfast also increases the likelihood of obesity and results in higher BMIs in adolescents age 9–11 years. In contrast, eating breakfast daily can help prevent inappropriate weight gain.[27] Breakfast should include at least three food groups, such as grains, dairy, and fruit. It is best to choose nutrient and fiber-rich food to maintain satiety and minimize hunger. Sometimes eating at home is not an option; encourage patients to prepare meals ahead of time or purchase ingredients that are easily portable to help meet the goal of eating breakfast. Combining fresh fruit and yogurt with high fiber dry cereal makes breakfast portable.

Infant Nutrition
Nutrition for the Premature Infant

Optimal nutrition is critical in the management of pre-term infants.[1] Although no standard exists for the precise nutritional needs of infants born prematurely, current recommendations are developed to simulate the *in-utero* growth rate. Breast milk or fortified breast milk is considered ideal for the pre-term infant. Human milk fortifiers can be added to breast milk for the pre-term infant to provide additional calories, protein, zinc, calcium, phosphorous, DHA, and folic acid. Powdered formula can be used to fortify breast milk once the infant is discharged home. Breast milk provides many advantages to pre-term infants in the form of growth factors, immunity to infection, support for the developing gastrointestinal tract, and enhanced calcium and phosphorus profiles. Infants who are formula fed should receive specialized pre-term formulas in the nursery and be discharged on pre-term follow-up formulas to allow continued catch-up growth and improvement in bone mineral density during the first year of life (Table 5-4).[9] It is suggested that these special formulas be used until 9–12 months corrected age (based on estimated date of confinement [EDC], not birth date).

Iron should be supplied to human milk-fed pre-term babies at 1 month of age (2 mg/kg/day) until one year.[1] Formula-fed pre-term infants may also benefit from an iron supplement (1 mg/kg/day) in addition to the iron present in pre-term infant formulas, through the first year of life.[1] All infants who are breast-fed should be supplemented with vitamin D (400 IU/kg/day) to support bone formation. Human milk powdered fortifiers and special formulas for pre-term infants supply between

---

Case 1: Premature Infant

An African-American female whose chronological age is 4 months presents for a well-child visit. PMH: 28-week gestation with retinopathy of prematurity (ROP), followed by ophthalmic care. Birth weight: 1300 g. Present weight is 2.7 kg. She is consuming Neosure Expert Care 22/cal/oz, 3 oz every 3 hours.
- What is your recommendation for feeding and the introduction of solid food?
- How would you plot her weight?
- Would you draw any labs?

APPROACH: First adjust for prematurity: Months Chronologic Age minus Months Premature equals Months Corrected Age (4 months – 3 months = 1 month Corrected) *Full term = 40 weeks, 4 weeks = 1 month.

Use WHO growth chart ≤2 years of age and correct for prematurity. Introduction of solid food is recommended at 4–6 months. Corrected age is 1 month so wait until 4 months corrected age or 7 months chronologic age. Screen for anemia at 4 months chronological age; CBC with reticulocytes or H/H with reticulocytes. Premature babies are at risk for anemia due to low iron stores (80% of an infant's iron stores develop in the third trimester), rapid growth, and frequent blood sampling in the NICU.

Table 5-4 Indications and Types of Infant Formulas

Formula	Indications	Unique Properties	Examples
Milk-based	Breast milk substitute for term infants	+/− Iron Ready to feed, powder, or liquid concentrate Variable whey casein (20 kcal/oz) Contains DHA/ARA	Enfamil Lipil Similac Advance Enfamil Lactofree Similac Lactose-free Enfamil AR (pre-thickened) Good Start Supreme
Soy-based	Breast milk substitute for infants with lactose intolerance or milk protein allergy*	Lactose-free, may contain sucrose or corn-free (20 kcal/oz) May contain fiber	Prosobee, Isomil Good Start Soy Essentials Isomil DF
Premature	Breast milk substitute for low-birth-weight, hospitalized pre-term infants	Low lactose Whey: casein 60:40 High calcium and phosphorus (20 and 24 cal/oz) Contains DHA/ARA	Enfamil Premature Lipil Similac SpecialCare Advance Similac HMF Enfamil HMF
Human Milk Fortifiers	Fortification of breast milk for pre-term infants	Increases calorie, protein, and vitamin/mineral content of breast milk	Similac HMF Enfamil HMF
Premature–transitional	Breast milk substitute for pre-term infants >2.5 kg or discharge formula for pre-term infants	22 kcal/oz ready to feed or powder Contains DHA/ARA	Enfacare Lipil Neosure Advance
Older Infant	Transition to whole milk	Varies	Good Start Essentials 2 Enfamil Next Step, & w/Soy
Hypoallergenic	Milk or soy protein allergy	Hydrolyzed protein Sucrose-free Lactose-free	Nutramigen
Predigested	Malabsorption Short bowel syndrome Allergy	Lactose-free Hydrolyzed protein or free amino acids	Alimentum Pregestamil Neocate Elecare
Fat-modified	Defects in digestion, absorption, or transport of fat	Contains increased calories as MCT	Portagen (no longer recommended for infants) Alimentum Pregestamil
Carbohydrate-modified	Simple sugar intolerance	Requires addition of complex carbohydrate to be complete	RCF 3232 A
Amino acid-modified	Inborn errors of metabolism	Low or devoid of specific amino acids that cannot be metabolized	Multiple products
Electrolyte and/or mineral modified	Renal disease requiring decreased electrolyte and mineral content	Decreased potassium content Decreased calcium and phosphorus content	Similac PM 60/40

*Children allergic to milk protein may also be allergic to soy protein.
Source: Sue Konek, MA, RD, CNSC, CSP, LDN, The Children's Hospital of Philadelphia, 2012. Used with Permission.

> ### Key Points for Pre-Term Infants
>
> - Breast milk or fortified breast milk is considered ideal for the pre-term infant.
> - Breast or formula fed pre-term infants may benefit from iron supplementation in addition to formula in the first 12 months of life.
> - All breast-fed pre-term infants should be supplemented with 400 IU vitamin D.
> - Pre-term infants are at high risk for rickets due to inadequate calcium intake: alkaline phosphatase, calcium, and phosphorous levels should be monitored.

400 IU/day vitamin D.[1,28] Pre-term infants are at high risk for rickets of prematurity due to inadequate calcium intake early in life. Therefore, alkaline phosphatase, calcium, and phosphorous levels should be monitored. When plotting the pre-term infant on the WHO growth chart after discharge from the hospital, correction for gestational age should be continued until age 2 years for linear growth and until age 3 years for weight and head circumference.

Nutrition for the Term Infant
Advocating Breastfeeding
The WHO and the American Academy of Pediatrics (AAP) strongly recommend exclusive breastfeeding infants for the first 6 months of life.[29,30] Successful lactation depends on the knowledge and supportive attitude of Nurse Practitioners on both in pediatric and obstetric services, and hospital policies and practices conducive to the initiation and maintenance of breastfeeding. Many mothers will require support to successfully breastfeed their infants. Breast milk is the most complete form of nutrition for infants, with a positive impact on health, growth, development, and immunity. Additionally, breastfeeding has been shown to improve maternal health, promote faster maternal weight loss to pre-pregnancy weight, and decrease the risk of maternal breast cancer. At 6 months post-partum, the target goal is 60.6%; 43.5% of infants born in 2006 were breast-fed at 6 months.[18] At 1 year the target is 34.1%; however, 22.7% of infants born in 2006 were breast-fed at 1 year.[18] *Healthy People 2020* target goals state that 81.9% of mothers should breastfeed their babies in the early post-partum period.[18] The most recent CDC data state that three out of every four new mothers in the US start out breastfeeding in the first few weeks after birth. However, rates of breastfeeding at 6 and 12 months, as well as rates of exclusive breast-feeding at 3 and 6 months, remain low.[31] The Breastfeeding Report Card Outcome Indicators that collect data on initiation and duration of breastfeeding, report that 75% of infants have been breast-fed, 33% exclusively breast-fed at 3 months, 13.3% exclusively breast-fed at 6 months (43% receiving some breastfeeding), and 22.4% partially breast-fed at 12 months.[31]

Benefits of Breastfeeding
Human milk is unique in its components and dynamic nutrient composition. Composition changes throughout lactation and provides a higher protein, more

digestible mixture for pre-term infants. Its whey:casein ratio of 70:30 makes it more digestible than the 18:82 content of cow's milk. Human milk contains the omega-3 fatty acids arachidonic acid (ARA) and docosahexanoic acid (DHA) which are essential for visual function and neurodevelopment in infants. Carbohydrates, in the form of lactose and oligosaccharides, are easily digested, and supported by the presence of the digestive enzyme lactase. Calcium and phosphorus, though present in lower levels than in cow's milk formulas, are more bioavailable in breast milk to support bone growth. Other micronutrients are adequate to meet the infant's nutritional needs until age 6 months when iron-fortified infant cereal should be introduced. Human milk contributes to the maturation of the gastrointestinal tract and provides a host of bioactive factors, including secretory IgA, lactoferrin, lysozyme, nucleotides, all supporting the immunity of the child.[24] Human milk protects against Crohn's disease, lymphoma, and type 1 diabetes mellitus. Exclusive breastfeeding in the first half-year of life may prevent the early development of allergic disease in early childhood.[32]

Adequacy of Breast Milk

The best way to be sure that infants are receiving adequate amounts of breast milk is to monitor their growth and development. Thus, all infants should be seen regularly by their primary care provider. Milk production works on the principle of supply and demand. The more frequently an infant nurses, the more milk is produced by the mother. Frequent nursing in the first few days of life (every 1–3 hours), helps to stimulate initial milk production. Nurse Practitioners can encourage parents to estimate appropriate intake at home by monitoring to ensure their baby has at least six wet diapers a day and a minimum of three stools per day if they are breastfeeding, or two-to-three stools per day if they are drinking formula. Although breast-fed infants consume less milk than formula-fed infants over a 24-hour period, and therefore have a lower energy intake, they are more energy efficient. By year three, breast-fed infants have a lower percentage of body fat and are rarely overweight. The breast-fed infant can control the flow of milk and this may help to explain why breast-fed infants are less likely to overfeed than formula-fed infants. The breast-fed infant adjusts feeding quantity according to its hunger and level of satiety, while bottle-fed infants are often fed until the bottle is empty.

Mothers who breastfeed rely on the infant to self-regulate intake. This ability helps a growing child eat enough, but not excessively, which may improve self-regulation of food intake later in childhood. Breastfeeding also promotes good jaw and tooth development in the infant. For these reasons, human milk is considered the best source of nutrition for infants. Even so, there are some cautions that should be stated regarding breastfeeding. Women who are infected with HIV should not breastfeed.[1] A second area of caution involves a breastfeeding mother who is a strict vegetarian or a vegan. Several cases have been reported in the literature of infants with vitamin B_{12} deficiency who were breast-fed by vitamin B_{12} deficient mothers with an extended history of vegan diets.[33,34] Infants of vegan mothers should be monitored for signs of vitamin B_{12} deficiency which include lethargy, failure to thrive, developmental delay, or macrocytic anemia.

Formula Feeding

Full-term infants who do not receive human milk can be adequately nourished with iron-fortified infant formulas during the first year of life. These formulas, designed to mimic human milk, have been greatly improved over the last 70 years.[1] Standard cow's milk-based formulas are the feeding of choice when breastfeeding is not used. Modification of the whey:casein ratio to increase the whey content has improved protein digestibility. As in human milk, lactose is the major carbohydrate. Only iron-fortified formulas should be offered to infants, as iron has a critical role in brain growth. In the past, low iron formulas were recommended for infants with constipation. However, well-controlled studies have consistently failed to show any increase in the prevalence of fussiness, cramping, colic, or constipation with the use of iron-fortified formulas.[1] In 1999, the AAP stated there was "no role for the use of low-iron formulas in infant feeding and recommends that all infant formulas be fortified with iron"[1] Standard infant formulas contain a caloric density of 67–70 kcal/dL (20 kcal/oz). The usual intake of 150–200 mL/kg/day will provide 100–135 kcal/kg/day. The fat composition of formula has changed with the recent addition of ARA and DHA. Whether addition of these omega-3 fatty acids will have a long-term effect on growth, visual development, information processing skills, or IQ, is not known.[35] Infant formulas other than standard cow's-milk-based formulas may be indicated for some infants.

Soy protein formulas are lactose-free and constitute approximately 25% of all formulas sold. Soy protein-based formulas are not recommended for pre-term infants of less than 1800 g to reduce the risk of osteopenia.[1] Phytates in soy protein bind calcium, resulting in decreased bioavailability for bone mineralization. Soy formulas are successfully used by vegetarians and indicated for infants with a cow's milk allergy. Soy formulas are also appropriate for the rare infant with lactase deficiency or galactosemia. Soy formulas may be used for secondary lactose deficiency following a prolonged gastroenteritis. Infants with these symptoms should be rechallenged with their regular formulas within 1 month.

Special formulas have been developed for babies with unique requirements. Protein hydrolysate formulas provide nutrition for infants who cannot digest or are intolerant of intact cow's milk protein. These are the preferred formulas for infants with cow's milk and soy protein intolerance and for those with gastrointestinal or hepatobiliary diseases such as biliary atresia or protracted diarrhea. These formulas may contain varying amounts of medium-chain triglycerides (MCTs) to facilitate fat absorption. Formulas containing free amino acids are also available for infants with extreme protein hypersensitivity who cannot tolerate hydrolyzed formulas. These formulas are very expensive and should be used only when needed. Cow's milk of any kind, as well as goat's milk, evaporated milk, or other milks should *not* be used during the first 12 months of life. The protein in cow's milk can cause chronic gastrointestinal blood loss and subsequent iron deficiency anemia. The higher content of protein, sodium, potassium, and chloride in cow's milk provides an inappropriately high renal solute load. The level of essential fatty acids, vitamin E, and zinc in cow's milk are inadequate for infants. Skim milk should not be given to infants younger than 2 years due to its excessive protein and inadequate fat content. The wide variety of formulas available, both standard and specialized, are reviewed in Table 5-4.

Key Points for Term Infants

- Support and encourage breastfeeding as part of the newborn infant assessment.
- Carefully monitor growth and development to ensure adequate breast milk intake.
- Only iron fortified formulas should be offered to term infants.
- Cow's milk and goat's milk should not be used during the first 12 months of life.
- Complementary foods should be initiated between 4 and 6 months of age.

Complementary Foods (Solid Foods)

Recommendations for the introduction of complementary (solid) foods have changed over the years.[36] In the past, health care professionals recommended that children be introduced to solid foods as early as the first month of life. Today, the consensus among pediatric clinicians is to delay introducing solid foods until the child is between 4 and 6 months of age. This recommendation is supported by both the AAP and the WHO. Both organizations support exclusively breastfeeding for the first 6 months. Introduction of solid foods earlier than 4–6 months may result in the development of food allergies. Furthermore, infants are not physiologically ready to accept solid foods from a spoon until their protrusion reflex becomes extinguished at approximately 4 months. The development of head and neck control and coordination of oral musculature at 3–4 months will also prepare the infant for solids after this time. A firm consensus on the progression of complementary foods does not exist. Review of practices in developed countries reveals a wide variety of recommendation for beginning foods. Guidelines on how to feed infants as they transition to solid food are shown in Table 5-5.

Eating Habits of Children

Knowledge of current intake patterns can assist in providing guidance to families on how to feed their toddlers in order to improve their nutritional intake. The 2002 Feeding Infants and Toddlers Study (FITS) surveyed 3022 US families with infants and toddlers age 4–24 months to see how nutrition in these children compared with current recommendations and DRIs.[37–41] This randomized survey was conducted through phone interviews using a 24-hour recall. Findings indicated that solid foods starting at the appropriate time and early introduction of whole cow's milk (<6 months) was uncommon. By 24 months some infants drank little or no milk. It was suggested that this might set the stage for decreased milk consumption into childhood and adolescence. Toddlers as a group had energy intakes greater than that recommended by the DRIs. Of concern, 18–33% of infants and toddlers between ages 7 and 24 months did not consume any vegetables and 25% did not consume any fruits.[38] French fries emerged as a commonly eaten vegetable, even in children as young as 9 months.

Also of concern was that almost 50% of 7–8 month old infants were already consuming sweets, desserts, and sweetened beverages, which increased through 24 months. After the first year of life, family eating patterns came into play.[37] For this reason, family-based approaches to food guidance are needed. The researchers of the FITS study recommended that parents be encouraged to offer a wide variety of

Table 5-5 How to Feed Your Infant During the First Year of Life

Age in months	Breast milk or iron-fortified infant formula	Cereals and breads	Fruits and fruit juices*	Vegetables	Protein foods	Dairy foods
0–4	5–10 feedings/day 17–24 fl oz/day (510–720 mL/day)	None	None	None	None	None
4–6	4–7 feedings/day 24–32 fl oz/day (720–960 mL/day)	Rice or barley infant cereals (iron fortified). Mix cereal with formula or breast milk until thin. Start with 1 tbsp at each feeding for a few days, and increase to 3–4 tbsp/day. Feed with small baby spoon (don't expect baby to eat much at first).	None	None	None	None
7–8	4–5 feedings/day 24–32 fl oz/day (720–960 mL/day)	Single grain infant cereals—rice, oatmeal, barley (iron fortified) in the morning 3–9 tbsp/day, mixed with breast milk or infant formula. Two feedings a day. Oven-dried toast or teething biscuits, crackers, or toast strips.	Strained or mashed fruits (fresh or cooked), mashed bananas, apple sauce. Infant 100% fruit juices (4 oz/day) < 4 oz/day mixed with water and served in a cup.	Strained or mashed, well-cooked: dark yellow or orange (not corn), dark green vegetables. Start with mild vegetables such as green beans, peas, o squash 1/2–1 jar or 1/4–1/2 cup/day.	Smooth preparations of single meats: lamb, veal, chicken, may be started in small quantities (up to 2 tbsp/day).	Cottage cheese, yogurt.

(Continued)

Table 5-5 How to Feed Your Infant During the First Year of Life (*Continued*)

Age in months	Breast milk or iron-fortified infant formula	Cereals and breads	Fruits and fruit juices*	Vegetables	Protein foods	Dairy foods
8–9	3–4 feedings/day 24–32 fl oz/day (720–960 ml/day)	Infant cereals or plain hot cereals mixed with breast milk or formula. Toast, bagels, crackers, teething biscuits. Small pieces of cooked noodles, potatoes.	Peeled soft fruit wedges: bananas, peaches, pears, oranges, apples (skin removed). 100% fruit juices including orange and tomato juices 4–6 oz/day.	Cooked, mashed vegetables.	Well cooked, strained, ground or finely chopped chicken, fish, and lean meats: 2–3 tbsp/day (remove all bones, fat, skin). Cooked dried beans. Egg yolks only, no whites.	Cottage cheese, yogurt, bite-size cheese strips.
10–12	3–4 feedings/day 24–32 fl oz/day (720–960 mL/day) by cup or bottle	Infant or cooked cereals mixed with breast milk or formula. Unsweetened cereals, white/wheat breads. Mashed potatoes, rice, noodles, spaghetti.	All fresh fruits peeled and seeded or canned fruits packed in water. 100% fruit juices 4–6 oz/day.	Cooked vegetable pieces. Some raw vegetables: tomatoes, cucumbers.	Small tender pieces of chicken, fish or lean meat. Cooked beans, Pasta.	Cottage cheese, yogurt, bite-size cheese strips.

These are general guidelines. Feeding schedules vary somewhat between children.
*There is no specific need for juice in an infant's diet.
Source: Lisa Hark, PhD, RD, 2012. Used with permission.

vegetables and fruits on a daily basis. This recommendation should emphasize inclusion of dark green, leafy, and deep yellow vegetables as well as colorful fruits. Sweets and desserts should be offered only occasionally, instead offering nutrient-dense food for dessert such as fruit, cheese, yogurt, and cereals. Beverages should consist of water, limited amounts of 100% fruit juice, and low-fat milk for children over 2 years of age. The practice of offering toddlers several snacks daily was commonly observed. Because toddlers received about 25% of their calories from snacks, the importance of providing planned nutrient-rich foods at snack-time becomes apparent. Five servings (serving = 1 tablespoon/year of age) of fruit and vegetables daily as well as three servings of dairy foods should remain a goal for toddlers.[42]

Introducing New Foods

In order to detect a potential food allergy, new foods should be introduced to infants one at a time with at least 3 days between new items. Dietary recommendations for children in families with a history of food allergies or asthma suggest avoidance of dairy products until 1 year of age, avoidance of eggs until age 2, and avoidance of peanuts, tree nuts and fish/shellfish until age 3. High risk children are those with parents or siblings with any allergies, including hay fever or pet allergies (FAAN).[43] The Food Allergy and Anaphylaxis Network (FAAN) is an excellent resource for families with food allergies. When preparing foods, it is important that salt and sugar not be added, to prevent infants from developing a preference for these tastes. Babies often prefer foods warmed to room temperature. If a microwave is used to warm foods, the food should be mixed well and temperature tested to avoid burning the infant's mouth. Table 5-6 outlines important feeding tips for infants and young children. Although there is no consensus on the exact order for the introduction of complementary foods, the following order is commonly used.

Table 5-6 Tips on Feeding Your Infant

- Avoid laying your baby down with a bottle to prevent ear infections and tooth decay.
- Introduce only one new food every 3 days to detect sensitivities or allergies.
- Avoid overfeeding. Stop feeding when baby turns away from food or shows disinterest.
- Use a baby spoon to feed cereal and other foods. Do not put cereal in the bottle.
- Feed only breast milk for the first 6 months, formula until 4–6 months — no solid foods.
- Throw away unused formula from a bottle after each feeding.
- Use formula or breast milk, not cow's milk, until your baby's first birthday.
- Limit juice intake to less than 4–6 oz/day beginning after 6 months and dilute with water.
- Avoid offering sweet desserts, candy, soft drinks, fruit-flavored or sweetened drinks, or sugar-coated cereal to infants and children.
- Avoid adding sugar or salt to baby's food. Check labels for added sugar and salt.
- Feed baby food from a bowl, not from the jar.
- Avoid hard and round pieces of food that can cause choking (whole grapes, raw carrots, popcorn, hot dogs, peanuts).
- At 1 year of age, initiate whole cow's milk. Encourage milk in a cup rather than a bottle.
- Consider offering vegetables before fruit to avoid setting up a preference for sweets.
- Avoid adding honey to baby food, as it may contain bacteria, which can cause botulism in infants. Honey may be used after 1 year of age.

Source: Lisa Hark, PhD, RD, 2012. Used with permission.

Cereals In the US, the most common initial solid food is iron-fortified rice cereal. It is recommended that this and other foods not be started before 4 months of age. Rice cereal, fortified with iron, is unlikely to cause allergies and is usually well tolerated. It is common practice to give one or two tablespoons of rice cereal, mixed with breast milk or infant formula, in the morning. There is no absolute with regard to the introduction of solid foods and various cultures and ethnic groups vary in this practice. The cereal should be mixed to a consistency similar to that of apple sauce, with adjustments made for the child's preference. Cereal should always be fed from a small spoon. Eating is a new skill which may take the infant a few weeks to master. The practice of putting cereal in a bottle of formula should be avoided. Studies show this does not help children to sleep through the night and may lead to over-feeding and possibly choking, especially if a larger hole is cut into the nipple. Oat or barley infant cereal may be tried after allowing 4 days to detect any allergic reaction. Wheat and mixed infant cereals should not be given to young infants, as wheat is a common allergen. These cereals can be added later in the first year.

Vegetables Cooked, strained vegetables, without salt or spices, either homemade or purchased baby food, are appropriate to start at 6–8 months of age. There is no evidence to support introducing foods in a particular order.[1] Even so, some practitioners believe that vegetables should be introduced before fruits to prevent the infant from developing a preference for sweets. Salt and spices should be avoided in infant feeding, especially for families preparing homemade infant foods. Raw vegetables that are soft may be introduced at one year. Some hard vegetables, such as carrots, should be avoided until the eruption of top and bottom molars, to prevent choking.

Fruits Cooked, strained, and pureed fruits, purchased as baby food or homemade, (without sugar) may be started after rice cereal. Fresh, mashed bananas can also be introduced at this time. Peeled, soft fruits such as pears and peaches may be cut into small pieces and started at 8–10 months of age. As with vegetables, hard fruits such as apples should be delayed until the child can easily chew harder foods. Juices, such as apple, made from 100% fruit, may also be offered, but in small quantities — less than 4–6 oz/day until 1 year is recommended by the AAP.[1] Excess juice consumption can lead to diarrhea due to high fructose and sorbitol content of fruit juices, as well as excessive weight gain.

Eggs Cooked egg yolks may be introduced to infants without a history of food allergies. Egg whites should be delayed until 1 year of age because of the potential risk of inducing egg allergy in younger infants. (Allergy to egg may delay or limit administration of vaccines that are produced with eggs.)

Meats Ground and finely chopped chicken, meats, and fish, either homemade or purchased as baby food, are generally introduced after fruits and vegetables are well tolerated. Meat is a rich source of iron and zinc, nutrients that are limited in human milk alone.

Starch/carbohydrate Children enjoy pasta, spaghetti and dry cereals, and these can be added to the diet later in the first year. These foods should not be used in place of more nutrient-rich foods, such as fruits and vegetables. Suggest whole wheat breads and pastas and whole grain pastas to help children learn to acquire a taste for these early on.

Iron Fortified Cereals The prevalence of iron deficiency in the US has decreased over the last 20 years due to increased iron supplementation of infant cereals and formulas and supplemental food programs for low-income families, such as the Women, Infants and Children (WIC) program. Even so, *Healthy People 2020* reported that 9% of children aged 1–2 years, and 40% of children aged 3–4 years are iron deficient.[18] Altered behavior and brain function, including learning difficulties, have been reported in iron-deficient infants and toddlers.[44] Some studies have questioned whether iron supplementation before 6 months would benefit breast-fed infants. Friel and colleagues found better visual acuity in breast-fed infants who were supplemented with iron.[45] Even small amounts of iron may be of benefit to the developing brain. Though practice change is not warranted in this regard at present, it is critical that iron-rich foods be among the initial foods introduced during the first year. Iron-rich foods, including iron-fortified cereals, red meat, dark-green leafy vegetables, and dried fruit such as raisins and prunes, should also be consumed regularly throughout childhood. Raisins should be soaked in hot water, cooled, and mashed for young children to reduce the risk of choking.

Fats Children under 2 years of age need a high-calorie diet to help ensure normal brain development and to support rapid growth. Fat in the diet allows young children to achieve their caloric goals. Essential fatty acids are especially important for normal brain development. Therefore, the AAP recommends that dietary fat should not be limited prior to age 2.[1] After 2 years of age, low-fat dairy products (1% or 2% milk and low-fat yogurt and cheese) and limited consumption of high fat foods (such as fried foods, ice cream, and pizza) are part of a strategy to help prevent children from becoming overweight or developing cardiovascular risk.

Special care to avoid choking During the first year of life and up to age 4, foods should be prepared to promote swallowing without the risk of aspiration. In addition, parents should not leave children alone when eating meals or snacks to guard against choking events (Table 5-7).

Table 5-7 Foods to Avoid Before Age 3–4 to Prevent Choking

- Carrots (unless cooked until very soft).
- Chewing gum.
- Chunks of meat.
- Hard candy.
- Nuts.
- Popcorn.
- Raw apples or pears.
- Seeds.
- Whole grapes (may be cut into small pieces).
- Whole or large sections of hot dogs.

Source: Lisa Hark, PhD, RD, 2012. Used with permission.

Detecting Food Allergies

Food allergies and food hypersensitivity reactions occur in 2–8% of children less than 3 years of age.[1] Approximately 2.5% of infants will experience allergic reactions to cow's milk in the first 3 years of life, 1.5% to eggs and 0.6% to peanuts. Approximately 85% of these will later become tolerant to milk and eggs (within the first 5 years of life). Even peanut allergy may be "outgrown" by 20% of children.

The gradual introduction of new foods (one new food every 3 days) starting after the age of 6 months, may reduce allergy risk and allow for the identification of foods which fit the definition of food hypersensitivity. Parents should be aware that swelling of the lips and face, skin rash, vomiting, or diarrhea are symptoms associated with food allergy. Once identified, strict avoidance of an offending food is the only way to prevent the allergic response. The challenge of treating food allergies occurs when children are allergic to many foods, sometimes requiring avoidance of whole groups of foods.[36]

Definitions of Food Allergies

Adverse reaction: Clinically abnormal response believed to be caused by an ingested food or food additive.

Food hypersensitivity (allergy): Immunologic reaction resulting from the ingestion of a food or food additive.

Food anaphylaxis: Classic allergic hypersensitivity reaction to food or food additives involving IgE antibody and release of chemical mediators.

Food intolerance: General term describing an abnormal physiologic response to an ingested food or food additive; can include idiosyncratic, metabolic, pharmacologic, or toxic responses.

Source: American Academy of Allergy and Immunology Committee on Adverse Reactions to Foods. 2010

Key Points for Children with Food Allergies

- Eight foods account for 90% of all food allergies: peanuts, tree nuts (such as walnuts or almonds), eggs, milk, fish, shellfish, soy, and wheat.
- Allergies to milk, wheat, or eggs require careful avoidance of many foods, as these ingredients may be "hidden" in many foods.
- Soy protein is also widely used in prepared foods.
- Children who are allergic to the foods that make up critical groups, such as dairy, may benefit from consultation with a dietitian to identify inadequacies and help plan a diet that meets all of their nutrient requirements while avoiding the offending foods.

Vitamin and Mineral Supplements

If children eat a varied diet, they should not require supplements. A very picky eater may benefit from a daily multi-vitamin/mineral supplement. At certain times during childhood, a few vitamins and minerals may be insufficient including calcium, vitamin D, vitamin K, fluoride, and iron.

Calcium Children who consume the recommended amounts of dairy foods for their age (milk, yogurt, cheese) will receive adequate calcium. Those who do not consume three servings of dairy foods everyday may require a calcium supplement. Calcium needs are particularly high for adolescents who increase height by 20% and gain 50% of adult skeletal mass during this period. Food sources of calcium are shown in Appendices G and H.

Vitamin D The AAP recommends that all babies, including those who are exclusively breast-fed, receive vitamin D within the first 2 months of life. Infant formulas provide adequate vitamin D.[28,29] Breast-fed infants should receive 400 IU/daily in a supplement. Vitamin D intake through the use of fortified dairy products should continue through childhood, and especially adolescence, to support development of a healthy skeletal structure. Food sources of vitamin D are show in Appendix B.

Vitamin K Newborn babies are given vitamin K, in injection form, soon after birth for prophylaxis against hemorrhagic disease of the newborn, now called vitamin K deficiency bleeding (VKDB).

Fluoride A supplement of fluoride is recommended for infants 6 months or older who are breast-fed or living in an area without fluoridated water. Infants aged 7–12 months require 0.5 mg/day, 1–2 years: 0.7 mg/d, 3–8 years: 1 mg/d. Primary care Nurse Practitioners should determine fluoride levels in their communities to guide adequate dosing of fluoride for children.

Toddler and Preschool Nutrition

After the rapid growth spurt of the first year of life, the normal decrease in food intake of 2 year-olds associated with a slowed growth rate may cause concern in uninformed parents. Toddlers' intake will vary depending on the timing of their growth spurts. In order to meet the nutritional needs of children between 2 and 5 years of age, small nutrient-rich meals and snacks are needed. It is recommended that a small snack be given between each meal and at bedtime. Parents need to know that a smaller appetite, varying from day to day, is normal for children at this age.

Portion Sizes for Toddlers

My Plate provides excellent guidance regarding portion sizes of all foods and a wealth of information on meal planning for people of all ages, based on age, sex, and activity level.[21] For toddlers, it provides an interactive tool that allows parents and clinicians to estimate calorie needs based on physical activity level. These calorie needs are then used to choose the appropriate sample meal plan based on a specific number of serving sizes for each food group. Sample menus are also available for a range of calorie levels.

Beverages

The healthiest drinks for young children over the age of 3 years are low-fat milk (1%) and water. Many parents allow children to drink large amounts of fruit juice,

---

Sample Menu: 1–2 years old

Breakfast: 2 mini whole grain waffles with low-sugar syrup, 4 oz of fruited yogurt, and 4 oz of dilute orange juice (half juice, half water)
Snack: 1/2 cup fruit salad and 4 oz of whole milk
Lunch: 1/2-1 cup of macaroni and cheese with green beans, 4 oz milk, and 1/2 banana
Snack: 2 graham crackers and 4 oz dilute apple juice
Dinner: 2 oz white-meat chicken with 1/2 cup cooked brown rice, 1/2 cup soft broccoli florets, 2 slices of cucumber, and 4 oz of whole milk

(Note: After 2 years, low-fat milk should be used instead of whole milk.)

Source: Darwin Deen, MD, MS, and Lisa Hark, PhD, RD, 2012. Used with permission.

Sample Menu: 3–5 years old

Breakfast: 1/2 cup low-sugar whole grain cereal with low-fat milk and 1/2 sliced banana
Snack: Apple with a slice of low-fat cheese and 8 oz of water
Lunch: Turkey slices on whole wheat bread and a peach with 6-8 oz low-fat yogurt
Snack: 4 graham crackers, mandarin oranges in own juice, and 4 oz low-fat milk
Dinner: 3 meatballs in tomato sauce with string beans and tomatoes and 4 oz low-fat milk
Snack: 1/2 cup seedless grapes

Source: Darwin Deen, MD, MS, and Lisa Hark, PhD, RD, 2012. Used with permission.

---

fruit-flavored drinks, sweetened beverages, or soda. This practice contributes to excessive weight gain, poor dental health, and inadequate vitamin and mineral intake. The AAP recommends limiting juice to 4–6 oz/day for 1–5 year-olds.[1] Fresh fruits should be recommended, as fruit has added nutrients and fiber. Only pasteurized juices should be offered to children. Nurse Practitioners should discourage parents from offering children sweetened beverages, soda, sports drinks, and any fruit drinks that are not 100% juice. Nurse Practitioners may suggest the use of non-nutritive sweeteners (aspartame, sucralose, acesulfame potassium, etc) in some scenarios. The American Dietetic Association supports the use of non-nutritive sweeteners as part of a varied diet and recognizes their role in reducing the percentage of total caloric intake from refined carbohydrates. In an era where toddlers and children are consuming above the maximum recommended 25% of total caloric intake from sugar, non-nutritive sweeteners may help to reduce caloric intake from sugars without the concern for adverse health effects.

Importance of Role Modeling

Parents must realize the important role they play in shaping the food habits of their children. The influence of family eating patterns is seen in children aged 2–4 years and may become more pronounced with increasing age.[12] Parental modeling does impact children's food choices. Research by Hart, Raynor and Jelalian demonstrates that role modeling may begin as early as the introduction of complementary foods, indicating the importance of parent modeling on children's diets.[46]

> ## Key Points for Toddler and Preschool Nutrition
>
> - Decrease in oral intake is appropriate and corresponds to a slowed growth rate in comparison to infancy.
> - Smaller appetites and varying eating patterns are common and normal.
> - Parents are important role models and should choose and prepare healthful foods while the child decides how much they should eat.
> - Family meals are important to develop lifelong communication skills as well as healthy eating habits.
> - Picky eating does not usually lead to nutritional problems; toddlers are good at intuitively balancing caloric intake with output. Parents should not become short-order cooks to meet the needs of toddlers.
> - Nurse Practitioners should be concerned about picky eating when a child is not gaining weight or growing appropriately, or when significant food refusal continues for more than 1 month.

Family Meals

Eating together as a family is important for many reasons: children learn that mealtime is a structured setting where healthy foods are served and family meals help children to develop both communication skills and healthy eating habits. Meals eaten together are the perfect opportunity for parents to serve as role models for good nutrition. Habits such as eating nutritionally balanced meals can be more easily established when parents and children do this together. Meals also offer an opportunity to relate as a family and talk about the day's events.

Teaching Toddlers About Food

Teaching toddlers about food, how it is prepared and how it helps their bodies grow, can increase their interest in eating a varied and healthy diet. Taking toddlers to the grocery store, farmers' markets, or to a working farm will increase their knowledge and curiosity about food and how it nourishes their bodies. Encourage parents to shop for and prepare healthy foods with their toddlers. Even younger toddlers can help prepare snacks and develop motor skills by spreading peanut butter on crackers and toast or mixing vegetable dip. Involvement in meal and snack preparation can help them enjoy nutritious foods even more.

Managing the "Picky Eater"

The "picky eater" typically presents when a child is between the ages of 1 and 3 years, and can last up to age 5. Picky eating during childhood is very common and does not typically lead to nutritional problems. Studies show that most toddlers who skip meals will meet their nutritional needs and are good at intuitively regulating caloric intake[47] Offering a new food once is not enough, parents should be advised that repeated exposures to new foods (up to 15 times) may be needed for their acceptance.[48] Parents' responsibility is to determine what foods will be presented and when.[22]

Table 5-8 Encouraging Healthy Eating Habits in Preschool Children

- Serve fruits and vegetables every day, at meals and snacks. Keep canned fruit such as pineapple, peaches, and mandarin oranges in their own juice on hand for quick snacks.
- Provide milk (low-fat for children over 2 years) and water for meals or snacks. Limit juice to 4–6 oz/day.
- Do not be afraid to say no to junk food, chips, soda, candy, or sweets.
- Serve small portions on small plates and small cups. Let the child regulate his or her own intake. Serving large portions and insisting on a "clean plate" can lead to overeating and the loss of self-regulation.
- Do not use dessert as a reward ("finish your vegetables or you won't have dessert") — dessert is part of the meal and should be no more desired than the meal itself. Serve healthy desserts when possible.
- When a child says they have finished, allow them to take their plate to the sink and return to the table while parents finish. Appropriate activities or books will allow the child to enjoy this time.
- Keep a cabinet full of healthy snacks for the child's choosing at snack time.
- Try to dine as a family whenever possible.
- Limit TV/computer time to less than 2 hours a day.
- Encourage your child to be physically active (children need at least one hour of activity/day).
- Offer family activities to promote exercise.

Source: Sue Konek, MA, RD, CNSC, CSP, LDN. The Children's Hospital of Philadelphia, 2012. Used with permission.

Parents must trust that the child can self-regulate energy intake. It is also important for parents to not strictly force or prohibit foods, as research has shown strict dietary control results in both increased intake when not under parental control as well as outright refusal of forced foods.[48]

During the second year of life, the decrease in growth velocity may result in appetites that seem to wax and wane. Children who are allowed to "graze" or drink juice between meals may not be hungry at mealtime. Snacks should be planned, leaving a reasonable time period before meals (2–3 hours). It is important for Nurse Practitioners to convey to parents that children have small stomachs. Portion sizes should be small, served on small plates with small cups. Food jags, in which only a few foods will be eaten over several weeks or months, are common. These periods are often a sign of developmentally appropriate increasing independence. The less pressure that parents impose for children to eat specific foods, the greater the likelihood that this phase will pass. Tips for coping with a picky eater are shown in Table 5-8. Children that demonstrate difficulty gaining weight or decline in percentiles on the growth chart are a concern and require further medical evaluation.

When to Be Concerned

Parents are often concerned about possible nutrient deficiencies in their children who refuse to eat fruits and vegetables. While certainly a theoretical concern, it rarely becomes a health problem.[1] Nurse Practitioners should be concerned about the picky eater when the child is not gaining weight or growing appropriately, or when significant food refusal continues for more than 1 month. If the diet is markedly restrictive so that macro-and/or micro-nutrient intake is very low (calcium, protein, iron), consultation with a registered dietitian is useful to guide families and determine the need

---

Case 2

A 24-month-old boy presents for a well-child visit. His mother is concerned that he doesn't eat and states he will only eat macaroni and cheese. He will not eat vegetables. He sometimes skips meals. The mother says she tries to force him to eat but he refuses. PMH: SVD, Full-term. He is at the 50th percentile for height and weight and 40th percentile for head circumference. His growth has been consistent.

APPROACH: Reassure the mother that her child is growing normally by showing her his growth chart. Explain that it is normal to have food jags. Suggest offering a different food, for example, a vegetable with his favorite food (macaroni and cheese). Remind her not to force him to eat and to reduce focusing all her attention on him during meal time. This will reduce the overall tension and stress that has been created at meal time. Assess his juice and milk intake. Make sure he is not having a snack right before a meal. Toddlers have small stomachs. Educate about appropriate portion sizes. Suggest that the mother write down what he eats for one week. Follow up as needed.

---

for supplements. Referral to a Feeding Team Program may also be appropriate if the food refusal and pickiness requires behavioral modification treatment. Toddlers that demonstrate difficulty gaining weight or are crossing or declining in percentiles on the growth chart require further medical evaluation.

Setting the Stage for Healthy Eating
Supporting Healthy Self-Regulation for Toddlers and Preschool Children

At this stage in their development, children become increasingly aware of the environment in which they eat and the social aspects of eating. Fostering independence, while promoting healthy eating habits, becomes vitally important. In these formative years, the division of responsibility for nutrition should be set.

- The parents and caregivers are responsible for providing a varied and healthy diet, in age-appropriate amounts. This should be done in a consistent and calm setting and with minimal distraction or television. Whenever possible, children should eat with family members.
- The child is responsible for deciding how much to eat at a given meal and to select which of the foods presented to eat. After an adequate amount of time (15–20 minutes), they should be allowed to leave the table and have an opportunity to eat again at the next planned meal or snack.
- Dessert and other sweets, should not be used as a bribe to get children to eat their vegetables or finish everything on their plate.

Nutrition for School-age Children

Nurse Practitioners have the opportunity to provide anticipatory guidance for school-aged children (ages 6–12). They continue to need nutritious foods and snacks and are now are able to help with meal preparation. Children at this age have a steady but slow rate of growth, and usually eat four to five times a day, including snacks. Many food likes and dislikes are established during this time, and their eating habits are influenced by family, friends, and television. School-aged children are often willing to eat a wider variety of foods. It is important for them to eat healthy after-school snacks because these snacks may contribute up to one-third of the total calorie intake for the day. School-age children require enough fuel to get them through the day and to support attentiveness and brain development.

Serving Sizes for School-aged Children

School-aged children need to eat three meals and at least one snack each day. Breakfast is important to start every day while lunch is most often the meal consumed outside the home. Review menu choices with children to help them with their selection of healthy meals. Packing lunch can also help children to select healthy food. Snack time is the perfect opportunity to serve fruits and vegetables to help children to achieve the goal of three to four servings per day. Dinner is an opportunity to allow children to select from a variety of healthy choices. My Plate (www.choosemyplate.gov) provides excellent guidance regarding portion sizes of all foods and a wealth of information on meal planning for people of all ages, based on age, sex, and activity level.[21] *My Plate* guidelines for children 6–12 are as follows:

- Grains: 5–6 oz/day - make half whole grains.
- Vegetables: 2–2½ cups/day.
- Fruits: 1½–2 cups/day.
- Dairy: 3 cups/day.
- Meat and beans: 5–5½ oz/day.

Physical Activity

The CDC recommends at least 60 minutes of moderately intense physical activity most days of the week for all children and adolescents. Aerobic activity should make up most of the 60 or more minutes of physical activity each day. Include muscle strengthening activities, such as gymnastics or push-ups, at least 3 days per week as part of the 60 or more minutes. Include bone strengthening activities, such as jumping rope or running, at least 3 days per week as part of the 60 or more minutes. The role

---

Sample Menu: 6 years old

Breakfast: 1 cup low sugar whole grain cereal with 1/2 cup 1% milk, 1/2 banana sliced onto cereal, and 4 oz orange juice
Snack: 1/2 whole wheat bagel with 1 teaspoon margarine (soft tub) and 4 oz apple juice
Lunch: 1 cup cheese ravioli with sauce, 1 slice whole wheat bread with margarine, 6 baby carrot sticks with low-fat ranch dressing, 4 oz fruit cocktail canned in its own juice, and 1/2 cup 1% milk
Snack: 4 graham cracker pieces and 1 cup 1% milk
Dinner: 1 baked chicken leg, 1 baked potato with margarine, 1/2 cup steamed broccoli, 1 slice whole wheat bread, 1/2 orange sliced in quarters, and 1 cup 1% milk

Source: Darwin Deen, MD, MS, and Lisa Hark, PhD, RD. 2012. Used with permission.

> ## Key Points for School-Aged Children
>
> - Breakfast is the most important of the three meals each day school children consume.
> - 1–2 snacks usually complete daily nutritional requirements.
> - The CDC recommends at least 60 minutes of moderately intense physical activity most days of the week for children and adolescents.

of physical activity in balancing the energy equation in order to prevent children from becoming overweight cannot be overstated.[11] As with food and eating, parents must set a positive example by leading an active lifestyle, and making physical activity part of the family's daily routine. Physical activity should be fun and can include team sports, individual sports, walking, running, skating, bicycling, swimming, jumping rope, and playground activities. Activity should be age-appropriate and safety should be ensured with helmets, wrist pads, and kneepads.

The AAP recommends restricting sedentary activity to 2 hours or less each day.[1] Parents should be advised that children under the age of 2 years should not watch television. By limiting screen time which includes television, video games, and computers, children have been shown to engage more in active play. Active play will assist with weight control.

Nutrition During Adolescence

Teenage Specific Needs

Children aged 11–18 years have increased needs for nutrients as they progress through puberty, the second major growth period of life. During puberty, energy needs increase to allow attainment of the individual's growth potential. Though boys and girls have different energy requirements, both need extra protein, calcium, and iron. The greater influence of peers with a variety of dietary patterns, the increased frequency of meals consumed away from home, and the adolescents' need for control, profoundly impact their food choices. Nurse Practitioners can help teens and their parents focus on physical activity as a method of weight control rather than calorie reduction. Emphasis on including key nutrients (calcium and iron are at the greatest risk for deficiency) rather than restricting intake gives teens the opportunity to practice independence by choosing what foods they would like to eat, rather than setting up a power struggle with food dynamics.

Serving Sizes

Serving sizes of each food group (e.g. 1 cup milk = 1 serving) for teenagers are identical to that of adults. The number of servings per day are calculated based on caloric need, which is determined by body size and physical activity levels. Most male teenagers will need to eat from the 2800 calorie food pattern while most females will meet requirements with the 2200 calorie food pattern. Choosemyplate.gov can help teens and Nurse Practitioners determine the correct servings sizes of each food group that are appropriate to meeting the needs for growth.[21]

Risk of Calcium Deficiency

Adolescents with a poor diet may be at increased risk for vitamin and mineral deficiencies, most notably riboflavin, calcium, and iron. Bone mineral content peaks in adolescence and young adulthood, then declines with age. Maximizing peak bone mineral density early in life can help prevent osteoporosis with advancing age.[49] Many teenage girls are not meeting their calcium requirement of 1300 mg per day during adolescence. The inclusion of four servings of low-fat dairy foods each day in a teen's diet should be discussed with both the parent and the patient themselves. Food sources of calcium are shown in Appendices G and H.

Risk of Iron Deficiency

The rapid growth rate during puberty increases iron requirements for males and females. Vigorous exercise, such as running and dancing, further increases requirements. Teenage girls require additional iron due to menarche, with those from ages 12 to 18 requiring 15 mg of iron daily. To achieve this intake, Nurse Practitioners should encourage consumption of lean red meat, iron-rich fruits such as dried fruits (raisins), vegetables such as fresh spinach, and iron-fortified breakfast cereal. Vitamin C enhances non-heme iron absorption when consumed together with iron-rich foods. Food sources of iron are shown in Appendix L.

Teenage Pregnancy

Teenagers who become pregnant require the calories and nutrients needed for adolescent growth, as well as additional key nutrients needed during pregnancy (folate, vitamins A, D and C, magnesium). It is especially important for Nurse Practitioners to spend time counseling teen mothers on nutritional issues as most teenage women are deficient in at least one key nutrient (see Chapter 4).

Teenagers and Exercise

The teen athlete requires increased calories and protein, depending on the activity. With normal appetites, most adolescents will eat enough to meet their energy requirements. The most essential and often neglected nutrient requirement in an athlete's diet is water.[1] Hydration is especially important for those involved in endurance

---

Key Points for Adolescent Nutrition

- Adolescents aged 11–18 years have increased needs for nutrients as they progress through major growth periods.
- Greater influence of peers with varied dietary patterns, increased frequency of meals consumed away from home and adolescent need for control impacts adolescent food choices.
- Adolescents are extremely high consumers of refined carbohydrates through added sugars. Nutrition counseling should focus on decreasing intake of soft drinks and other high sugar beverages.
- Adolescents are also at risk for calcium and iron deficiencies. Dietary counseling should target appropriate intake of these nutrients.

sports during hot weather. An athlete exercising in hot/humid weather may lose more than $1.0\,l/m^2/h$ through sweating. Water with simple sugars (2.5–5%) or glucose polymers is sufficient to restore fluid losses from sweat. Cold fluids have the advantage of helping to cool the body and may be more readily consumed. Recommended fluid intake during exercise is about 4–8 oz for every 15 minutes of physical activity. Small amounts of electrolytes, mostly sodium and chloride, may be lost in sweat during exercise. Most of these losses can be replaced in the diet. Sports drinks may be used, but the average teenage athlete is not losing electrolytes at amounts that would be needed to be supplemented in the diet. Additionally, sports drink consumption results in increased sugar consumption, caloric intake, and often leads to unwanted weight gain.

Weight Loss in Athletes

Teens involved in gymnastics, ballet, cross-country track, diving, wrestling, and figure skating may feel pressure to reduce weight. If appropriate, this can be accomplished, but gradual loss (no more than 1–2 lb per week) should be the goal. Rapid weight loss may result in loss of muscle tissue. Increased emphasis on weight loss and exercise can lead to disordered eating, unhealthy relationships with food and weight as well as distorted body image. Nurse Practitioners should focus counseling on nutrition with athletes by using food as fuel to maintain optimal athletic performance, rather than focus on weight loss.

Eating Disorders: Anorexia Nervosa and Bulimia

While overweight and obesity are a growing problem among children and adolescents, for some adolescent girls eating disorders are a serious concern. These disorders are more often found in industrialized cultures, and occur in all socioeconomic levels and across all major ethnic groups. Dancers, long-distance runners, figure skaters, actors, models, wrestlers, gymnasts, and jockeys are at higher risk for the development of eating disorders. Studies suggest that about 20% of teenagers engage in abnormal eating behavior, while about 5% of high-school-aged women have a diagnosed eating disorder.[49] Eating disorders primarily occur in adolescents and college-aged women.

Anorexia Nervosa

Teenagers with anorexia nervosa typically have an altered perception of their own body image that causes them to see themselves as overweight. This altered perception leads to severe restriction of calories and a drop in body weight to below-normal levels for age and height (less than 85% expected weight). According to the American Psychiatric Association[50] diagnostic criteria for anorexia nervosa include:

- Refusal to maintain body weight at or above the lower limit of normal or failure to make expected weight gain during growth, which leads to a BMI <17.5.
- Intense fear of gaining weight or becoming fat, despite being thin.
- Disturbance in the way in which one's body weight or shape is experienced, undue influence of body shape and weight on self-evaluation, or denial of the seriousness of current low body weight.
- In females, absence of at least three consecutive menstrual cycles when otherwise expected to occur. This condition is referred to as amenorrhea.

- People who have anorexia are also classified as restrictive type or binge eating purging type (see below).

Restricting type During the episode of anorexia nervosa, the person *does not* regularly engage in binge eating or purging behavior (i.e. self-induced vomiting or the misuse of laxatives or diuretics).

Binge eating/purging type During the episode of anorexia nervosa, the person regularly engages in binge eating or purging behavior (i.e. self-induced vomiting or the misuse of laxatives or diuretics).

Bulimia Nervosa

A second type of eating disorder, bulimia nervosa, is characterized by frequent episodes of binge-eating followed by purging (self-induced vomiting or ingestion of laxatives or cathartics to induce diarrhea or vomiting). Adolescents with bulimia nervosa tend to be of normal or increased weight. Purging behavior may be associated with both anorexia nervosa and bulimia nervosa. According to the American Psychiatric Association[50], diagnostic criteria for bulimia nervosa include:

- Recurrent binge eating at least twice a week for a minimum of 3 months.
- Binge eating refers to eating in a discrete period of time (e.g. within any 2-hour period an amount of food that is definitely larger than most people would eat during a similar period of time in similar circumstances; and, having a sense of lack of control over eating during the episode, such as a feeling that you cannot stop eating or control what or how much you are eating).
- May compensate for overeating by self-inducing vomiting, misusing laxatives, diuretics, or other medications, fasting or exercising excessively.
- Excessive preoccupation with body weight or shape. The disturbance does not occur exclusively during episodes of anorexia nervosa.

Treatment Recommendations for Eating Disorders

Treating eating disorders requires a team approach that combines medical management, psychological interventions, and nutritional counseling. Eating disorders are psychiatric conditions, but can lead to physical complications. Assessment and treatment by a psychologist or psychiatrist familiar with eating disorders is crucial in establishing a diagnosis, evaluating the risk of suicide, and assessing the severity of the psychological symptoms as well as other related conditions such as depression, anxiety, substance abuse, or personality disorders. To improve, a teenager with an eating disorder needs to recognize the problem, address his/her perceived body image, and set and achieve nutritional and weight goals. A multidisciplinary team composed of a dietitian experienced with eating disorders should provide guidance for nutritional rehabilitation and education, and an experienced physician or Nurse Practitioner must monitor the patient for medical complications.

Vegetarianism

Many adolescents experiment with their dietary patterns as a developmentally appropriate form of self discovery. The decision to become a vegetarian may be influenced by health-related or philosophical reasons as well as social and societal influences. Vegetarianism is the accepted dietary practice of many cultures in the world and can be healthful when appropriately planned to be nutritionally adequate. A vegetarian diet is defined as one that does not include meat, fish or fowl and may exclude dairy foods and eggs. Nutrients that are at risk for decreased or deficient intake include: protein, iron, zinc, calcium, vitamin D, riboflavin, vitamin B_{12}, vitamin A, omega-3 fatty acids, and iodine. There are two distinct patterns of vegetarianism: lacto-ovo vegetarians, and vegans.

Lacto-ovo Vegetarians
Lacto-ovo vegetarians eat dairy foods, and eggs in addition to vegetable products. A diet including dairy and eggs provides adequate intake of most nutrients.

Vegans
Vegetarians who are vegan omit all animal products from the diet. Removing dairy and eggs from the diet decreases the availability of many important nutrients, most notably vitamin B_{12}. These diets require the inclusion of a wide variety of vegetables, fruits, grains, and oils. It may be necessary to include grain products that are fortified, especially with iron, on a regular basis. Supplementation with B_{12} is recommended for all vegans. Vitamin B_{12} supplements come in the form of sublingual daily pills, quarterly injections or nasal spray. Soy milk fortified with vitamin B_{12} may be recommended on a daily basis. Achieving adequate calcium intake is also a challenge for many vegans. Calcium needs can be met with the inclusion of fortified soy products (fortified soy milk/tofu) as well as calcium-fortified juices. Calcium supplements can augment daily intake to meet nutritional requirements. A varied diet is the key to adequate nutrition for all vegetarians, especially vegans, with examples listed in Table 5-9.

Table 5-9 Meeting Nutrient Needs in Vegan Diets

Protein: Legumes, whole grains, soy products, nuts and seeds, fruits, and all vegetables.

Iron: Iron-fortified breakfast cereals, iron-fortified grain products, dried beans, and peas. (Eat with food high in vitamin C to increase absorption.) Iron supplement.

Zinc: Yeast-fermented whole grain breads and zinc-fortified cereals.

Calcium: Calcium-fortified soy products, calcium-fortified cereals and orange juice, dark leafy green vegetables (chard, broccoli, kale and mustard greens), nuts, calcium-set tofu, and calcium supplements.

Vitamin D: Cod liver oil and menhaden oil if these are acceptable and vitamin/mineral supplements containing vitamin D. Soy products that are supplemented with vitamin D.

Riboflavin: B-vitamin fortified grain products and cereals.

Vitamin B12: Supplement for vegans.

Vitamin A: Supplementation or inclusion in the diet of beta-carotene in the form of yellow vegetables.

Omega-3 fatty acids: Available in flax and other seeds, as well as walnuts and soybeans.

Iodine: Iodine-fortified salts, sea salts.

Source: Lisa Hark, PhD, RD, 2012. Used with permission.

Summary: Role of Nurse Practitioners

Nurse Practitioners have an important responsibility to support and guide families in the health and normal growth of their children. Nurse Practitioners can help children lead healthier lives by advocating for just a few lifestyle changes and have the tools needed to do so. Primary care Nurse Practitioners are among the first to note deviations from normal growth and can provide early intervention to allow correction and facilitate return to healthy growth patterns. Referral to specialists when indicated, including registered dietitians, will provide families the support they require to achieve normal growth and development of their children.

References

1. Kleinman RE (Ed.). *Pediatric Nutrition Handbook*. 6th edition. American Academy of Pediatrics, Committee on Nutrition. AAP, Illinois, 2009.
2. Gilluly K, Johnson L, Rossiter K. Effect of educational preparation on the accuracy of linear growth measurement in pediatric primary care practices: results of a multicenter nursing study. *J Pediatr Nurs* 2005;20:64–74.
3. Centers for Disease Control and Prevention. National Center for Health Statistics 2000. CDC Growth charts: United States. www.cdc.gov/growth charts. Accessed 2012.
4. Koplan JP, Liverman CT, Kraak VI (Eds). *Preventing Childhood Obesity: Health in the Balance*. Institute of Medicine. The National Academies Press, Washington DC, 2005.
5. Ogden CL, Carroll MD, Curtin LR, et al. Prevalence of high body mass index in US children and adolescents, 2007–2008. *JAMA* 2010;303:242–249.
6. Trasande L, Chatterjee S. The impact of obesity on health service utilization and costs in childhood. *Obesity* 2009;17:1749–1754.
7. Barlow SE, Expert Committee. Expert Committee Recommendations Regarding the Prevention, Assessment, and Treatment of Child and Adolescent Overweight and Obesity: Summary Report. *Pediatrics* 2007;120(Suppl 4):S164–S192.
8. Owen CG, Martin RM, Whincup PH, et al. Effect of infant feeding on the risk of obesity across the life course: a quantitative review of published evidence. *Pediatrics* 2005;115: 1367–1377.
9. Carver JD, Wu P, Hall RT, et al. Growth of pre-term infants fed nutrient enriched or term formula after hospital discharge. *Pediatrics* 2001;107:683–689.
10. Dietz W, Lee J, Wechsler H, et al. Health plans' role in preventing overweight in children and adolescents. *Health Aff* 2007;26:430–440.
11. United States Department of Agriculture (USDA). http://www.letsmove.gov/learnthe facts.php. Accessed 2012.
12. Berkowitz, RI, Stallings VA, Maislin G, et al. Growth of children at high risk of obesity during the first 6 years of life: implications for prevention. *Am J Clin Nutr* 2005;81: 140–146.
13. Christian JG, Bessesen DH, Byers TE, et al. Clinic-based support to help overweight patients with type 2 diabetes increase physical activity and lose weight. *Arch Intern Med* 2008;168: 141–146.
14. The HEALTHY Study Group. A School-Based Intervention for Diabetes Risk Reduction. *N Engl J Med* 2010;363:443–453.
15. American Diabetes Association Statistics. Standards of medical care in diabetes—2009;32 (suppl.1):S15.

16. Daniels SR, Greer FR. Lipid screenings and cardiovascular health in childhood. *Pediatrics* 2008;122:198–208.

17. USDA Center for Nutrition Policy and Promotion. *Dietary Guidelines for Americans, 2010.* Policy Document. www.cnpp.usda.gov. Accessed 2012.

18. *Healthy People 2020.* Department of Health and Human Services. www.healthypeople.gov

19. Baker RD, Greener DR. Diagnosis and prevention of iron deficiency and iron deficiency anemia in infants and young children. *Pediatrics* 2010;126:1040–1050.

20. Institute of Medicine Food and Nutrition Board, Institute of Medicine. *Dietary Reference Intakes for Energy and Protein.* National Academy of Science. National Academies Press, Washington, DC, 2005.

21. *United States Department of Agriculture's (USDA) MyPlate.* http://www.choosemyplate.gov. Accessed 2012.

22. Krugman DS, Dubowitz H. Failure to thrive. *Am Fam Physician* 2003;68:879–886.

23. Niedbala B, Swanson M. Failure to thrive. In: Ekvall SW, Ekvall VK (Eds). *Pediatric Nutrition in Chronic Diseases and Developmental Disorders: Prevention, Assessment, and Treatment (2nd Edition).* Oxford University Press, USA, 2005.

24. Markowitz R, Duggan C. Failure to thrive: malnutrition in the pediatric outpatient setting. In: Walker WA, Watkins JB, Duggan C (Eds), *Nutrition in Pediatrics.* 3rd Edition. BC Decker Inc., Hamilton, London, 2003.

25. Rampersaud GC, Pereira MA, Girard BL, et al. Breakfast habits, nutritional status, body weight, and academic performance in children and adolescents. *J Am Diet Assoc* 2005;105:743.

26. Pereira MA, Erickson E, McKee P, *et al.* Effect of breakfast frequency and quality on glycemia and appetite in adults and children. *J Nutr* 2011;141:163–8.

27. Hill, JO. Can a small-changes approach help address the obesity epidemic? *Am J Clin Nutr* 2009;89:477–484.

28. Wagner CL, Greer FR. American Academy of Pediatrics Section on Breastfeeding; American Academy of Pediatrics Committee on Nutrition. Prevention of rickets and vitamin D deficiency in infants, children, and adolescents. *Pediatrics* 2008;122:1142–1152.

29. American Academy of Pediatrics. Breastfeeding and the use of human milk. http://aappolicy. aappublications.org/cgi/content/full/pediatrics;115/2/496. Accessed 2012.

30. World Health Organization. Exclusive Breastfeeding. http://www.who.int/nutrition/topics/ exclusive_breastfeeding/en/. Accessed 2012.

31. Centers for Disease Control and Prevention. National Center for Health Statistics. National Health and Nutrition Examination Survey (NHANES). www.cdc.gov/nchs/nhanes.htm. Accessed 2012.

32. Kull I, Wickman M, Lilja G, et al. Breast feeding and allergic diseases in infants — a prospective birth cohort study. *Arch Dis Child* 2002;87:478–481.

33. Roschitz B, Plecko B, Huemer M, et al. Nutritional infantile vitamin B12 deficiency: patho-biochemical considerations in seven patients. *Arc Dis Child* 2005;90:F281–FF282.

34. Zschocke J, Schindler S, Hoffman GF, et al. Nature and nurture in vitamin B12. *Arch Dis Child* 2002;87:75–76.

35. Thorpe M. Infant formula supplemented with DHA: are there benefits? (Editorial.) *J Am Diet Assoc* 2003;103:551–552.

36. Khakoo GA, Lack G. Introduction of solids to the infant diet. (Commentary.) *Arch Dis Child* 2004;89:295.

37. Dwyer JT, Suitor CW, Hendricks K. FITS: new insights and lessons learned. *J Am Diet Assoc* 2004:104:(1 Suppl 1):S5–S7.

38. Fox MK, Pac S, Devaney B, et al. Feeding infants and toddlers study: what foods are infants and toddlers eating? *J Am Diet Assoc* 2004;104(1 Suppl 1):S22–S30.

39. Briefel RR, Reidy K, Karwe V, et al. Toddlers' transition to table foods: impact on nutrient intakes and food patterns. *J Am Diet Assoc* 2004;104:S38–S44.

40. Skinner JD, Ziegler P, Pac S, et al. Meal and snack patterns of infants and toddlers. *J Am Diet Assoc* 2004;104:S65–S70.

41. Devaney B, Ziegler P, Pac S, et al. Nutrient intakes of infants and toddlers. *J Am Diet Assoc* 2004;104:S14–S21.

42. United States Department of Agriculture (USDA). *My Plate*. http://www.choosemyplate.gov. Accessed 2012.

43. The Food Allergy and Anaphylaxis Network. www.foodallergy.org. Accessed 2012.

44. Georgieff MK. The role of iron in neurodevelopment: fetal iron deficiency and the developing hippocampus. *Biochem Soc Trans* 2008;36:1267–1271.

45. Friel JK, Aziz K, Andrews WL, et al. A double-masked, randomized control trial of iron supplementation in early infancy in healthy term breast-fed infants. *J Pediatr* 2003;243:554–556.

46. Hart CN, Raynor HA, Osterholt KM, et al. Eating and activity habits of overweight children on weekdays and weekends. *Int J Pediatr Obes* 2011;6:467–472.

47. Galloway AT, Fiorito L, Lee Y, et al. Parental pressure, dietary patterns and weight status among girls who are "picky eaters". *J Am Diet Assoc* 2005;105:541–548.

48. Satter E. *How to Get Your Kid to Eat but Not Too Much*. Bull Publishing Company, Boulder, CO, 1987.

49. Rappaport EB, Thorpe J, Tershakovec AM. Infants, children, and adolescents. In: Hark L, Morrison G.(Eds), *Medical Nutrition and Disease*. 4th Edition. Wiley-Blackwell, Malden, MA, 2009.

50. American Psychiatric Association. *Diagnostic and Statistical Manual of Mental Disorders*, 4th Edition. Text Revision. American Psychiatric Association, Washington, DC, 2000.

6 Nutrition for Older Adults

Cecilia Borden, EdD, MSN, RN
Christine Conner, MPA-HAS, BSN, RN
Lisa Hark, PhD, RD

OBJECTIVES

- Identify the physiological changes associated with aging and describe the impact on nutrient requirements, absorption, and metabolism.
- List common factors associated with poor nutritional status in older adults.
- Utilize the RDA macronutrients and minerals for adults ≥ 51 years of age.
- Understand the instruments utilized for nutritional and oral assessments in older adults.

Introduction

Approximately one in every eight Americans is over the age of 65. By 2030, 72.1 million individuals will be 85 years or older, representing 19% of the population, or more than 9.6 million Americans.[1] Hispanics, Asians/Pacific Islanders, Native Americans, and African Americans are projected to represent approximately 25% of the elderly population by 2030, and women will continue to outnumber men. For older adults, nutrition involves eating habits, eating ability, managing meals, relationships, culture, financial resources, and social support. Nutrition-related concerns for the older adult include chronic disease, depression, dementia, dysphagia, obesity, cachexia, and nutritional frailty. Nutrition programs have to be more diverse and flexible to meet the needs of this ever-growing and diverse older population.[2] This chapter reviews the impact of aging on nutritional needs and details appropriate interventions for many important nutrition-related concerns for the older adult. The chapter also focuses on the impact of aging on nutritional needs, appropriate interventions, and the role of Nurse Practitioners in caring for and influencing the nutritional status of older adult patients.

The Nurse Practitioner's Guide to Nutrition, Second Edition. Edited by Lisa Hark, Kathleen Ashton and Darwin Deen.
© 2012 John Wiley & Sons, Inc. Published 2012 by John Wiley & Sons, Inc.

Alterations in Nutritional Needs

Alterations in nutritional needs of older adults are related to the physiological and metabolic changes associated with normal aging. According to the Healthy Eating Index Scores among adults 60 years of age and over, 17% had diets that were rated "good", approximately 14% reported diets rated "poor", and 67% consumed diets that "needed improvement".[3] Metabolically, caloric needs decline with age. Therefore, in order to determine who is at risk, a comprehensive nutritional assessment, including past medical history, vital signs, review of systems, physical exam, and biochemical data is critical to ascertain, as outlined in Chapter 2. The following section discusses the concerns of older adults, including social and economic considerations, cultural and health literacy issues, fluid and hydration, and physiological and metabolic changes to meet nutritional requirements.

Social and Economic Considerations

Economic hardship may limit financial resources for adequate nutrition.[4] Deficits in physical functioning contribute to food insecurity, defined as uncertain ability to acquire nutritionally adequate and safe foods, and/or lack of appropriate nutrition in older adults. Many older adults who eat alone make poor decisions and eat the same food day after day. Reduced social contact and eating meals alone impacts dietary intake, as will inadequate assistance with shopping and preparing food. This is often insufficient to meet dietary needs and places the individual at increased risk for malnutrition.[5] These risk factors may go unrecognized by healthcare providers, family, and friends. Nurse Practitioners need to inquire about these issues and refer patients with social and economic issues to social workers and community agencies that can intervene.

Cultural Issues

Food habits in older adults are the product of ethnic origin and cultural norms imparted at an early age. Food preferences can vary depending on where people grew up, in rural or urban settings, which give meaning and value to our food habits. Food can provide a means for communication of love or disapproval in families.[6] For older adults, cultural values may be challenged because of economic decline, stressors, or chronic illness. Nurse Practitioners should consider these unique issues and the challenges they present when assessing a patient's nutritional status.

Health Literacy

It is important for older adults to understand health information in order to navigate through the health system. To do this, patients need the capacity to process health information and understand the health services that are available to them. This allows them to make better judgments regarding health care services.[7] Education does not guarantee the ability to read. Age-related cognitive decline and past learning experiences impact literacy and this may determine a patient's ability to interpret food labels, choose proper nutrients, take medications, and achieve better health outcomes.[7,8]

One way to address this is by using illustrations to improve patients' understanding of heath information and ensure greater compliance with health regimens. Setting up a medication schedule that is easier to follow will also ensure greater adherence. Research shows that patients with low literacy rates do not use a standardized medication regimen even if they are taking medications up to 7 times/day.[9] Another study found that low health literacy was significantly associated with higher all-cause mortality in patients with heart failure.[10]

Fluid and Hydration

Fluid and hydration are especially important to the health of older adults. Older adults often have a poor thirst response and therefore are at increased risk of dehydration as well as urinary tract infections. Individuals with impaired cognition are also at risk for dehydration. Therefore, it is imperative that Nurse Practitioners teach patients to drink fluids on a regular basis. Six to eight glasses of fluid every day will provide sufficient hydration for the healthy older adult; however, it is often difficult to reach this level.[11] Additional drinks such as tea and juices, especially cranberry juice, may be helpful to older adults who need to consume more fluids.[11–13]

However, patients with certain conditions, such as chronic heart failure and kidney disease, require decreased fluid intake. In addition, there are potential negative effects of excessive water consumption that can lead to dilutional hypernatremia (water intoxication) and increased nocturia.

Macronutrients

Energy

Body composition changes with age. Lean body mass declines, body fat mass increases, and a lack of physical activity results in lower energy expenditure, all leading to a reduction in metabolic rate.[14] Therefore, caloric needs typically decline as people advance in age unless they are physically active to maintain their muscle mass and hence, their metabolic rate. Unfortunately, as described in Chapter 7, at least one in three Americans are overweight, due to this energy imbalance. However, later in life, negative energy balance (caloric malnutrition) may result due to changes in taste, dentition, cognitive impairment, and depression.

Protein

The current RDA for protein (0.8 g/kg/day) is the same for adults of all ages, although there is evidence that a higher protein intake could help counteract sarcopenia (loss of muscle mass) by enhancing hypertrophic response to strength conditioning in the older adult.[14] The oldest age groups are most at risk for protein deficiency, especially when health problems or other stresses are manifested and when patients are institutionalized, hospitalized, or reside in long-term care facilties.

Lipids, Carbohydrates, and Fiber

There is a decrease in the intake of fat and cholesterol with age. There is also a reduction in the percentage of calories coming from fat. While absolute intake of carbohydrate typically decreases with age, carbohydrate as a percentage of calories increases slightly due to the reduction of calories coming from fats. Most adults, including the elderly, consume less fiber than the recommended of 25–35 g/day. Increasing dietary fiber helps prevent constipation as well as age-related chronic diseases, such as coronary heart disease, and is beneficial for those with diabetes, hyperlipidemia, and gastrointestinal conditions, as described in Chapter 8, 9, and 10.[15]

Vitamins
Vitamin A
The RDA for vitamin A is 900 µg/day for men and 700 µg/day for women and requirements do not change with age. The tolerable upper intake level for adults is 3000 µg/day. Concentrations of vitamin A decrease during aging and lack of dietary or micronutrient intake of vitamin A may further exacerbate this deficiency. Many times individuals who face economic decline frequently do not consume foods sufficient in vitamin A.[16] Retention of this vitamin seems enhanced in aging, especially in older adults who consume large amounts from supplements and fortified food. There are implications that vitamin A may be helpful in age-related immune dysfunction, though has this not been concluded definitively.[17] Foods sources of vitamin A are listed in Appendix A.

Vitamin D
The RDA for vitamin D in men and women 51 years and older is 600 IU/day, and for those over 70, requirements increase to 800 IU/day. In clinical practice, higher doses may be prescribed without apparent undue effects. The tolerable upper intake level for adults is 2000 IU/day. There is an increased need for vitamin D in older adults due to age-related changes. In North America, it is estimated that 50% of the older population is vitamin D deficient.[18] Vitamin D status can also be negatively impacted by use of sunscreen, being home-bound, and northern latitude. The NIH Office of Dietary Supplements defines a mild to moderate deficiency as a serum level of 25(OH)D level of 30–50 nmol/L and optimal vitamin D levels as 75 nmol/L.[18] Vitamin D deficiency results not only in impaired bone metabolism, but also muscle weakness predominantly in the proximal muscles group.[18, 19] Vitamin D supplementation in vitamin D-deficient older adults improved muscle strength, walking distance, and functional ability, and resulted in a reduction in falls and non-vertebral fractures.[19] Studies also show a protective relationship between sufficient vitamin D status and lower risk of colorectal cancer.[20]

Vitamin D status should be routinely assessed and supplements prescribed when food intake is inadequate to maintain optimal health status.[21] Foods sources of vitamin D are listed in Appendix B. It is important for Nurse Practitioners to teach patients that sunlight (UVB) exposure from 5–15 minutes twice a week helps maintain appropriate levels of vitamin D. After 15 minutes of sun exposure, sunscreen can be used as a protective measure against skin cancer.[18] This fact should to be impressed upon the older adult patient, as many do not obtain adequate sun exposure and skin synthesis to the active form of vitamin D from sunlight declines with age.

Vitamin E
The RDA for vitamin E in adults is 15 mg (22.4 IU) and does not change with age. Alpha tocopherol is the most bioavailable form of vitamin E. Vitamin E absorption

and utilization does not change with age, but dietary intake of vitamin E has been shown to be below recommended levels in older adults.[22] A possible explanation is a reduction in high-fat foods containing vitamin E, such as vegetable oils and nuts. For optimal antioxidant function, vitamin E dietary intake needs to be supported with adequate intake of vitamin C, niacin, selenium, and glutathione. However, obtaining vitamin E via supplementation is not recommended. A recent meta-analysis concluded that high doses of supplemental vitamin E, more than 150 IU /day, may be linked with increased all-cause mortality, and supplements exceeding this amount should be avoided.[23] Foods sources of vitamin E are listed in Appendix C.

Vitamin C

The RDA for vitamin C is 90 mg/day for men and 75 mg/day for women and requirements do not change with age. The tolerable upper intake level for adults is 2000 mg/day. Intake of vitamin C is highly variable among older adults. While most older adults consume generous amounts of vitamin C and achieve nutritional adequacy, some groups have been identified as having increased risk of deficiency, such as those with dental problems, dementia, and those in hospitals and nursing homes. Aging does not alter the absorption or metabolism of vitamin C, so low levels are generally attributed to poor intake or increased requirements. The clinical significance of vitamin C deficiency, other than scurvy, has not definitively been concluded.[19] However, one study found that severe or marginal vitamin C deficiency was significantly associated with all-cause mortality.[24] A meta-analysis of individuals taking vitamin C supplements found that 500 mg daily of vitamin C for a minimum of 4 weeks demonstrated a significant decrease in serum LDL-cholesterol and triglyceride concentrations.[25] HDL-cholesterol levels remained unchanged with vitamin C supplementation. Even with modest changes, the beneficial effect of vitamin C may be helpful in coronary heart disease.[25] Foods sources of vitamin C are listed in Appendix E.

Thiamin, Riboflavin and Niacin

Thiamin (vitamin B_1), riboflavin (vitamin B_2), and niacin (vitamin B_3) function as coenzymes in energy metabolism. This may lead to the notion that requirements for these vitamins diminish with declining energy requirements in older adults.[26] However, available evidence suggests that requirements for these nutrients are unchanged with age. Potential causes of low blood levels include chronic alcohol use (thiamin) and low consumption of dairy products (riboflavin). Niacin status is likely to be adequate, although older patients with food insecurity have been reported to have low intake levels of B vitamins.[27]

Folate

The RDA for folate in men and women 51 years and older is 400 μg/day. The tolerable upper intake limit for folate has been set at 1000 μg/day. Requirements for folate do not change with age; however, inadequate folate status contributes to hyperhomocysteinemia, which may increase the risk of coronary disease, and other chronic diseases common in older adults. A reduction in stroke events was observed in the *Heart Outcomes Prevention Evaluation-2* study, but there were no significant effects on death rates and non-fatal myocardial infarction in patients receiving folate supplements.[28]

A reduction in the stroke mortality rate was seen in North America after folic acid fortification. Folate intake has increased due to food fortification programs to the point of raising concerns about excessive intake in older adults who consume a large amount of fortified foods such as breakfast cereals, breads, and products made from enriched flours. The concern is that this may mask a vitamin B_{12} deficiency, allowing the neurological sequelae to progress even though the anemia associated with this deficiency resolves. Also, high folate levels may reduce the response to anti-folate drugs used in the treatment of rheumatoid arthritis, psoriasis, malaria, and some forms of cancer. As a result, higher folic acid intake may not benefit some patients. It is therefore recommended that Nurse Practitioners prescribe both folate and vitamin B_{12} supplements to older adults. Foods sources of folate are listed in Appendix F.

Vitamin B_{12}

The RDA for vitamin B_{12} for men and women 51 years and older is 2.4 μg/day. Requirements for vitamin B_{12} do not increase with age, but low stomach acid secretion, secondary to atrophic gastritis, may seriously impair the absorption of vitamin B_{12} in those over age 50. To assure nutritional adequacy, supplements containing vitamin B_{12} or good food sources of vitamin B_{12}, such as animal and dairy foods, as well as foods supplemented with vitamin B_{12} (soy milk), should be consumed daily. Widespread use of vitamin B_{12} injections is no longer necessary if the free form of B_{12} is given as an oral supplement at 2000 μg/day.[29] Patients taking metformin have been shown to have poor vitamin B_{12} absorption.[30] Serum and red blood cell vitamin B_{12} levels should be checked and vitamin B_{12} should be prescribed when levels are borderline or below normal.[30]

See Appendices S and T for all Dietary Reference Intake (DRI) tables.

Minerals
Calcium

The RDA for calcium in men and women 51 years and older is 1200 mg/day. The tolerable upper intake level for calcium is 2000 mg/day. Osteoporosis is a major health risk for older women and men. Calcium recommendations are set at levels associated with maximum retention of body calcium since bones that are calcium rich are known to be less susceptible to fractures.[31] Calcium supplements should be considered for those whose dietary intake of calcium is deficient. More than 70% of men and 78% of women may have low calcium intakes.[31] The disparity between the dietary requirement for calcium and the amount that is actually consumed by the older adult population is the most dramatic of any known essential nutrient, especially in older women. Foods sources of calcium are listed in Appendices G and H.

Iron

The RDA for iron is 8 mg/day in both men and women 51 years and older. The tolerable upper intake level for both men and women in this age group is 45 mg/day. Iron is essential for the function of normal human physiology. It is also an important component of proteins that transport oxygen. Iron deficiency limits the amount of oxygen that is delivered to the cells. This results in a lack of energy and a decrease in immunity. An excess of iron can cause toxicity and death.[32] Approximately 11% of men and 10% of women aged 65 and older in the United States are anemic. Rates of anemia rise to 50–60% for those living in nursing homes. Poor outcomes from anemia include frailty, increased fall rates, impaired cognition, and death.[33]

Dietary iron is composed of two forms, heme and non-heme. Heme iron is found in red meats, fish and poultry; non-heme iron is found in plant form, e.g. in lentils and beans. Non-heme iron is added to iron-enriched and iron-fortified foods. Although heme-iron is better absorbed that non-heme iron, most dietary iron is non-heme iron. Nurse Practitioners need to assess iron levels and encourage patients to increase their intake of protein, iron, and vitamin C (to provide nutrients needed for hemoglobin production), prescribe the appropriate amount of iron, and provide patients with information regarding their nutritional needs. Foods sources of iron are listed in Appendix L.

Magnesium

The RDA for magnesium is 420 mg/day for men and 320 mg/day for women and requirements do not change with age. The tolerable upper intake level for magnesium supplementation is 350 mg/day, the upper limit for magnesium represents intake from a pharmacological agent only and does not include intake from food and water.[34] Magnesium is an essential nutrient for bone health and functions in conjunction with vitamin D and calcium.[35] It also serves other critical roles such as nerve and muscle function, since it is an integral component to the sodium/potassium pump and required for potassium to enter the cell.[35] Magnesium status has been linked to bone mineral density in both men and women. With age, magnesium absorption decreases, urinary losses increase, and low magnesium intake is often observed. Food sources rich in magnesium include fruits and vegetables (bananas, apricots, avocados green leafy vegetables), halibut, nuts (almonds, cashews), peas, beans, legumes, seeds, soy products (soy flour, tofu), and whole grains (brown rice, millet).[34]

Zinc

The RDA for zinc is 11 mg/day for men and 8 mg/day for women. The tolerable upper intake level for zinc is 40 mg/day. Aging effects on zinc requirements are not completely understood, but it is likely that zinc needs increase with age. Reduced zinc status in older adults has been linked with decreased immunity and poor response to vaccinations.[36] Zinc supplementation reduces susceptibility to infections and has been shown to enhance wound healing.[36] Studies show that older adults are oxidatively stressed and that zinc is an effective anti-inflammatory as well as an antioxidant.[36] Supplemental doses of zinc should not exceed 40 mg/day unless patients are under regular medical supervision, as high doses can induce copper deficiency and/or immune suppression.[37] Foods sources of zinc include oysters, wheat germ, red meats, liver, dark chocolate and roasted pumpkin seeds.

Identifying Individuals at Risk for Malnutrition

It is a considerable challenge for Nurse Practitioners to achieve optimal balance of nutrient needs in the care of older adults. Older adults who are hospitalized for serious illnesses, nursing home patients, and homebound older adults are at risk for malnutrition.[38] The prevalence of malnutrition increases for those over the age of 70 years and is more likely to occur in individuals living in an urban setting.[39] Overweight and obesity also have pronounced detrimental effects on the health and quality of life of older adults. Evidence is growing that nutritional interventions can improve overall function and quality of life for older adults. Nurse Practitioners are ideally placed to appropriately screen, diagnose, and treat malnutrition in older adults in order to minimize the risk for malnutrition and optimize nutritional needs.

Nutrition Assessment of Older Adults

The purpose of a brief nutrition assessment is to identify patients at risk for poor or excessive nutritional intake. Nutrition assessment includes the past medical, family, and social history, diet and exercise history, vital signs, review of systems, physical exam, and biochemical data and should be incorporated into routine primary care visits. The importance of nutritional screening is paramount when caring for older patients because culturally, older adults do not typically share their nutritional concerns. This lack of communication may be related to their loss of independence, fear of dementia, or shame associated with their chronic disease. Recognizing individuals at risk for malnutrition is a greater challenge than actually diagnosing the condition once it occurs. Various screening tools have been developed to help clinicians identify patients at risk for malnutrition[40]. The Nutrition Screening Initiative (NSI) can be filled out by the patient and used not only to identify those at risk, but also identify potential contributing factors for malnutrition (Figure 6-1).[41] NSI is a broad, inter-professional effort of the American Academy of Family Physicians, The American Dietetic Association, and a coalition of more than 25 national health, aging, and medical organizations with the goal of promoting the integration of nutrition screening and intervention into health care for older adults. Another commonly used screening measure for older adults is the Mini Nutrition Assessment (Figure 6-2). This tool is completed by Nurse Practioners while interviewing patients and/or family members.[42]

Oral Health Assessment

Oral health assessment is integral to the health and nutritional status of older adults. Factors that can contribute to oral health problems include tooth decay, disease, ill-fitting dentures, endentulism, pain, disease states, and medication which may alter taste. There is a strong connection between oral health and a person's general health status. An association has been noted between periodontal disease and myocardial infarction.[43] It has also been reported that endentulous older adults consume fewer servings of fruits and vegetables and more soft foods, often leading to decreased fiber intake. There is a growing need for a community-based coalition of health care providers to ensure adequate oral health care for older adults in assisted living facilities, nursing homes, and home health agencies. A number of these facilities have on-site dentists and dental hygientists to improve the oral health of their residents. Use of the Kayser-Jones BOHSE oral screening instrument is an appropriate tool to utilize for the oral assessment of older adults (Figure 6-3).[44] Table 6-1 also lists soft foods to suggest for patients with chewing difficulty.

The Warning Signs of poor nutritional health are often overlooked. Use this Checklist to find out if you or someone you know is at nutritional risk.

DETERMINE YOUR NUTRITIONAL HEALTH

Read the statements below. Circle the number in the "yes" column for those that apply to you or someone you know. For each "yes" answer, score the number in the box. Total your nutritional score.

	YES
I have an illness or condition that made me change the kind and/or amount of food I eat.	2
I eat fewer than 2 meals per day.	3
I eat few fruits or vegetables or milk products.	2
I have 3 or more drinks of beer, liquor or wine almost every day.	2
I have tooth or mouth problems that make it hard for me to eat.	2
I don't always have enough money to buy the food I need.	4
I eat alone most of the time.	1
I take 3 or more different prescribed or over-the-counter drugs a day.	1
Without wanting to, I have lost or gained 10 pounds in the last 6 months.	2
I am not always physically able to shop, cook and/or feed myself.	2
	TOTAL

Total Your Nutritional Score. If it's –

0-2   Good! Recheck your nutritional score in 6 months.

3-5   You are at moderate nutritional risk. See what can be done to improve your eating habits and lifestyle. Your office on aging, senior nutrition program, senior citizens center or health department can help. Recheck your nutritional score in 3 months.

6 or more   You are at high nutritional risk. Bring this Checklist the next time you see your doctor, dietitian or other qualified health or social service professional. Talk with them about any problems you may have. Ask for help to improve your nutritional health.

Remember that Warning Signs suggest risk, but do not represent a diagnosis of any condition. Turn the page to learn more about the Warnings Signs of poor nutritional health.

These materials are developed and distributed by the Nutrition Screening Initiative, a project of:

AMERICAN ACADEMY OF FAMILY PHYSICIANS

THE AMERICAN DIETETIC ASSOCIATION

THE NATIONAL COUNCIL ON THE AGING, INC.

The Nutrition Screening Initiative • 1010 Wisconsin Avenue, NW • Suite 800 • Washington, DC 20007
The Nutrition Screening Initiative is funded in part by a grant from Ross Products Division of Abbott Laboratories, Inc.

Figure 6-1 Determine Your Nutritional Health (Nutrition Screening Initiative)[41]

Physical Examination (also see Chapter 2)

It is important for Nurse Practitioners to begin a physical exam by measuring the height and weight of all patients. This allows calculation of the body mass index = weight [kg]/height [m]^2 (BMI), which reflects weight in relationship to height. The association between BMI and mortality follows a U-shaped curve, with increased mortality being associated with BMIs both above and below the ideal range. The nadir of the U-shaped curve increases with age, with the best BMI for older

Mini Nutritional Assessment
MNA®

Nestlé
Nutrition**Institute**

Last name:		First name:	
Sex:	Age:	Weight, kg:	Height, cm:	Date:

Complete the screen by filling in the boxes with the appropriate numbers. Total the numbers for the final screening score.

Screening

A   Has food intake declined over the past 3 months due to loss of appetite, digestive problems, chewing or swallowing difficulties?
0 = severe decrease in food intake
1 = moderate decrease in food intake
2 = no decrease in food intake   ☐

B   Weight loss during the last 3 months
0 = weight loss greater than 3 kg (6.6 lbs)
1 = does not know
2 = weight loss between 1 and 3 kg (2.2 and 6.6 lbs)
3 = no weight loss   ☐

C   Mobility
0 = bed or chair bound
1 = able to get out of bed/chair but does not go out
2 = goes out   ☐

D   Has suffered psychological stress or acute disease in the past 3 months?
0 = yes 2 = no   ☐

E   Neuropsychological problems
0 = severe dementia or depression
1 = mild dementia
2 = no psychological problems   ☐

F1 Body Mass Index (BMI) (weight in kg) / (height in m²)
0 = BMI less than 19
1 = BMI 19 to less than 21
2 = BMI 21 to less than 23
3 = BMI 23 or greater   ☐

IF BMI IS NOT AVAILABLE, REPLACE QUESTION F1 WITH QUESTION F2.
DO NOT ANSWER QUESTION F2 IF QUESTION F1 IS ALREADY COMPLETED.

F2 Calf circumference (CC) in cm
0 = CC less than 31
3 = CC 31 or greater   ☐

Screening score   ☐☐
(max. 14 points)

12-14 points: ☐   Normal nutritional status
8-11 points: ☐   At risk of malnutrition
0-7 points: ☐   Malnourished

Save
Print
Rest

® Société des Produits Nestlé, S.A., Vevey, Switzerland, Trademark Owners. © Nestlé, 1994, Revision 2009. N67200 12/99 10M.
For more information: www.mna-elderly.com

Figure 6-2 Mini Nutrition Assessment[42]

adults (~25) being higher than the best BMI for younger adults. A BMI of less than 22 kg/m² indicates that an older patient is underweight and further assessment is warranted.[45] Obtaining a correct BMI may be difficult to determine, due to alterations in height caused by kyphosis or the inability to stand for measurement. Patients can therefore be measured in bed in a supine position using a tape measure. This possibility makes it important to systematically monitor a patient's weight over time.

The Kayser-Jones Brief Oral Health Status Examination (BOHSE)

Resident's Name _____   Date _____

Examiner's name _____   TOTAL SCORE_____

CATEGORY	MEASUREMENT	0	1	2
LYMPH NODES	Observe and feel nodes	No enlargement	Enlarged, not tender	Enlarged and tender*
LIPS	Observe, feel tissue and ask resident, family or staff (e.g. primary caregiver)	Smooth, pink, moist	Dry, chapped, or red at corners*	White or red patch, bleeding or ulcer for 2 weeks*
TONGUE	Observe, feel tissue and ask resident, family or staff (e.g. primary caregiver)	Normal roughness, pink and moist	Coated, smooth, patchy, severely fissured or some redness	Red, smooth, white or red patch; ulcer for 2 weeks*
TISSUE INSIDE CHEEK, FLOOR AND ROOF OF MOUTH	Observe, feel tissue and ask resident, family or staff (e.g. primary caregiver)	Pink and Moist	Dry, shiny, rough red, or swollen*	White or red patch, bleeding, hardness; ulcer for 2 weeks*
GUMS BETWEEN TEETH AND/OR UNDER ARTIFICIAL TEETH	Gently press gums with tip of tongue blade	Pink, small indentations; firm, smooth and pink under artificial teeth	Redness at border around 1-6 teeth; one red area or sore spot under artificial teeth*	Swollen or bleeding gums, redness at border around 7 or more teeth, loose teeth; generalized redness or sores under artificial teeth*
SALIVA (EFFECT ON TISSUE)	Touch tongue blade to center of tongue and floor of mouth	Tissues moist, saliva free flowing and watery	Tissues dry and sticky	Tissues parched and red, no saliva*
CONDITION OF NATURAL TEETH	Observe and count number of decayed or broken teeth	No decayed or broken teeth/roots	1-3 decayed or broken teeth/roots*	4 or more decayed or broken teeth/roots; fewer than 4 teeth in either jaw*
CONDITION OF ARTIFICIAL TEETH	Observe and ask patient, family or staff (e.g. primary caregiver)	Unbroken teeth, worn most of the time	1 broken/missing tooth, or worn for eating or cosmetics only	More than 1 broken or missing tooth, or either denture missing or never worn*
PAIRS OF TEETH IN CHEWING POSITION (NATURAL OR ARTIFICIAL)	Observe and count pairs of teeth in chewing position	12 or more pairs of teeth in chewing position	8-11 pairs of teeth in chewing position	0-7 pairs of teeth in chewing position*
ORAL CLEANLINESS	Observe appearance of teeth or dentures	Clean, no food particles/ tartar in the mouth or on artificial teeth	Food particles/tartar in one or two places in the mouth or on artificial teeth	Food particles,tartar in most places in the mouth or on artificial teeth

Upper dentures labeled: Yes _____ No _____ None_____   Lower dentures labeled: Yes _____ No _____ None _____

Is your mouth comfortable? Yes _____ No _____ If no, explain: _____

Additional comments: _____

Underlined* -refer to dentist immediately

Copyright © The Gerontological Society of America. Reproduced by permission of the publisher.

Figure 6.3 Oral Health Assessment Tool (Kayser Jones,[44] with permission)

Percent Weight Change

Weight loss is common in patients who are hospitalized or who reside in nursing homes. Weight loss is also frequently seen in older adults with significant changes in appetite due to acute illness, chronic disease, or gastrointestinal problems secondary to surgery, chemotherapy, or radiation (Chapter 12). It is important to take a diet history and determine the percent weight change using the patient's current weight and usual weight. Malnutrition is diagnosed by clinically significant, unintentional weight loss of 5% weight change in a 1-month period or 10% weight change over 6 months is generally considered a significant weight change that needs further evaluation.[46]

Table 6-1 Soft Foods to Suggest for Patients with Chewing Problems

- Apple sauce
- Baked beans
- Boiled vegetables
- Broiled fish
- Canned fruit in natural juice
- Chopped and pureed foods
- Cooked prunes
- Cottage cheese
- Ground meat
- Ice cream
- JELLO
- Juices
- Mashed potatoes
- Oatmeal
- Pudding
- Potato salad
- Scrambled eggs
- Shakes
- Soft bread with melted cheese
- Soups
- Tuna fish
- Yogurt

Source: Lisa Hark, PhD, RD, 2012. Used with permission.

Other Signs and Symptoms

Other aspects of the physical exam may reveal many conditions that can contribute to malnutrition, as well as frank malnutrition, e.g. muscle wasting, in particular temporal muscle wasting (sunken temples), ill-fitting dentures, and mouth sores or abscesses that limit oral intake.[48] It is particularly important to examine patients with cognitive impairment, since they may not be able to verbally report conditions such as constipation, urinary retention, or abdominal discomfort. A brief cognitive screening test, such as the Mini-Mental Status Exam, will help to uncover cognitive deficits that may be contributing to poor dietary intake and lead to malnutrition.[42] Figure 6-4 provides an algorithm to assist Nurse Practitioners in assessing, identifying, and treating weight loss and nutritional frailty in older adults.

Nutritional Frailty

Nutritional frailty is a condition that occurs in older adults and is characterized by low functional reserve, decreased muscle strength, and increased susceptibility to diseases. This is due to sarcopenia (loss of lean muscle mass), which reflects a progressive decrease in anabolism, increased catabolism, and a reduced muscle generation capacity.[47] These changes lead to decreased overall physical functioning, increased frailty, falls risk, and eventually loss of independence. Disease processes, medications, and physical de-conditioning can play a role in the development of nutritional frailty. These factors are elucidated in Figure 6-5.

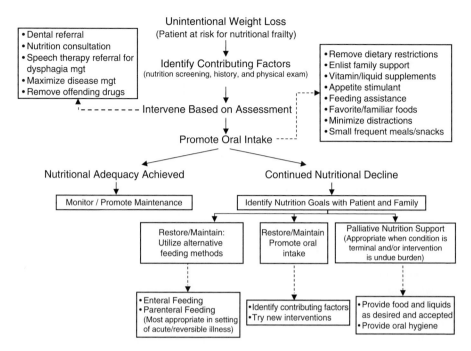

Figure 6-4 Algorithm to Address Unintentional Weight Loss and Nutritional Frailty in Older Adults Living in the Community
Source: Connie Bales, PhD, RD, 2012. Used with permission.

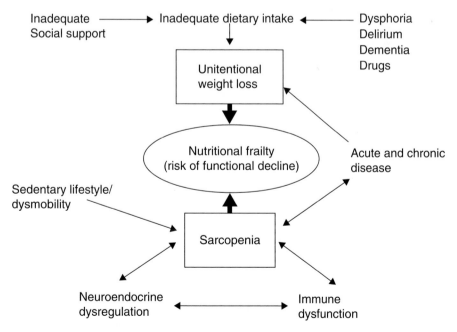

Figure 6-5 Dimensions of Nutritional Frailty
Source: Connie Bales, PhD, RD, 2012. Used with permission.

Etiology of Malnutrition

Decreased oral intake may result from poverty, poor dentition, gastrointestinal pathology, pain, anorexia, dysphagia, depression, social isolation, and pain from eating.[47] Increased nutrient losses can occur secondary to glycosuria, bleeding in the digestive tract, diarrhea, malabsorption, nephrosis, draining fistula, or protein-losing enteropathy. Additionally, any hypermetabolic state or excessive catabolic process can result in increased nutrient requirements. Surgery, trauma, fever, wound healing, burns, severe infection, malabsorption syndromes, and critical illness can also dramatically increase nutrient requirements.[47]

Chronic Diseases

Chronic disease is an important risk factor for malnutrition. However, it is important to recognize and address malnutrition as a separate treatable condition from chronic illness. Cancer cachexia has been largely related to the effects of pro-inflammatory cytokines on metabolic processes, causing excessive muscle turnover and wasting syndromes.[48] Reversal of these processes is often difficult, even with adequate nutritional support. Tumor burden, including location and size, can cause symptoms such as dysphagia, early satiety, abdominal pain, and intestinal obstruction that negatively impact nutritional status (Chapter 12). Cardiac cachexia is marked by the loss of lean muscle mass and metabolic disturbances that may result from altered cytokine levels. Weight loss is a common clinical feature of chronic obstructive pulmonary disease (COPD). This is likely related to increased resting energy expenditure from the increased work load of breathing and total daily energy expenditure, despite the inactivity associated with the disease process. Similarly, those with cancer[49], cardiac cachexia, and COPD can have elevated cytokine levels and catabolic processes that lead to muscle wasting. Symptoms such as dyspnea and fatigue may also interfere with caloric intake. Corticosteroids used in the treatment of COPD contribute to reduced muscle mass, reduced bone density, and negative nitrogen balance.[48] Patients with chronic illness may also experience depression. Rates of major depression are particularly high among hospitalized patients with acute illness or those living in nursing homes. Depression often goes unrecognized and untreated, and can affect nutritional status either by an increasing or decreasing appetite.[50]

Cognitive dysfunction is another important cause of unintentional weight loss and malnutrition among older adults. Numerous studies have confirmed the tendency for patients with Alzheimer's disease to lose weight early in the disease process. Weight loss and subsequent malnutrition can lead to serious consequences, including increased mortality. There are two primary physiologic mechanisms that might explain anorexia and therefore decreased caloric intake in Alzheimer's disease: taste and smell dysfunction, and the effect of inflammatory mediators (e.g. cytokines) on appetite.[51]

Medications

Medication can have a profound impact on nutritional status. Many older adults take multiple medications, both prescribed and non-prescribed. Multi-drug regimens are even higher among nursing home residents. Medications can alter nutritional status in a variety of ways, including alteration or loss of taste and smell, nausea, anorexia, dry mouth, diarrhea, reduced feeding ability or increased appetite. Non-prescription and recreational drugs should not be overlooked, since they can contribute to the overall problem.

Table 6-2 Recommendations to Improve Appetite

Make Eating an Enjoyable Experience
- Eat by the window or outside.
- Light a few candles.
- Make the food look good by varying colors and textures.
- Put flowers on your table.
- Set the table with placemats.
- Use your holiday place settings.
- Use good china and silverware.

Invite Company or Engage In Group Activities
- Go out for dinner weekly.
- Invite someone over for a meal.
- Join senior citizen groups.
- Take part in senior activities and gatherings.
- Talk to your neighbors.

Make Eating a Priority and As Easy as Possible
- Cook in quantity and pack/freeze the leftovers for later.
- Eat at appropriate times to avoid missing meals.
- Keep frozen vegetables on hand for quick side dishes.
- Keep meal time consistent and eat something even if you are not hungry.
- Try to include all food groups at lunch and dinner.
- Learn how to use the microwave.

Source: Lisa Hark, PhD, RD, 2012. Used with permission.

Dietary Modifications

When calorie and protein intake are inadequate, it is appropriate to remove traditional dietary restrictions related to disease processes, a position strongly supported by the American Dietetic Association.[52] For example, low sodium and low cholesterol diets have a profound negative impact on the taste and smell of food, and limit overall food intake. On a positive note, flavor and caloric enhancement, such as butter, margarine, oil, and powdered milk, have been shown to increase food intake and maintain weight in nursing home residents. Additionally, having someone else to eat with has been shown to significantly increase food consumption among homebound older adults.[53] Some facilities offer older adults a glass of wine before dinner to help stimulate their appetite and provide a social event such as "happy hour." Table 6-2 lists recommendations to tell patients to help improve dietary intake and appetite.

Dysphagia

Dysphagia can contribute to weight loss among frail older adults. Many neurological conditions effect the enervation of muscles which control swallowing and cause dysphagia. Esophageal muscle dysphagia is more often due to mechanical abnormalities such as stricture, webs, carcinoma, or extrinsic compression.[54] Symptoms of dysphagia usually include coughing, coryza, and aspiration pneumonia. It is important for Nurse Practitioners not only to ask about difficulty swallowing, but also coughing or watering of the eyes with meals and intolerance to solids or liquids. Swallowing studies are indicated if any of these symptoms are present.

For optimal patient care, Nurse Practitioners need to refer to a speech pathologist for these swallowing studies. A speech pathologist consultation can assist in diagnosing dysphagia, developing a treatment plan and educating patients and caregivers. In older adults diagnosed with dysphagia, altering food and liquid consistency can minimize the risk of aspiration and reduce weight loss. The Nurse Practitioner's role is to re-educate as needed for compliance with techniques to minimize the risk of aspiration, such as positioning the patient upright during mealtime and for 30 minutes after meals, tucking the chin during swallowing, and swallowing multiple times with each bolus of less than one teaspoon.[54]

Interventions for Malnutrition and Nutritional Frailty

Much of the research and guidelines for assessing and managing frailty in older adults has been done in the context of nursing home patients. In the nursing home environment, it is easier to monitor closely nutritional status and the resources to intervene, including the availability of dietitians. Many of the interventions applied in nursing homes can be applied in the outpatient primary care settings. It is important for Nurse Practitioners caring for older adults in these outpatient settings to be knowledgeable about the potential benefits, risks, and costs of specific interventions.

Supplements for Nutritional Frailty

When adequate nutrition cannot be achieved from *ad libitum* (self-regulated) meals, commercially prepared (usually liquid) nutritional supplements are often prescribed to increase total nutrient and caloric intake.[55] These products provide a good source of shelf-stable nutrients in appropriate amounts. However, some products may be low in protein and/or fiber content and they may be misused as meal replacements rather than taken in addition to a meal. Timing of liquid nutrition supplements can be a major determinant of their effectiveness. These drinks should not be given with meals, but in between meals and/or at bedtime. The chance of electrolyte and carbohydrate overload in chronic renal insufficiency and diabetes should be considered. A meta-analysis of 55 supplementation trials showed that hospitalized subjects (more than 65 years) and/or malnourished subjects benefited the most and had fewer complications and decreased mortality from using these supplements.[56] In the community setting, liquid protein/calorie supplements may benefit those patients with limitations in their oral food intake, such as food intolerances, and inability, or unwillingness to eat, and the more severely malnutritioned.[57]

Appetite Stimulants and Antidepressants

Orexigenic agents are often considered in the treatment of weight loss and malnutrition in older adults. In an effort to enhance food intake, megestrol acetate has been studied in undernourished older adults as a means to improve oral nutrition. The effects of megestrol take several months to have an impact on appetite and weight status.[58] Side effects include adrenal suppression, fluid retention, deep vein thrombosis, confusion, and impotence. Other agents that have been used to stimulate appetite include cyroheptadine, dronabinol, testosterone, growth hormone, oxandrolone, and steroids, but there is little data regarding their use.

The disease process is also important to consider when deciding to prescribe these medications since benefits may be less in conditions such as advanced dementia than in other disease processes where the improved sense of well-being has been a meaningful and measurable outcome with orexigenic agents. Patients with advanced dementia or terminal cancer are not likely to benefit.[58] In the situation of otherwise unexplained weight loss, the diagnosis of depression must be considered. Even when the diagnosis is uncertain, a trial of an antidepressant medication may be reasonable. Tricyclic antidepressants frequently result in weight gain in younger patients, but they may not produce weight gain in frail older adults.[59] Side effects including constipation, dry mouth, orthostatic hypotension, and urinary retention, make tricyclic antidepressants less desirable than the selective serotonin reuptake inhibitors (SSRIs, e.g. sertaline and citalopram). Initial concern that SSRIs may produce weight loss in older adults has not been substantiated. In many instances of depression, weight gain may represent improvement in depression.

Summary: Role of Nurse Practitioners

Nurse Practitioners are in unique positions to influence the health and well-being of their older adult patients by recognizing threats to nutritional adequacy and maximizing nutritional health. Nurse Practitioners also have the responsibility in guiding older adults toward appropriate nutritional choices. Nurse Practitioners should be able to identify, screen, inform, and intervene, as well as refer patients to registered dietitians when appropriate. Alterations in nutrient requirements for older adults should be discussed with patients and family members to optimize nutrient intake and avoid excessive consumption of calories. The status of hydration, protein, carbohydrates, lipids, and fiber needs cannot be assumed or ignored, especially in frail older adults with multiple chronic illnesses. Nurse Practitioners should align with physicians, dietitians, speech pathologists, dentists, and pharmacists in a multidisciplinary team approach. Most of all, Nurse Practitioners can assist their patients in setting realistic goals for their nutritional health and support them in achieving these goals by utilizing evidence-based practice to implement appropriate nutritional interventions.

Role of Nurse Practitioners

- Assess dietary intake for adequacy of energy, protein, fiber, vitamins and minerals.
- Assess nutritional status to diagnose overweight, underweight and malnutrition.
- Evaluate the potential benefit or harm regarding vitamins and herbal supplements.
- Evaluate food/medication interactions and over the counter medications.
- Recommend nutritional supplements when food intake is inadequate.
- Counsel patients regarding the benefit of healthy eating and fortified foods.
- Refer to registered dietitians for additional guidance and follow-up.

Source: Cecilia Borden, EdD, MSN, RN and Lisa Hark, PhD, RD, 2012. Used with permission.

Case 1

Benjamin is an 85-year-old man who is brought to his Nurse Practitioner by the local Older Americans Transportation Service. He had missed his two prior scheduled office visits due to a fractured hip. Ben seems to be withdrawn and much more frail than on previous visits. His wife died 3 months ago. He admitted that in addition to the loss of his wife, he has been experiencing financial hardship. Ben is 5'8" tall and weighs 140 lb. His usual weight has been 160 lb, and his weight before his surgery 6 months ago was 150 lb. His dentures are not fitting properly, he has a sore beneath the bottom plate, and he has cracks at the corners of his mouth. Ben currently takes medicine for depression and an iron supplement for anemia three times per day. He also uses over-the-counter laxatives and glycerin suppositories for his constipation, which he attributes to his iron tablets. The nurse practitioner needs to assess Ben and evaluate his needs.

HISTORY: Ben tripped on steps 2 months ago and fractured his hip, which required surgery to repair the fracture. He underwent in-patient rehabilitation for 10 days after discharge from the surgical service, and then returned to his, two-story home where he lives alone. He uses a cane and can climb stairs with difficulty. He was diagnosed with depression while in the hospital, and was started on antidepressant medication. His son and daughter both live out of state. Ben now shows little interest in going to the senior center and attending church, activities he previously enjoyed when his wife was alive. His appetite has decreased considerably, and his diet is low in calories, protein, fiber, fluids, vitamins, and minerals. He states that food does not have much taste and he complains of constipation.

PROBLEM: Although Ben can feed himself, he has trouble chewing because of his loose dentures and the sore in his mouth. Ben also has poor mobility. He walks with a cane, has difficulty with stairs, and fears falling since his hip fracture. Ben dislikes eating alone. Since his injury, he has been afraid to go outside. Ben reports a very limited social life; since his wife's death he has avoided church, community programs, and the senior center. He dislikes cooking just for himself. Ben has lost weight within the past 6 months, which increases his risk of malnutrition. Unfortunately, his son and daughter have not been in touch with him.

PLAN: The Nurse Practitioner needs to do the following:
- Assess Ben's dietary, vitamin, and mineral needs
- Develop a dietary plan based on his nutritional needs
- Prescribe needed macro and micronutrients
- Make referrals to interdisciplinary health team, which include:
  - Area Agency on Aging
  - Home care nursing assistance
  - Occupational therapist for a home assessment
  - Physical therapist to assess his mobility needs
  - Dentist to evaluate Ben's need for new dentures
  - Social Services for community resources, financial needs, psycho-social needs, wheels on meals, and contacting family

References

1. Department of Health and Human Services Administration on Aging. *A Profile of Older Americans: The Older Population 2010.*

2. Shrestha LB, Heisler JE. Congressional Research Service. *The Changing Demographic Profile of the United States.* March 31, 2011. www.fas.org/sgp/crs/misc/RL32701.pdf.

3. Ervin B. Healthy eating index scores among adults, 60 years of age and over, by sociodemographic and health characteristics: United States, 1999–2002; *Advance Data* 2008;395:1–16.

4. Crimmins EM, Kim JK, Seeman TE. Poverty and biological risk: The earlier "aging" of the poor. *J Geront* 2009; 64A:286–292.

5. Ramic E, Pranjic N, Batic-Mujanovic O, et al. The effect of loneliness on malnutrition in elderly population. *Med Arch* 2011;65:92–95.

6. Burns C. Seeing food through older eyes: the cultural implications of dealing with nutritional issues in aged and ageing. *Nutr Diet* 2009;66:200–201.

7. Rajda C, George N. The effect of education and literacy on health outcomes of the elderly. *J Nurse Pract* 2009;2:115–119.

8. Baker E, Metzler M, Galea S. Addressing social determinants of health inequities: learning from doing. *Am J Public Health* 2005;95:553–555.

9. Wolf MS, Curtis LM, Waite K, et al. Helping patients simplify and safely use complex prescriptions regimens. *Arch Intern Med* 2011;47:300–305.

10. Patterson PN, Shetterly SM, Clarke CL, et al. Health literacy outcomes in assessing patients with heart failure. *JAMA* 2011;305:16:1695–1701.

11. Popkin BM, D'anci KE, Rosenberg IH. Water hydration and health. *Nutr Rev* 2010;68: 439–458.

12. Howell AB, Foxman B. Cranberry juice and adhesion of antibiotic-resistant uropathogens. *JAMA* 2002;287:3082–3083.

13. Kontiokari T, Laitinen J, Jarvi, L, et al. Dietary factors protecting women from urinary tract infections. *Am J Clin Nutr* 2003;77:600–604.

14. Wernette C, White D, Zizza C. Signaling proteins that influence energy intake may affect unintentional weight loss in elderly persons. *J Am Diet Assoc* 2011;111:864–873.

15. Bruchert E, Rosenbaum D. Increased dietary fiber intakes are associated with significant lower prevalence of cardiovascular disease and lower cholesterol of about 5–10%. *Curr Opin Lipid* 2011;22:43–48.

16. West K, Sucheta M. Vitamin A intake and status in populations facing economic stress. *J Nutr.* 2010;140:201S–207S.

17. Minet-Quinard R, Farges C, Thivat E, et al. Neutrophils are immune cells preferentially targeted by retinoic acid in elderly subjects. *Immun Aging* 2010;7:1–16.

18. Pearce SH, Cheetham TD. Diagnosis and management of vitamin D deficiency. *Br Med J* 2010;340:B5665.

19. Shinchuk L, Holick M. Vitamin D and rehabilitation: improving functional outcomes. *Nutr Clin Pract* 2007;22:297–304.

20. Touvier M, Chan DS, Lau R, et al. Meta-analysis of vitamin D intake, 25-hydroxybitamin D status receptor polymorphisms, and colorectal cancer risk. *Cancer Epid Biomar Prev* 2011; 20:1003–1016.

21. Food and Nutrition Board, Institute of Medicine, Dietary Reference Intakes (DRIs) for Vitamins, Minerals and Trace elements. National Academies Press. Washington, DC. 1997–2004.

22. Capuron L, Moranis A, Combe N, et al. Vitamin E status and quality of life in the elderly: influence of inflammatory process. *Br J Nutr* 2009;102:1390–1394.

23. Miller E, Pastor-Barriuso R, Dolal D, et al. Meta-analysis: high-dosage vitamin E supplementation may increases all-cause mortality. *Ann Intern Med* 2005;142:37–46.

24. Lykkesfeldt J, Poulsen H. Is vitamin C supplementation beneficial? Lessons learned from randomised controlled trials. *Br J Nutr* 2010;103:1251–1259.

25. McRae M. Vitamin C supplementation lowers serum low-density lipoprotein cholesterol and triglycerides: a meta-analysis of 13 randomized controlled trials. *J Chiropr Med* 2008;7:48–58.

26. Fattal-Valveski A. Thiamine (Vitamin B1). *J Evidence-Based Complem Altern Med* 2011; 16:12–20.

27. Nord M, Andrews M, Carlson S. Household food security in the United States. *United States Department of Agriculture/Economic Research Service.* 2009.

28. Bleie O, Strand E, Ueland P, et al. Coronary blood flow in patients with stable coronary artery disease treated long term with folic acid and vitamin B12. *Coronary Artery Disease* 2011; 22:270–278.

29. Kripke C. Is oral vitamin B12 as effective as effective as intramuscular injection? *Am Fam Phys* 2006;73:65.

30. Butler C, Vidall-Alaball J, Cannings J, et al. Oral vitamin B12 vs IM vitamin B12 for vitamin B12 deficiency: a systematic of randomized control trials. *Family Practice* 2006;3:279–285.

31. Reid I, Ames R, Mason B, et al. Effects of calcium supplementation on lipids, blood pressure, and body composition in healthy older men: a randomized controlled trial. *Am J Clin Nutr* 2010;91:131–139.

32. Dietary Supplement Fact Sheet: Iron. Office of Dietary Supplements. National Institutes of Health. http://ods.od.nih.gov.factsheets/Iron. Accessed 2012.

33. Price E, Mehra R, Holmes T, et al. Anemia in older persons: etiology and evaluation. *Blood Cells Mol Dis* 2011;46:159–165.

34. Dietary Supplement Fact Sheet: Magnesium. Office of Dietary Supplements. National Institutes of Health. http://ods.od.nih.gov/factsheets/magnesium. Accessed 2012.

35. Carvil P, Cronin J. Magnesium and implications on muscle function. *Stren Condit J* 2010; 32:1:48–54.

36. Zorilla P, Salido JA, Lopez-Alfonso A, et al. Serum zinc as a prognostic tool for wound healing in hip hemiarthroplasty. *Clin Orthop Rel Res* 2004;420:304–308.

37. Prasad A, Beck F, Bao B, et al. Zinc supplementation decreases incidence of infections in the elderly: effect of zinc on generation of cytokines and oxidative stress. *Am J Nutr* 2007;85:837–844.

38. Landi F, Liperoti R, Fusco D, et al. Prevalence and risk factors of sarcopenia among nursing home older residents. *J Gerontol A Biol Sci Med Sci* 2011. doi:10.1093/Gerona/glr035.

39. Wham C, Teh R, Robinson M, et al. What is associated with nutritional risk in very old age? *J Nutr Healthy Aging* 2011;15:247–251.

40. Donini L, Savina C, Rosano A, et al. Systematic review of nutrition status evaluation and screening tools on the elderly. *J Nutr Health Aging* 2007;11:421–432.

41. Nutrition Screening Initiative: www.aafp.org/x16081.xml. Accessed 2012.

42. Kaiser MJ, Bauer JM, Ramsch C, et al. Validation of the Mini Nutritional Assessment Short Form (MNA®-SF): A practical tool for identification of nutritional status. *J Nutr Health Aging* 2009;13:782–788.

43. Baily R, Gueldner S, Ledikwe J, et al. The oral health of older adults: an interdisciplinary mandate. *J Gerontol Nurs* 2005;7:11–17.

44. Kayser-Jones J, Bird W, Paul S, et al. An instrument to assess the oral health status of nursing home residents. *Gerontologist* 1995;35:814–824.

45. Ahmed T, Haboubi N. Assessment and management of nutrition in older people and its importance to health. *Clin Interven Aging* 2010;5:207–216.

46. Florida Dietetic Association. Christie C (Ed), *Manual of Medical Nutrition Therapy* 2011; A1–6.

47. Lang T, Streeper T, Baldwin K, et al. Sarcopenia: etiology, clinical consequences, intervention, and assessment. *Osteopor Int* 2010;21:4:543–559.

48. Andrew I, Kirkpatrick G, Holden K, et al. Audit of symptoms and prescribing in patients with the anorexia-cachexia syndrome. *Pharmacy World Science* 2008;30:489–496.
49. Ritchie CS, Bales CW. Sarcopenia and nutritional frailty. Diagnosis and intervention. In: Bales CW, Ritchie CS (Eds), *Handbook of Clinical Nutrition and Aging*. Humana Press Inc, Totowa, NJ, 2004:309–333.
50. Chan-Quan H, Xue-Mei Z, Bi-Rong D, et al. Health status and risk for depression among the elderly: a meta-analysis of published literature. *Age and Aging* 2010;39:23–30.
51. Hansen ML, Waldorff FB, Waldemar G. Prognostic factors for weight loss over a 1 year period in patients recently diagnosed with mild Alzheimer Disease. *Alzheimer Dis Assoc Disord* 2011;25:269–275.
52. The American Dietetic Association. Position of the American Dietetic Association: Nutrient supplementation. *J Am Diet Assoc* 2009;109:2073–2085.
53. German L. Depressive symptoms are associated with food insufficiency and nutritional deficiencies in poor community-dwelling elderly people. *J Nut Health Aging* 2011;15:1–8.
54. Corrigan M, Escuro A, Celestin J, et al. Nutrition in the stroke patient. *Nut Clin Prac* 2011;26:242–245.
55. Palesty J, Dudrick S. Cachexia, malnutrition, the refeeding syndrome, and lessons from Goldilocks. *Surg Clin N Am* 2011;91:653–673.
56. Klek S, Szybinski P, Sierzega M, et al. Commercial enteral formulas and nutrition support teams improve the outcome of home enteral tube feeding. *J Parent Ent Nutr* 2011;35:380–385.
57. Mudge A, Ross L, Young A, et al. Helping understand nutritional gaps in the elderly (HUNGER): a prospective study of patient factors associated with inadequate nutritional intake in older medical patients. *Clin Nutr* 2011;30:320–325.
58. Rudolph D. Appetite stimulants in long term care: a literature review. *Internet J Adv Nurs Prac* 2010;11:1. Accessed 2012.
59. Rigler SK, Webb MJ, Redford L, et al. Weight outcomes among antidepressant users in nursing facilities. *J Am Geriat Soc* 2001;49:49–55.

Section 3
Nutrition in the Clinical Setting

7   Obesity and Bariatric Surgery Care

Lisa Hark, PhD, RD
Darwin Deen, MD, MS
Dory Ferraro, MS, APRN-CS

OBJECTIVES

- Identify the medical complications associated with overweight and obesity.
- Describe the diagnosis, prevalence, health consequences, and etiology of obesity.
- Explain the treatment methods currently available for patients who are overweight and obese.
- Summarize the dietary guidelines for bariatric surgery patients.
- Discuss the recommendations for management of micronutrient deficiencies following bariatric surgery.

Introduction

Obesity is a complex, multi-factorial condition associated with increased morbidity and premature mortality.[1,2] Obesity is an increasingly common problem faced by Nurse Practitioners working in both outpatient and inpatient settings.[2-4] The National Heart, Lung, and Blood Institute's (NHLBI) *Clinical Guidelines on the Identification, Evaluation, and Treatment of Overweight and Obesity in Adults* states, "next to smoking, obesity is the second leading cause of preventable death in the US today".[5] The life expectancy of a moderately obese person could be shortened by 2–5 years, while the life expectancy of an obese man with a body mass index (BMI) greater than $40 \, kg/m^2$ is likely to be reduced by almost 13 years.[6] This chapter aims to provide Nurse Practitioners with the tools to assess and manage overweight and obese patients, including those considering bariatric surgery.

Health Consequences of Obesity

According to the National Institutes of Health (NIH),[7] obese individuals have a 50–100% increased risk of premature death from all causes compared with normal weight individuals due to the associated medical complications (NHLBI). Rising prevalence of obesity is also a worldwide health concern because excess weight gain

---

The Nurse Practitioner's Guide to Nutrition, Second Edition. Edited by Lisa Hark, Kathleen Ashton and Darwin Deen.
© 2012 John Wiley & Sons, Inc. Published 2012 by John Wiley & Sons, Inc.

Table 7-1 Potential Co-morbidities of Obesity

Vascular	**Endocrine**
Hypertension	Type 2 diabetes
Dyslipidemia	Insulin resistance
Coronary artery disease	Polycystic ovarian syndrome
Congestive heart failure	Metabolic syndrome
Left ventricular hypertrophy	
Deep vein thrombosis	**Musculoskeletal**
Pulmonary embolism	Degenerative disc and joint disease
Venous stasis disease	Chronic back pain
	Gout
Women's Health	Plantar fasciitis
Gestational diabetes	
Infertility	**Neurological/Psychiatric**
Miscarriage	Depression
Fetal abnormalities and infant mortality	Anxiety
	Stroke
Pulmonary	Pseudotumor cerebrii
Asthma	Migraine headache
Obesity hypoventilation syndrome	
Obstructive sleep apnea	**Gastrointestinal**
Pulmonary hypertension	Gallstones
	Abdominal hernia
Genitourinary	Gastroesophageal reflux disease
Stress incontinence	Nonalcoholic fatty liver disease (NASH)
Urinary tract infection	

Source: Darwin Deen, MD, MS, 2012. Used with permission.

increases the burden from several diseases, most notably cardiovascular diseases, diabetes, and cancers as shown in Table 7-1. The World Health Organization (WHO) predicts that deaths from diabetes complications associated with obesity will increase 50% worldwide in the next 10 years.[8] Trend analysis reports indicate that by 2030, the prevalence of obesity in the US will rise from 26% to 35–48%.[9-11] Consequently an additional 6–8.5 million cases of diabetes, 5.7–7.3 million cases of heart disease and stroke, 492 000 to 669 000 additional cases of cancer, and 26–55 million quality-adjusted life years forgone in the US.[9] By 2030, the combined medical costs associated with treatment of these preventable diseases are estimated to increase by $48 to $66 billion/year in the US.[9,11] Currently, US businesses spend $45 billion annually in medical expenses and lost productivity related to obesity.[12] The NIH estimates costs for obesity treatment to be approximately $117 billion, accounting for 5–7% of national health expenditures in the US.[7,13] Even a modest 1% reduction in BMI would substantially reduce the number of obesity-related diseases and their costs, therefore, the role of Nurse Practitioners is extremely important in the prevention and treatment of the obesity epidemic.

Prevalence of Overweight and Obesity

According to the Centers for Disease Control (CDC),[14,15] more than one-third of US adults or 72 million Americans are obese.[16-18] This translates into an obesity prevalence rate of 32.2% among adult men and 35.5% among adult women.[16] The WHO states that more than 1.6 billion adults worldwide (ages 15 years and older) are overweight, and at least 400 million are obese.[19] Although the CDC's Behavioral Risk Factor Surveillance System (BRFSS) has tracked an increase in the prevalence of obesity over the past few decades, rates have not continued to increase at the same rate over the past 10 years, particularly among women.[16,17,20] Age-adjusted prevalence of overweight or obesity in racial and ethnic minorities is higher among non-Hispanic black and Mexican-American women than among non-Hispanic white women.[16,17,21]

Etiology of Obesity

Overweight and obesity result from an imbalance in energy intake and energy expenditure. At a basic level, eating too many calories and not getting enough physical activity contributes to obesity; however, body weight is also determined by genes, metabolism, behavior, environment, culture, and socio-economic status.[22,23] Behavior and environment significantly contribute to the development of overweight and obesity and these are the most important areas for prevention and treatment strategies.[24] The environment and a sedentary lifestyle may be the dominant contributing factors in the development of late onset obesity in adults, while genetic factors may exert a greater influence in young children who develop obesity.[25–27] Figure 7-1 summarizes the multiple dietary and lifestyle factors that have been linked to the increased prevalence of overweight and obesity across populations.

Excess Energy Intake

According to the National Health and Nutrition Examination Survey III (NHANES), Americans are eating 220 more calories per day compared with 20 years ago.[28,29] This increase in calories can be partially attributed to a combination of increased portion sizes, sweetened beverages, snacks, eating more meals outside the home, and greater frequency of eating fast foods as shown in Figure 7-1. According to the Health Professional Follow-up Study, foods most associated with adding weight over a 4-year

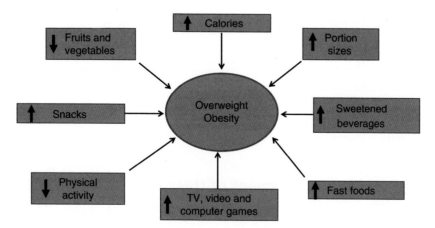

Figure 7-1 Dietary and Lifestyle Factors Associated with Overweight and Obesity
Source: Lisa Hark, PhD, RD, 2012. Used with permission.

period were french fries, potato chips, sugar-sweetened drinks, meats, desserts and refined grains.[30] Those who ate more fruits, vegetables, yogurt, nuts, and whole grains were more likely to lose weight or maintain their weight over time.[30]

Decreased Physical Activity

The dramatic increase in sedentary activities as a result of labor-saving devices, such as sitting at the computer, watching television, using the remote control, taking escalators, elevators, or moving sidewalks, using drive-through windows to pick up food, and using garage door openers, has reduced the amount of energy we expend as a society.[31,32] Studies from the National Weight Control Registry have indicated that regular physical activity is the single best predictor of long-term weight control in overweight and obese individuals who have lost weight.[33,34] Regular physical activity modestly contributes to caloric expenditure, reduced abdominal fat, and increased cardio-respiratory fitness. Therefore, increasing physical activity should be strongly encouraged in children and adults, along with a reduced calorie diet, to improve the health of overweight and obese patients.

Genetics

In humans, 426 variants of 127 different genes have been associated with obesity.[27] According to the latest update of the Human Obesity Gene Map, single mutations in 11 genes were strongly implicated in 176 cases of obesity worldwide (Genome NIH). Additionally, 50 chromosomal locations have been mapped that contain genes that may be related to obesity. According to the CDC, "recently, several independent population-based studies reported that a gene of unknown function, referred to as fat mass and obesity-associated gene (FTO), may be responsible for up to 22% of all cases of obesity. Interestingly, the FTO gene also shows a strong association with diabetes. The mechanism by which FTO operates is currently under investigation".[27]

Family history reflects genetic susceptibility and environmental exposures shared by close relatives. Genetic studies over the past several decades investigating adopted twins and their biological and adoptive parents show that adoptees' weight correlates most strongly with their biological parents' weight.[35] Additional research has shown that children of one overweight parent have a 40% chance of becoming overweight as adults. This risk increases to 80% if both parents are overweight.

Environment

Regardless of the strong evidence for genetic influences on human obesity, genetics accounts for no more than one-third of the variance in body weight. Experts agree that since there has been no change in the gene pool over the past three decades, the dramatic increase in the prevalence of obesity in both children and adults in the US likely reflects the diet and lifestyle factors shown in Figure 7-1.[27,36]

Diagnosis and Assessment of Overweight and Obesity

Body Mass Index (BMI)

As described in detail in Chapter 2, BMI provides a more accurate measure of total body fat than body weight alone (Figure 7-2).[5]

To calculate BMI using metric units:

BMI = weight (kg)/height (m²)

To calculate BMI using Imperial units:

BMI = weight (lb) × 703 height (in²)

Figure 7-2 Calculation of BMI
Source: NHLBI 2000.[5]

Table 7-2 International Classification of Adult Underweight, Overweight, and Obesity
According to BMI

	BMI (kg/m²)	
Classification	**Principal Cut-off Points**	**Additional Cut-off Points**
Underweight	< 18.50	< 18.50
Severe thinness	< 16.00	< 16.00
Moderate thinness	16.00–16.99	16.00–16.99
Mild thinness	17.00–18.49	17.00–18.49
Normal range	18.50–24.99	18.50–22.99
		23.00–24.99
Overweight	≥ 25.00	≥ 25.00
Pre-obese	25.00–29.99	25.00–27.49
		27.50–29.99
Obese	**≥ 30.00**	**≥ 30.00**
Obese class I	30.00–34.99	30.00–32.49
		32.50–34.99
Obese class II	35.00–39.99	35.00–37.49
		37.50–39.99
Obese class III	≥ 40.00	≥ 40.00

Source: WHO.[8]

The World Health Organization classifies BMI as shown in Table 7-2. Individuals with a BMI of 25 kg/m² or greater begin to experience complications, such as elevated low-density lipoprotein cholesterol (LDL-C) levels, hypertension, and pre-diabetes.[37,38]

Waist Circumference

Waist circumference is an independent measure of risk in normal weight patients, as well as overweight and obese patients.[5,39] Excess visceral adipose tissue located in the abdominal area is reflected by the waist circumference measurement.[40,41] Waist circumference is a predictor of morbidity, and is considered an independent risk factor for diabetes, dyslipidemia, hypertension, and cardiovascular disease even when BMI is not markedly increased.[5,42] Measuring waist circumference is recommended in patients with a BMI less than 35 kg/m^2 and is particularly important for patients with a family history of diabetes and those who may be considered borderline overweight.[43] These values also represent one of the diagnostic criteria of metabolic syndrome (Chapter 8). Since waist circumference may decrease without significant weight loss, this measure is an important tool to evaluate patients' progress.[43]

Measuring Waist Circumference

In order to obtain an accurate waist circumference measurement, patients should be standing in only their underwear. A horizontal mark should be drawn just above the uppermost lateral border of the right iliac crest, which should then be crossed with a vertical mark in the mid-axillary line. The measuring tape is placed in a horizontal plane around the abdomen at the level of this mark on the right side of the trunk. The plane of the tape should be parallel to the floor and the tape should be snug but not tight. High risk waist circumference values are shown in Table 7-3.

Table 7-3 High Risk Waist Circumference Values

Men > 40 inches (102 cm)
Women > 35 inches (88 cm)

Source: NHLBI.[5]

Treatment of Overweight and Obesity

There is strong evidence that a modest weight loss of 10% of body weight will result in a reduction of blood pressure and fasting glucose and lipid levels, thereby reducing the risk of developing diabetes and heart disease.[44,45] The incidence of other health problems associated with obesity, such as sleep apnea, metabolic syndrome, and osteoarthritis, also decreases with moderate weight loss.[43,46]

Behavior and Lifestyle Change

As described in Chapter 3, lifestyle changes often require many attempts, large and small, over many years. In making changes, patients move through a series of steps: Precontemplation, Contemplation, Preparation, Action, Maintenance, and Relapse.[47] Nurse Practitioners can identify which stage the patient is experiencing and help them move from one stage to another. Key questions to ask overweight and obese patients are shown in Table 7-4. Reviewing barriers to change, the circumstances and experiences of previous behavior change attempts and relapses, and motivation to change can also provide useful insights to overweight and obese patients.[48] Key nutritional recommendations for patients who are overweight and obese are listed in Table 7-5.

Table 7-4 Key Questions To Ask Overweight and Obese Patients

Initial Visit
- How many meals and snacks do you eat every day?
- Do you feel that you eat a healthy balanced diet? Why or why not?
- What do you like to drink during the day?
- Do you drink alcohol? What kind and how much?
- How often do you eat fruits and vegetables?
- How often do you eat dairy products? Low-fat or regular type?
- How often do you eat out? What kinds of restaurants?
- Do you usually finish what is on your plate?
- How often do you exercise, including walking?

Follow-Up Visit
- How have you changed your diet or exercise since the last visit?
- What problems did you encounter in making these changes?
- Do you feel confident that you can maintain the changes you have made?
- What changes would you still like to make in your diet or exercise pattern?
- How can I help you with these changes?

Source: Lisa Hark, PhD, RD and Darwin Deen, MD, MS, 2012. Used with permission.

Table 7-5 Key Nutritional Recommendations for Overweight and Obese Patients

- Focus on healthy eating rather than weight loss.
- Try to be as active as possible everyday.
- Eat more fruits and vegetables.
- Eat a healthy low-fat, high fiber breakfast everyday.
- Prepare healthy recipes when cooking.
- Drink more water and fat-free milk.
- Limit eating out, especially at fast food restaurants.
- Stop eating when you feel full.
- Reduce your portion sizes at lunch and dinner.
- Eat in the kitchen or dining room and not in front of the TV.
- Limit TV to less than 2 hours per day.
- Self-monitor by writing down what you eat and drink.
- Get involved in support groups, such as Weight Watchers.

Source: Lisa Hark, PhD, RD, 2012. Used with permission.

Weight Reduction Medications

- Prescription weight-loss medications may be appropriate for patients who are at increased medical risk because of their weight.[49] In addition, patients who have previously failed weight loss attempts with diet and physical activity may be candidates. However, according to the NHLBI guidelines, prescription weight-loss drugs are approved only for patients with:[5]
- BMI > 30 kg/m^2 or
- BMI > 27 kg/m^2 with an obesity-related condition, such as hypertension, type 2 diabetes, or hyperlipidemia.

Along with being overweight or obese, the conditions listed in Table 7-1 increase the risk for heart disease, cancer, and other ailments. Pharmacotherapy may improve weight loss effects of diet and exercise when diet and exercise alone are not sufficient.[50]

Case 1

LIFESTYLE: Jeffrey is a 30-year-old lawyer who eats most of his meals on the run since he doesn't have time to cook. He skips breakfast, snacks on donuts or pastries and juice at work and drinks four large cups of coffee with cream and sugar every day. Four out of five days a week Jeffrey eats in a fast-food restaurant for lunch where he orders a double cheese burger, large fries, and a large soda. On Fridays, he has two slices of pepperoni pizza with a large soda. Since he works late, he frequently orders take-out in his office for dinner from a variety of local restaurants. For Chinese meals, he orders Kung Pao chicken (breaded and fried), fried rice, and an egg roll. For Italian meals, he orders chicken parmesan and spaghetti with garlic bread or at a diner he likes a hot open faced turkey sandwich with gravy and a milkshake.

On weekends, he eats a bowl of cereal and milk for breakfast at home, he skips lunch and eats out for dinner with his friends at a local pub. He chooses appetizers, such as chicken wings or mozzarella sticks, and entrees such as prime rib, London broil or grilled chicken, and French fries for dinner. He rarely eats any vegetables. He usually drinks two beers on Friday and Saturday night at the pub. He does not smoke cigarettes and does not have time to exercise.

PROBLEM: Jeffrey has gained 15 lb since last year when he decided to change jobs and open up his own law firm. He has been complaining of feeling tired all of the time and has been drinking more coffee everyday to stay alert during the day. Because of his schedule, he has not had the time to exercise like he used to last year. He complains of constipation, fatigue, and requests assistance to lose weight. He has no other medical conditions.

ADVICE: Jeffrey's main complaints of constipation, fatigue, and weight gain are related to his diet and sedentary lifestyle. He does not eat fruits and vegetables, and his diet is very low in fiber. He has gained weight because he is taking in more calories than he burns. He has been eating most of his meals away from home, where larger portions are served and admits that he usually finishes everything on his plate. He can add more fiber to his diet by eating a bowl of cereal with milk at home before work, bringing fresh or dried fruit to work as an alternative to the midmorning pastry snack, and including vegetables with lunch and/or dinner. At dinner, he could order a side of vegetables or a salad with any entrée as well as minestrone soup at the Italian restaurant, which has beans, legumes, and vegetables.

If he is willing to order grilled chicken instead of high-fat burgers and fries at fast-food restaurants a few days a week, this would be a good start. He could opt for a vegetable topping or a slice of tomato pie with a salad instead of the pepperoni pizza. For dinner, he should choose broiled or grilled fish or chicken, and add a salad to the meal when he is eating out. Recommend regular chicken and vegetables with white rice, rather than fried at Chinese restaurants. Skip high-fat appetizers, when eating out. Finally, Jeffrey needs to schedule time to exercise such as walking to his client's offices. On the weekends, recommend he try to make time for biking, walking, running, and playing squash or other sports that he enjoys.

As the maintenance of weight loss becomes integral to treatment paradigms, long-term effects of medications become important criteria for success.[49] Therefore, to be approved by the Food and Drug Administration (FDA) medications for long-term weight loss, must show safety and efficacy for 2 years or more.[51] Currently there is only one drug approved for long-term use: orlistat (Xenical), a lipase inhibitor.[52,53]

Unlike other weight loss medications, orlistat (Xenical by Hoffman-LaRoche) is the first non-systemic weight loss medication, acting entirely on the gut, not the brain. Weight loss occurs because of reduced absorption of fat calories.[54] Approximately 30% of dietary fat is eliminated in the stool. Orlistat is prescribed in 120 mg doses to be taken three times per day, during meals. Since its mechanism of action is influenced by the amount of fat in the meal, patients are prescribed a low-fat diet to reduce side effects. If a low-fat diet is not consumed, side effects can be significant, and include flatulence, oily stools, severe diarrhea, and abdominal cramping. Orlistat, at 60 mg (half the dose of Xenical), is now approved by the FDA for over-the-counter (OTC) use in adults over 18 years of age.[51] The product, called Alli, is the first weight loss medication to be approved by the FDA for OTC use.[51]

The FDA has also approved exenatide (incretin mimetic) as adjunctive therapy to improve blood sugar control in patients with type 2 diabetes who have not achieved adequate control on metformin and/or a sulfonylurea. Exenatide is a synthetic protein (from the Gila monster) that mimics the activity of the naturally occurring hormone glucagon-like peptide-1 (GLP-1).[55] GLP-1 binds to pancreatic beta-cell receptors to stimulate the release of insulin. In response to food intake GLP-1 will stimulate the release of insulin by binding to the pancreatic beta-cell receptors.[29,56] In clinical trials, exenatide has been shown to improve blood sugar control by lowering both post-meal and fasting glucose levels, leading to better long-term control as measured by hemoglobin A1C. Weight loss appears to be an added benefit.[57] Exenatide has been shown to reduce weight through several actions, including the stimulation of insulin secretion only when blood sugar is high and by restoring the first-phase insulin response, an activity of the insulin-producing cells in the pancreas that is lost in patients who have type 2 diabetes. The major side effect from exenatide appears to be nausea. Nurse Practitioners need to understand that medications have been shown to reduce weight by 5–10% only when combined with diet and exercise.

Bariatric Surgery

The total number of bariatric surgeries increased almost tenfold, from 1998 to 2004.[58] Estimates suggest the number in 2010 will exceed 220,000.[59] Nurse Practitioners should know the indications, contraindications, and types of bariatric surgery and recognize their role during pre-operative and postoperative care. Surgery is more effective than conventional management for the individual with clinically severe obesity, but should only be considered when all other treatments have failed. Bariatric surgery consistently results in significant and sustained weight loss; patients typically lose more than 50% of their excess weight.[60] Co-morbid conditions markedly improve, reducing cardiovascular mortality and improving life expectancy. A Cochrane review of procedures performed in adults for weight reduction: gastric bypass, adjustable gastric banding, biliopancreatic diversion, sleeve gastrectomy, and vertical banded gastroplasty, concluded that surgical intervention in obese adults results in greater weight loss and reduction of co-morbidities compared with conventional treatment.[61]

Increasingly the evidence suggests that bariatric surgery may be among the most effective treatments for metabolic conditions and diseases such as type 2 diabetes, hypertension, hyperlipidemia, obstructive sleep apnea, and non-alcoholic fatty liver disease. A landmark study showed remission of type 2 diabetes (76.8%), resolution of hypertension (61.7%), and resolution of sleep apnea (85.7%) in a majority of the patients undergoing bariatric surgery.[62,63]

Table 7-6 Criteria for Bariatric Surgery

- Body mass index (BMI)$\geq 40\,kg/m^2$, or$\geq 35\,kg/m^2$ with serious obesity-related condition (type 2 diabetes, hypertension, heart disease, sleep apnea).
- Documented failure of non-surgical weight loss program.
- Willingness to adequately comply with the post-operative regimen.
- Acceptable operative risks.
- An understanding of the operation and the necessary lifestyle changes.

Source: NIH Consensus Development Program, NIDDK website.[7]

BMI Criteria for Bariatric Surgery

In 1991, the National Institutes of Health Consensus Development Panel established criteria for bariatric surgery eligibility (Table 7-6). Candidates must have a BMI $\geq 40\,kg/m^2$ and have failed conservative attempts at weight loss through diet and exercise. Approximately 10 million Americans (5% of the population) have a BMI $\geq 40\,kg/m^2$ (Class III obesity) and are therefore, potential surgical candidates.[17,64] Individuals with BMI $\geq 35\,kg/m^2$ may qualify when a life-threatening co-morbid condition, such as type 2 diabetes, hypertension, sleep apnea, or cardiovascular disease is present. Those who suffer obesity-related physical and functional impairment (debilitating joint disease, severe interference with ambulation, job performance, or family functions) may also be candidates for bariatric surgery.

Patients considering bariatric surgery must have acceptable surgical risk and have failed previous weight loss interventions. Bariatric surgery is safe in adolescents aged 12–18 years and associated with significant weight loss, correction of obesity co-morbidities, and improved self-image and socialization.[65,66] Contraindications to bariatric surgery include patients with untreated major depression or psychosis, binge eating disorders, those with ongoing drug and alcohol abuse, or those with cardiovascular disease with prohibitive operative risks, coagulopathy, or inability to comply with life-long, postoperative nutritional requirements and vitamin and mineral supplementation.

Therefore, prospective patients are evaluated by a multidisciplinary weight management team consisting of: a physician, Nurse Practitioner, registered dietitian, and bariatric psychologist. A thorough medical evaluation should be performed, including cardiac and pulmonary clearance to assess operative risk. Patients with severe cardiopulmonary disease, active substance abuse or severe psychopathology are generally not considered appropriate candidates for bariatric surgery.

Surgical Options

The field of bariatric surgery is dynamic with surgical procedures and techniques that are constantly being developed and refined.[67] Bariatric procedures reduce caloric intake through a number of mechanisms, which include appetite suppression, restriction of intake, nutrient diversion from the duodenum, and nutrient malabsorption.[68] It is hypothesized that bariatric surgery may also affect the gut-brain axis by altering the effects of gastrointestinal peptides, such as ghrelin, peptide YY, glucagon-like peptide, and pancreatic polypeptides, that regulate satiety and appetite.[69]

There are a number of procedures commonly performed for the treatment of severe obesity. These include purely restrictive procedures, such as laparoscopic adjustable gastric banding (LAGB) and sleeve gastrectomy, which induce weight loss by limiting caloric intake. Malabsorptive procedures, such as biliopancreatic diversion (BPD) with or without duodenal switch limit nutrient absorption, and combination procedures, such as the Roux-en-Y gastric bypass (RNYGB) combine both restriction and malabsorption. Generally, procedure selection is a shared decision between the physician and the patient.[70]

Gastric Bypass The RNYGB, which is considered the gold standard operation for weight loss in the US, combines both restrictive and malabsorptive components.[71] During a RNYGB, a gastric pouch (20–30 mL) is created with a small outlet (stoma) to the jejunum, and a Roux limb that reroutes approximately 100 cm of the alimentary tract to bypass the distal stomach and proximal small bowel. Food intake is restricted, and absorption of nutrients is limited. Patients experience marked loss of appetite with rapid, radical weight loss during the first 6 months following surgery. Weight loss generally plateaus between 12 and 18 months post-operatively. Potential complications include anastamotic leaks, pulmonary embolism, bleeding, vomiting caused by narrowing of the stoma, micronutrient deficiencies, and small bowel obstruction. Dumping syndrome can occur following ingestion of refined sugar, which is characterized by symptoms including rapid heart rate, nausea, diarrhea, and feeling faint.

Adjustable Gastric Banding The least invasive of all the bariatric surgical procedures is LAGB. An adjustable elastic band with an inflatable elastic collar is placed around the upper part of the stomach just below the gastroesophageal junction, creating a small upper gastric pouch. The band is adjustable through an access port placed subcutaneously in the upper abdomen; normal saline can be added or removed to tailor restriction to individual needs. Weight loss following LAGB results in generally 1–3 lb per week, and varies depending on patient adherence to diet and physical activity guidelines, as well as frequency of follow-up and periodic band adjustments.[72] Risks associated with LAGB include band slippage, band erosion, reservoir deflation/leak, vomiting, acid reflux, and failure to lose weight. When compared with the laparoscopic RNYGB, LAGB was found to have fewer and less severe complications.[73,74]

Sleeve Gastrectomy (SG) Once the first part of a two-stage procedure for high-risk patients, the SG has recently been considered an acceptable option as a primary weight loss procedure.[75] During a SG procedure the stomach is divided vertically, reducing its volume by about 80%, leaving the pylorus and normal digestive process intact. Risks include leaks, bleeding, and vomiting due to stenosis or overeating. Recent studies have shown the SG to be safe and effective, but due to its relatively new application, there are no long-term data.

Biliopancreatic Diversion (with or without duodenal switch) The BPD is primarily a malabsorptive procedure.[76] During a BPD, part of the stomach is resected to limit food intake, leaving a gastric pouch larger than that created during a GB. A long limb of the small intestine is bypassed with a short common alimentary channel of about 50 cm. An adaptation of this procedure, the BPD with duodenal switch (DS) is essentially a SG with the added component of a long limb bypass. The benefit of a BPD with DS is that the pylorus is preserved. Risks associated with BPD surgery (with or without DS) include anastamotic leak, anastamotic ulcers, protein malnutrition, frequent and foul-smelling stools and flatus, vitamin and mineral deficiencies, and alopecia.

Weight Loss After Bariatric Surgery

Weight loss after bariatric surgery varies with procedure and the individual patient, and is often expressed as the percentage of excess weight lost (defined as the number of pounds above ideal body weight). Mean weight loss is usually greatest with BPD/DS (70%), followed by GB (62%), SG (55%), and LAGB (48%) as shown in Table 7-7. The malabsorptive procedures generally result in a more rapid, radical weight loss compared with those procedures which solely rely on restriction. All procedures require patients be willing and able to make significant lifestyle changes, which include dietary and behavior modifications. The FDA recently approved use of the LAP-BAND System® (Allergan) for adults with BMI of 30–40 kg/m² and at least one obesity-related co-morbid condition. Several recent studies have shown that patients with BMI < 35 kg/m² derived benefits similar to those seen in patients who met the NIH criteria.[77]

Table 7-7 Percent Weight Loss After Bariatric Surgery

Type of Procedure	Mean Weight Loss (%)	Range (%)
Roux-en-Y Gastric Bypass	61.6	33–77
Biliopancreatic Diversion	70.1	62–75
Adjustable Gastric Banding	47.5	32–70
Sleeve Gastrectomy	55.4	33–85

Sources: Buchwald 2004,[62] Clinical Issues Committee of ASMBS 2010.[75]

Safety of Bariatric Surgery

The safety of bariatric surgery has long been a topic of discussion. With bariatric procedures being performed in increasing numbers, the level of scrutiny remains high. Improvements in technology, formal training programs, greater experience, rigorous clinical trials, an increasing body of knowledge and accrediting and credentialing activities have all contributed to a dramatic decrease in surgery-related morbidities and mortalities. Until recently, the risks and benefits of bariatric surgery had not been rigorously assessed with a large-scale, multicenter trial. A recent study of nearly 5000 patients found the overall risk of death (0.3%) and low major adverse outcomes (4.3%) after bariatric surgery, to be less than the long-term risk of dying from heart disease, diabetes, or other consequences of obesity.[78] In assisting patients to make appropriate choices, it is recommended that they be referred to accredited bariatric programs with an experienced multidisciplinary weight management team with the medical and psychosocial support that patients will need pre- and post-operatively.

Bariatric Surgery and Survival

Recent studies indicate that individuals who have had bariatric surgery have a survival advantage when compared with matched controls. Findings from the Swedish Obese Subjects study revealed an estimated 28% reduction in mortality in surgery groups when compared with control groups primarily due to fewer deaths from cardiovascular disease and cancer.[79] Adams compared 7,925 gastric bypass patients with age, BMI, and gender-matched controls and demonstrated the rate of death from all diseases (coronary artery disease, diabetes and cancer) was 52% lower in those who had bariatric surgery.[80] Perry reported a statistically significant improvement in survival rates in morbidly obese Medicare recipients who underwent bariatric surgery when compared with a similar non-surgical group.[81] This study also showed significant improvements in diabetes, sleep apnea, hypertension, hyperlipidemia, and coronary artery disease morbidity.

Pre-Operative Evaluation: The Team Approach

Patient evaluation for bariatric surgery should be performed by a multidisciplinary team, comprised of specially trained health professionals with expertise in surgical obesity management including a bariatrician, surgeon, Nurse Practitioner, dietitian, exercise physiologist, and psychologist or psychiatrist.[82] A thorough medical evaluation should be performed to rule out hormonal causes or genetic syndromes. The scope and focus of the medical exam should be designed to identify any co-morbid conditions and to assess for the acuity, stability, and any complications of these co-morbidities.[83]

Pre-Operative Nutrition Assessment

It is vital that Nurse Practitioners educate their patients about the post-operative nutrition therapy necessary before and after bariatric surgery prior to describing the type of procedure.[84,85] A pre-operative nutrition assessment will provide data to guide the pre- and post-operative management.[85] This assessment includes: (1) the patient's weight history and previous weight-loss strategies, (2) factors affecting weight issues such as work, social, and cultural information, (3) dietary patterns and alcohol intake, (4) nutritional and vitamin supplements use, (5) physical activity and limitations, and (6) readiness and motivation to make long-term lifestyle changes.[86,87] Pre-operative dietary goals should be created which form the foundation for post-operative meals and snacks.

Significant deficiencies of specific nutrients known to become deficient after bariatric surgery may also exist prior to surgery. In a retrospective study of 379 patients scheduled to undergo RYGB, deficiencies were noted in iron (44%), thiamin (29%), and 25-hydroxyvitamin D (68%) as reflected by low ferritin and hemoglobin levels.[88] Pre-operative testing of iron status (iron, total iron-binding capacity, ferritin, serum transferrin receptor), vitamin B_{12}, 25-hydroxyvitamin D, and parathyroid hormone is recommended, especially in patients undergoing a surgical procedure with a malabsorptive component.[83]

Pre-Operative Weight Loss Recommendations

Patients who lose 10% of their excess body weight prior to surgery have fewer surgical complications.[89] They also have shorter operative times and hospital stays, reduced blood loss compared with those who do not lose weight prior to surgery, and reduced intra-operative need for conversion to open surgical technique.[90] Additionally, patients who were able to lose weight prior to surgery may also have improved long-term weight loss results.[89,90] Key points to tell patients prior to surgery are listed below.

Key Points for Patients Prior to Bariatric Surgery

- Reduce intake of high-fat foods.
- Use meal replacement shakes for breakfast.
- Pack lunch instead of eating fast food.
- Reduce intake of sweets.
- Snack on fresh fruit.
- Substitute one half serving of a meal replacement shake instead of an evening snack.
- Take prescribed dietary supplements as directed by the pre-op nutritional and lab tests evaluations.

Source: Donna Kulick, MD, Lisa Hark, PhD, RD, Darwin Deen, MD, MS, 2012. Used with permission.

Post-Operative Nutrition Assessment

Post-operative nutritional goals are to maintain an adequate intake of essential macro- and micronutrients while producing a significant caloric deficit. Usually the more significant the component of malabsorption, the greater the amount of weight loss; however, nutritional deficiencies follow the same trend.[91] Malabsorption of protein may occur following BPD procedures but protein malnutrition may also occur after restrictive surgeries. Protein malnutrition presents with edema, alopecia, and low serum albumin levels (less than 3.5 g/dL). Monitoring serum albumin concentration is adequate to monitor protein nutritional status. Protein malnutrition is rarely seen as a complication of restrictive procedures (0–2%), but may affect up to 13% of patients after RYGB.[92,93]

Many vitamins and minerals are absorbed in the duodenum and proximal jejunum which can lead to deficiencies in patients who have undergone malabsorptive bariatric procedures. In those patients who have undergone restrictive procedures, dietary

Table 7-8 Routine Nutrient Supplementation After Bariatric Surgery

- Chewable multivitamin and minerals supplement: 1–2 tab twice daily.
- Calcium citrate: 1200–1500 mg/d.
- Vitamin D3: 1000–1400 IU/day.
- Vitamin B12: 500 µg/day orally or 1000 µg/mo intramuscularly.
- Folic acid: 400 µg /day.
- Elemental iron: 65–80 mg/day (preferably with vitamin C).

Source: Donna Kulick, MD, Lisa Hark, PhD, RD, and Darwin Deen, MD, MS, 2012. Used with permission.

changes associated with caloric restriction may lead to deficiencies. Iron is the most common deficiency seen after bariatric surgery but clinical manifestations of calcium, vitamin D, vitamin B_{12}, folic acid, and thiamin deficiencies have also been described.[94,95,96] The prevention of these problems depends upon a carefully selected diet to ensure adequate intake and clinical monitoring to identify potential deficiencies before symptoms occur. Table 7-8 describes routinely recommended vitamin and mineral supplementation to prevent and treat these various deficiencies.[87,97–99]

Post-Operative Nutrition Therapy

Post-operative recommendations for dietary advancement are outlined in Table 7-9. Although there are no strict dietary guidelines after bariatric surgery, the recommendations are to follow a meal progression pattern which calls for gradual progression of food consistency over weeks or months.[100,101] Patients are typically advised to follow a clear liquid diet for a few days after surgery and advance to full liquids while keeping the feeding volume small (no more than 1/4 cup four to six times per day) during the first week. During the second post-operative week, pureed foods, emphasizing higher protein foods may be added. Semi-solid/soft foods are added as tolerated, with the advice to take small bites and chew foods thoroughly. Foods not well tolerated during the first few months after surgery include red meat, chicken, and turkey (except when finely minced), white flour products, foods high in sugar or fat, and raw fruits and vegetables with high fibrous consistency (celery stalks, corn, artichokes, tomatoes, pineapple, oranges).

Key Points for Patients After Bariatric Surgery

- Keep portions small.
- No beverages 30 minutes before eating and 30–60 minutes after eating.
- Ingest at least 60 g of protein per day to avoid protein malnutrition.
- Eat at scheduled times and avoid snacking.
- Allow 30 minutes for each meal and chew food well.
- Incorporate physical activity on most days of the week.
- At 2-months post-operative, patients can eat approximately 1 cup of food per meal, averaging 60–80 g of protein every day and drink 48 oz of water.

Source: Donna Kulick, MD, Lisa Hark, PhD, RD, and Darwin Deen, MD, MS, 2012. Used with permission.

Table 7-9 Dietary Advancement Recommendations Post-Bariatric Surgery

Time Post-Op	Recommendation
Days 1–2	• Clear liquids (sugar-free, non-carbonated, caffeine-free). • Sip water as tolerated and advance to 48 fluid ounces/day. • Always avoid drinking liquids with a straw to reduce intake of air.
Days 3–7	• Continue clear liquids (sugar-free, non-carbonated, caffeine-free). • 48–64 fluid ounces/day (half as clear liquids). • Start full liquids (non-fat milk, soy milk, plain or blended yogurt, blended soups). • May add whey and soy protein powder to full liquids (Limit to < 20 g protein/serving). • Start chewable multivitamin mineral supplement (1 tablet twice daily).
Weeks 2–3	• Increase clear liquids to 48–64 fluid ounces/day. • Replace full liquids with solid, soft, moist, pureed, ground, low-fat, high protein foods (eggs, low-fat cottage cheese, fish, poultry, lean meat, cooked beans). • Consume four to six meals/day (limit portion size ~1/4 cup). • Consume protein first (at least 60 g/day).
Weeks 4–6	• Advance diet as tolerated: add well-cooked, soft, pureed vegetables, peeled, pureed fresh or frozen low fiber fruits, or canned fruits (no sugar added). • Add one soft, moist, solid food/meal/day as tolerated. • Consume four to six meals/day (limit portion size ~1/2 cup). • Consume protein first (60–80 g/day). • Avoid dehydration by consuming 48–64 fluid ounces/day of clear liquids (sugar-free, non-carbonated, caffeine-free). • No clear liquids within 30 minutes after meal. • Chew foods well.
Week 7 and beyond	• Daily caloric needs are based on height, weight, and age. • Advance to well-cooked, soft, pureed vegetables. • Advance to soft, peeled, pureed fresh or frozen low fiber fruits or canned fruits (no sugar added). • Avoid raw fruits and vegetables with high fibrous consistency (celery stalks, corn, artichokes, tomatoes, pineapple, orange). • Choose whole grains and avoid pasta, rice, and bread before consuming protein foods, vegetables, and fruits. • Consume three meals and two snacks/day (limit portion size ~1 cup). • Consume 48–64 fluid ounces/day of clear liquids (non-carbonated, calorie-free, caffeine-free). • No beverages 30 minutes before eating and 30–60 minutes after eating. • Chew foods well.

Source: Donna Kulick, MD, Lisa Hark, PhD, RD, and Darwin Deen, MD, MS, 2012. Used with permission.

Addressing Dumping Syndrome

Patients who complain of nausea, chills, diaphoresis, and diarrhea after eating are likely to have dumping syndrome, which initially occurs in 70–76% of patients with RYGB.[102] Dumping syndrome can be divided into early and late phases depending on the relationship of the symptoms to the time elapsed from the meal. Symptoms may occur within 10–30 minutes after eating. Early dumping results from accelerated gastric emptying of hyper-osmolar content into the small bowel and is associated with nausea, bloating, abdominal cramps, and diarrhea.[103] Alternatively, symptom onset may occur 1–3 hours after eating (late dumping), and consists of flushing, dizziness, palpitations, and lightheadedness associated with orthostatic blood pressure changes. Late dumping typically relates to hypoglycemia due to exaggerated release of insulin and affects 25% of dumping syndrome patients.[104,105] Specific dietary changes (reduction of carbohydrate intake) usually help resolve these symptoms. In addition, avoiding liquids for 30 minutes after a meal, and consuming smaller portions is recommended.

Case 2

Camilla is a 46-year-old female who had been obese most of her adult life. Several years ago, she reached an all-time high weight of 251 lb, and at a height of 62 inches, her BMI was 45.9 classifying her as morbidly obese. After multiple attempts at traditional weight loss methods, she elected to undergo laparoscopic Roux-en-Y gastric bypass. During the year following her surgery, Camilla lost 70 lb, nearly 60% of her excess weight. As a result of her surgery and subsequent weight loss, her glycosolated hemoglobin dropped from 8.2 to 6.0% and she no longer required medication for her type 2 diabetes. She reported she had been taking a multivitamin daily, but no other supplements. She had been feeling well until several months ago when she began feeling tired and noticed occasional episodes of lightheadedness. She also reported thinning of her hair.

PROBLEM: Laboratory evaluation revealed a hemoglobin of 9.9 g/dL, hematocrit: 31.4%, MCV: 72.6 (81–99), MCH: 22.9 (27–31), RDW: 20.8% (11–18), iron: 21 µg/dL (35–200), ferritin: 8 ng/mL (18–350), and zinc: 82 µg/dL (75–125). Camilla had developed an iron-deficiency anemia as a result of her lack of adherence to dietary supplementation recommendations. Camilla's iron stores are depleted and as a result she has developed functional impairment. Iron deficiency is the most common deficiency seen in bariatric patients postoperatively.

ADVICE: Camilla's iron deficiency anemia is likely the cause of her fatigue and light headedness. Following Roux-en-Y gastric bypass, micronutrient absorption is diminished. Without daily supplementation with multivitamins, iron, calcium, and vitamin B12, patients are at risk for developing deficiencies. Camilla was advised to begin iron repletion with elemental iron daily. She is to avoid taking any calcium supplements or consuming calcium rich foods for 2 hours before or after taking iron. Additionally, she was counseled on the importance of lifelong supplementation with a multivitamin, calcium, and B12.

Reports of thinning hair after bariatric surgery are common. Telogen effluvium, a diffuse loss of hair, can be precipitated by various stressors including major surgery, acute weight loss, and nutritional deficiencies such as low protein intake, iron, and zinc deficiencies. Because Camilla's hair loss did not occur until after her acute weight loss phase, it is more likely related to a nutritional deficiency rather than to her acute weight loss. In addition to iron repletion, Camilla's dietary intake of protein was found to be sub-optimal, and a meal plan was developed to include a total of 60 g of protein daily. Camilla needs to include five small servings of lean protein each day, such as low fat cottage cheese and yogurt, lean meats, and fish.

Table 7-10 Routine Blood Tests at Annual Post-operative Bariatric Surgery Visits

- CBC.
- Chemistry panel including liver enzymes.
- Lipid panel.
- HbA1c.
- Ferritin, Iron, TIBC, TIBC saturation.
- Vitamin B_{12}.
- 25-hydroxy Vitamin D.
- Intact parathyroid hormone.

Bone density scan and other laboratory tests should be done based on clinical judgment. Patients who have undergone gastric bypass are routinely prescribed supplements for the rest of their lives to aggressively prevent the associated nutrient deficiencies.

Source: Donna Kulick, MD, Lisa Hark, PhD, RD, and Darwin Deen, MD, MS, 2012. Used with permission.

Long-Term Nutritional Issues

Referral to a dietitian and behavioral therapist are recommended any time patients have difficulty maintaining their dietary goals or regain weight.[82] Annual primary care visits with Nurse Practitioners focus on building long-term healthy dietary behavior, continuing physical activity, and monitoring and correcting potential nutritional deficiencies.[82] Routine blood tests at those annual visits are listed in Table 7-10. Adherence with nutritional supplements should be assessed, as iron deficiency is common.

Summary: Role of Nurse Practitioners

Given the increasing prevalence of obesity and bariatric surgery procedures, care of patients who have undergone bariatric surgery is an important role for Nurse Practitioners. This field has the potential to create many new job opportunities and rewarding clinical experiences for Nurse Practitioners. Close post-operative follow-up and careful monitoring will improve the odds for successful surgical outcomes and Nurse Practitioners play a very important role in this process. Future research is needed to provide more evidence-based recommendations for best practice in the nutritional evaluation and management of the bariatric patient.

References

1. de Gonzalez BA, Hartge P, Cerhan JR, et al. Body mass index and mortality among 1.46 million white adults. *N Engl J Med* 2010;363:2211–2219.
2. Ogden CL, Carrol MD, McDowell MA, et al. Obesity among adults in the US — no statistical change since 2003–2004. *JAMA* 2007;1:1–6.
3. Rubenstein AH. Obesity: a modern epidemic. *Trans Am Clin Climatol Assoc* 2005;116: 103–113.
4. Christakis NA, Fowler JH. The spread of obesity in a large social network in the last 32 years. *N Engl J Med* 2007;357:370–379.
5. National Institute of Health, National Heart, Lung, and Blood Institute, North American Association for the Study of Obesity. The Practical Guide: Identification, Evaluation, and Treatment of Overweight and Obesity in Adults. *NIH Publication*. Number 00-4084, October 2000.

6. Stewart SS, Cutler DM, Rosen AB. Forecasting the effects of obesity and smoking on US life expectancy. *N Engl J Med* 2009;361:2252–2260.

7. National Institute of Health. Weight-control Information Network. Statistics Related to Overweight and Obesity. Available from win.niddk.nih.gov/statisics/index.htm#preval. Accessed 2012.

8. World Health Organization. Obesity and overweight. Fact sheet no. 311. 2011. Geneva: World Health Organization.

9. Wang CY, McPherson K, Marsh T, et al. Health and economic burden of the projected obesity trends in the USA and the UK. *The Lancet.* 2011;378:815–825.

10. Dietz WH. Reversing the tide of obesity. *The Lancet* 2011;378:744–746.

11. King D. The future challenge of obesity. *The Lancet* 2011;378:743–744.

12. Weights and Measures: What To Do About Obesity In Your Workforce. The Conference Board. *The Conference Board: Trusted Insights for Business Worldwide.* http://www.conference-board.org. Accessed 2012.

13. Finkelstein EA, Strombotne KL. The economics of obesity. *Am J Clin Nutr* 2010;91: 1520S–1524S.

14. Centers for Disease Control and Prevention. National Center for Health Statistics. Prevalence of overweight and obesity among adults: US, 2003–2004. Available from www.mm.gov. Accessed 2012.

15. Centers for Disease Control and Prevention. Vital and Health Statistics. Summary Health Statistics for US adults: National Health Interview Survey 2006. Available from http://www.cdc.gov. Accessed 2012.

16. Flegal KM, Carroll MD, Ogden CL, et al. Prevelance and trends in obesity among US adults, 1999–2008. *JAMA.* 2010;303:235–241.

17. Ogden CL, Carrol MD, Curtin LR, et al. Prevalence of overweight and obesity in the US, 1999–2004. *JAMA* 2006;295:1549–1555.

18. Hedley AA, Ogden CL, Johnson CL, et al. Prevalence of overweight and obesity among US children, adolescents, and adults, 1999–2002. *JAMA* 2004;291:2847–2850.

19. World Health Organization. Nutrition: global programming note 2005–2006. Available from www.who.int/nmh/donorinfo/nutrion/en/index.html. Accessed 2012.

20. Centers for Disease Control and Prevention. New CDC study finds no increase in obesity among adults; but levels still high. Available from www.cdc.gov/nchs/pressroom/07news releases/obesity.htm. Accessed 2012.

21. National Center for Health Statistics. Chartbook on Trends in the Health of Americans. Health, United States, 2006. Hyattsville, MD: Public Health Service, 2006.

22. Centers for Disease Control and Prevention. National Office of Public Health Genomics. Obesity and Genetics. Available from www.cdc.gov/Features/Obesity. Accessed 2012.

23. Bouchard C. Current understanding of the etiology of obesity: genetic and nongenetic factors. *Am J Clin Nutr* 1991;53:1561S–1565S.

24. French SA, Story M, Jeffery RW. Environmental influences on eating and physical activity. *Ann Rev Public Health* 2001;22:309–335.

25. Stunkard AJ, Sorensen TI, Hanis C, et al. An adoption study of human obesity. *N Engl J Med* 1986;314:193–198.

26. Maes HH, Neale MC, Eaves LJ. Genetic and environmental factors in relative body weight and human adiposity. *Behav Genet* 1997;27:325–351.

27. Bell CG, Walley AJ, Froguel P. The genetics of human obesity. *Nat Rev Genet* 2005;6: 221–234.

28. Centers for Disease Control and Prevention. Behavioral risk factor surveillance system. US Obesity Trends 1985–2009. Available from www.cdc.gov/obesity/data/trends.html. Accessed 2012.

29. Wright JD, Kennedy-Stephanson J, Wang CY, et al. Trends in intake of energy and macronutrients - United States, 1971–2000. *MMWR Morb Mortal Wkly Rep* 2004;53:80–82.

30. Mozaffarian D, Hao T, Rimm E, et al. Changes in diet and lifestyle and long-term weight gain in women and men. *N Engl J Med* 2011;364:2392–2404.

31. Bish CL, Blanck HM, Sedula MK, et al. Diet and physical activity behaviors among Americans trying to lose weight: 2000 Behavioral Risk Factor Surveillance System. *Obes Res* 2005;13:596–607.

32. Foster GD, Wyatt HR, Hill JO, et al. A randomized trial of a low-carbohydrate diet for obesity. *N Engl J Med* 2003;2082–2090.

33. Catenacci VA, Wyatt HR. The role of physical activity in producing and maintaining weight loss. *Nat Clin Prac Endocrin Metab* 2007;3:518–529.

34. Catenacci VA, Ogden LG, Stuht J, et al. Physical activity patterns in the National Weight Control Registry. *Obesity* 2008;16:153–161.

35. Stunkard AJ, Foch TT, Hrubec Z. A twin study of human obesity. *JAMA* 1986;256:51–54.

36. Walley AJ, Blakemore AIF, Froguel P. Genetics of obesity and the prediction of risk for health. *Hum Mol Genet* 2006;15:R120–R130.

37. Welborn TA, Dhaliwal SS. Body-mass index and mortality among white adults. *N Engl J Med* 2011;364:781–783.

38. Narayan KMV, Boyle JP, Thompson TJ, et al. Effect of BMI on lifetime risk for diabetes in the US. *Diabetes Care* 2007;30;1562–1566.

39. Price GM, Uauy R, Breeze E, et al. Weight, shape, and mortality risk in older persons — elevated waist-hip ration, not high body mass index, is associated with a greater risk of death. *Am J Clin Nutr* 2006;84:449–460.

40. Welborn TA, Dhaliwal SS. Preferred clinical measures of central obesity for predicting mortality. *Eur J Clin Nutr* 2007;61:1373–1379.

41. Katzmaryzyk PT, Janssen I, Ross R, et al. The importance of waist circumference in the definition of metabolic syndrome. *Diabetes Care* 2006;29:404–409.

42. Asia Pacific Cohort Studies Collaboration. Central obesity and risk of cardiovascular disease in the Asia Pacific Region. *Asia Pac J Clin Nutr* 2006;15:287–292.

43. Grundy SM, Cleeman JI, Daniels SR, et al. Diagnosis and management of the metabolic syndrome: an American Heart Association/National Heart, Lung, and Blood Institute Scientific Statement. *Circulation.* 2005;112:2735–2752.

44. Wadden TA, Berkowitz RI, Womble LG, et al. Randomized trial of lifestyle modification and pharmocotherapy for obesity. *N Engl J Med* 2005;353:2111–2120.

45. Yusuf S, Hawken S, Ôunpuu S, et al. Obesity and the risk of myocardial infarction in 27 000 participants from 52 countries: a case-control study. *Lancet* 2005;366:1640–1649.

46. Nonas CA. Clinical Monitoring. In: Foster GD, Nonas CA (Eds), *Managing Obesity: A Clinical Guide.* American Dietetic Association, Chicago, IL, 2004.

47. Prochaska JO, Norcross JC, DiClemente CC. *Changing for Good.* William Morrow, New York, NY, 1994.

48. Snow V, Barry P, Fitterman N, et al. Pharmacologic and surgical management of obesity in primary care: a clinical practice guideline from the American College of Nurse practitioners. *Ann Intern Med* 2005;142:525–531.

49. Department of Health and Human Services. Food and Drug Administration. Guidance on the Clinical Evaluation of Weight Control Drugs. FDA, 2004. www.fda.gov

50. Friedrich MJ. Better strategies sought against obesity. *JAMA* 2006;296:1577–1579.

51. Food and Drug Administration. Orlistat approved for over-the-counter use by FDA. January 2006. www.fda.gov

52. Hofbauer KG, Nicholson JR. Pharmacotherapy of obesity. *Exp Clin Endocrinol Diabetes* 2006;114:475–484.

53. Cooke D, Bloom S. The obesity pipeline: current strategies in the development of antiobesity drugs. *Nat Rev Drug Discov* 2006;5:919–531.

54. Davidson MH, Hauptman J, DiGirolamo M, et al. Weight control and risk factor reduction in obese subjects treated for 2 years with orlistat: a randomized controlled trial. *JAMA* 1999;281: 235–242.

55. Triplitt C, Chiquette E. Exenatide: from the Gila monster to the pharmacy. *J Am Pharm Assoc* 2006;46:44–52.

56. Barnett AH. Exantide. *Drugs Today* 2005;41:563–578.

57. Heine RJ, Van Gaal LF, Johns D. Exenatide versus insulin Glargine in patients with suboptimally controlled type 2 diabetes. *Ann Intern Med* 2005;143:559–569.

58. Zhao Y, Encinosa W. Bariatric Surgery Utilization and Outcomes in 1998 and 2004. Statistical Brief #23. January 2007. Agency for Healthcare Research and Quality, Rockville, MD. www.hcup-us.ahrq.gov/reports/statbriefs/sb23.pdf. Accessed 2012.

59. Santry HP, Gillen DL, Lauderdale DS. Trends in bariatric surgical procedures. *JAMA* 2005;294:1909–1917.

60. Brethauer S, Chand B, Schauer P. Risks and benefits of bariatric surgery: current evidence. *Clev Clin J Med* 2006;73:993–1007.

61. Colquitt J, Picot, J, Loveman E, Clegg A. Surgery for obesity. Cochrane Database of Systematic Reviews. 2009; (2). Available from www.mrw.interscience.wiley.com. Accessed 2012.

62. Buchwald H, Avidor Y, Braunwald E, et al. Bariatric surgery: a systematic review and meta-analysis. *JAMA* 2004;292:1724–1737.

63. Buchwald H, Estok R, Fahrbach K, et al. Trends in mortality in bariatric surgery: a systematic review and meta-analysis. *Surgery* 2007;142:621–632.

64. National Institute of Health. Consensus Development Conference Panel. NIH conference: Gastrointestinal Surgery for Severe Obesity. *Ann Intern Med* 1991;115:956–961.

65. Lawson ML, Kirk S, Mitchell T, et al. One-year outcomes of Roux-en-Y gastric bypass for morbidly obese adolescents: a multicenter study from the Pediatric Bariatric Study Group. *J Pediatr Surg* 2006;41:137–143.

66. Sugerman HJ, Sugerman EL, DeMaria EJ, et al. Bariatric surgery for severely obese adolescents. *J Gastrointest Surg* 2003;7:102–107.

67. Tice JA, Karliner L, Walsh J, et al. Gastric banding or bypass? A systematic review comparing the two most popular bariatric procedures. *Am J Med* 2008;121:885–893.

68. O'Brien PE. Bariatric surgery: mechanisms, indications and outcomes. *J Gastroent Hepat* 2010;25:1358–1365.

69. de Fatima, Haueisen Sander, Diniz M, de Azeredo, Passos VM, Diniz MT. Gut-brain communication: how does it stand after bariatric surgery? *Curr Opin Clin Nutr Metab Care* 2006;9:629–636.

70. Hell E, Miller KA, Moorehead MK. Evaluation of health status and quality of life after bariatric surgery: comparison of standard Roux-en-Y gastric bypass, vertical banded gastroplasty and laparoscopic adjustable silicone gastric banding. *Obes Surg* 2000;10:214–219.

71. DeMaria EJ. Bariatric surgery for morbid obesity. *N Engl J Med* 2007;356:2176–2183.

72. Cunneen SA. Review of meta-analytic comparisons of bariatric surgery with a focus on laparoscopic adjustable gastric banding. *Surg Obes Relat Dis* 2008;4(3 Suppl):S47–55.

73. Parikh MS, Laker S, Weiner M, et al. Objective comparison of complications resulting from laparoscopic bariatric procedures. *J Am Coll Surg* 2006;202:252–261.

74. Angrisani L, Lorenzo M, Borrelli V. Laparoscopic adjustable gastric banding versus Roux-en-Y gastric bypass: 5-year results of a prospective randomized trial. *Surg Obes Relat Dis* 2007;3:127–132.

75. Clinical Issues Committee of American Society for Metabolic and Bariatric Surgery. Updated position statement an sleeve gastrectomy as a bariatric procedure. *Surg Obes Relat Dis* 2010;6:1–5.

76. Marceau P, Hould FS, Simard S, et al. Biliopancreatic diversion with duodenal switch. *World J Surg* 1998;22:947–954.

77. Choi J, et al. Outcomes of laparoscopic adjustable gastric banding in low BMI patients. *Surg Obesity Related Dis* 2009;5(35 Suppl).

78. Flum DR, Belle SH, King WC, et al. Perioperative safety in the longitudinal assessment of bariatric surgery. *N Engl J Med.* 2009;361:445–454.

79. Sjostrom L, Narbro K, Sjostrom CD, et al. Effects of bariatric surgery on mortality in Swedish obese subjects. *N Engl J Med* 2007;357:741–752.

80. Adams, TD, Gress RE, Smith SC, et al. Long-term mortality after gastric bypass surgery. *N Engl J Med* 2007;357:753–761.

81. Perry CD, Hutter MM, Smith, DB, et al. Survival and changes in comorbidities after bariatric surgery. *Ann Surg* 2008;247:21–27.

82. McMahon MM, Sarr MG, Clark MM, et al. Clinical management after bariatric surgery: value of a multidisciplinary approach. *Mayo Clin Proc* 2006;81(10 Suppl):S34–S45.

83. Mechanick JI, Kushner RF, Sugerman HJ, et al. American Association of Clinical Endocrinologists, The Obesity Society, and American Society for Metabolic and Bariatric Surgery Medical Guidelines for Clinical Practice for the perioperative nutritional, metabolic, and nonsurgical support of the bariatric surgery patient. *J Surg Obes Relat Dis* 2008; 4(5 Suppl):S109–S184.

84. Collazo-Clavell ML, Clark MM, McAlpine DE, et al. Assessment and preparation of patients for bariatric surgery. *Mayo Clin Proc.* 2006;81(10 suppl):S11–S17.

85. Kushner RF, Roth JL. Assessment of the obese patient. *Endocrinol Metab Clin North Am* 2003;32:915–933.

86. Cunningham E. What is the registered dietitian's role in the preoperative assessment of a client contemplating bariatric surgery? *J Am Diet Assoc* 2006;106:163.

87. Kulick D, Hark L, Deen D. The bariatric surgery patient: a growing role for the registered dietitian. *J Am Diet Assoc.* 2010;110:593–599.

88. Flancbaum L, Belsley S, Drake V, et al. Preoperative nutritional status of patients undergoing Roux-en-Y gastric bypass for morbid obesity. *J Gastrointest Surg* 2006;10:1033–1037.

89. Alami RS, Hsu G, Safadi BY, et al. The impact of preoperative weight loss in patients undergoing laparoscopic Roux-en-Y gastric bypass. *Obes Surg* 2005;15:1282–1286.

90. Still CD, Benotti P, Wood GC, et al. Outcomes of preoperative weight loss in high-risk patients undergoing gastric bypass surgery. *Arch Surg* 2007;142:994–98.

91. Davies DJ, Baxter JM, Baxter JN. Nutritional deficiencies after bariatric surgery. *Obes Surg* 2007;17:1150–1158.

92. Coupaye M, Puchaux K, Bogard C, et al. Nutritional consequences of adjustable gastric banding and gastric bypass: A 1-year prospective study. *Obes Surg* 2009;19:56–65.

93. Song A, Fernstrom MH. Nutritional and psychological considerations after bariatric surgery. *Aesthet Surg J* 2008;28:195–199.

94. Vargas-Ruiz AG, Hernández-Rivera G, Herrera MF. Prevalence of iron, folate, and vitamin B12 deficiency anemia after laparoscopic Roux-en-Y gastric bypass. *Obes Surg* 2008;18: 288–293.

95. Matrana MR, Vasireddy S, Davis WE. The skinny on a growing problem: dry beriberi after bariatric surgery. *Ann Intern Med* 2008;149:842–844.

96. Compher CW, Badellino KO, Boullata JI. Vitamin D and the bariatric surgical patient: a review. *Obes Surg* 2008;18:220–224.

97. Goldner WS, Stoner JA, Lyden E, et al. Finding the optimal dose of vitamin D following Roux-en-Y gastric bypass: a prospective, randomized pilot clinical trial. *Obes Surg* 2009;19:173–9.

98. Malone M. Recommended nutritional supplements for bariatric surgery patients. *Ann Pharmacother* 2008;42:1851–1858.

99. Ledoux S, Larger E. Nutritional deficiencies after Roux-en-Y gastric bypass can be prevented by standard multivitamin supplementation. *Am J Clin Nutr* 2008;88:1176.

100. Stocker DJ. Management of the bariatric surgery patient. *Endocrinol Metab Clin North Am* 2003;32:437–457.

101. Kushner R. Managing the obese patient after bariatric surgery: a case report of severe malnutrition and review of the literature. *J Parenter Enteral Nutr* 2000;24:126–132.

102. Mallory GN, Macgregor AM, Rand CS. The influence of dumping on weight loss after gastric restrictive surgery for morbid obesity. *Obes Surg* 1996;6:474–478.

103. Deitel M. The change in the dumping syndrome concept. *Obes Surg* 2008;18:1622–1624.

104. Goldfine AB, Mun EC, Devine E, et al. Patients with neuroglycopenia after gastric bypass surgery have exaggerated incretin and insulin secretory responses to a mixed meal. *J Clin Endocrinol Metab* 2007;92:4678–4685.

105. Kellogg TA, Bantle JP, Leslie DB, et al. Postgastric bypass hyperinsulinemic hypoglycemia syndrome: characterization and response to a modified diet. *Surg Obes Relat Dis* 2008; 4:492–499.

8   Cardiology Care

Frances Burke, MS, RD
Lisa Hark, PhD, RD

OBJECTIVES

- Identify patients at risk for coronary heart disease using the National Cholesterol Education Program and American Heart Association guidelines and determine appropriate LDL-C goals.
- Given a patient's medical, social, dietary history, and laboratory data, propose an optimal set of lifestyle goals using the National Cholesterol Education Program and American Heart Association guidelines for nutrition and exercise to reduce risk for coronary heart disease.
- Describe the parameters of the National Cholesterol Education Program's Therapeutic Lifestyle Changes diet.
- Summarize the dietary recommendations of the DASH diet for the hypertensive patient.
- Prioritize nutritional goals for the patient with heart failure.

Introduction

According to the National Center for Health Statistics and the American Heart Association (AHA), about one third of Americans have cardiovascular disease (CVD).[1,2] Nurse Practitioners working in the majority of acute and chronic care settings will be taking care of patients who are either at risk for CVD or who have CVD. It is well-known that nutrition plays a critical role in the prevention and treatment of various types of CVD, particularly those most common in the American population – coronary heart disease (CHD) and hypertension.[3,4] Recognition of the important role of nutrition in CHD prevention and treatment has heightened with growing awareness of metabolic syndrome, in which elevated triglyceride and reduced high-density lipoprotein cholesterol (HDL-C) levels, insulin resistance, and hypertension combine with abdominal obesity to increase the potential for morbidity and mortality from heart disease.[5,6] Therefore, it is imperative that Nurse Practitioners gain knowledge and skills in this area and be able to provide appropriate nutritional guidance and evidence-based practice to their patients.

The Nurse Practitioner's Guide to Nutrition, Second Edition. Edited by Lisa Hark, Kathleen Ashton and Darwin Deen.

Evidence-Base for Diet and Heart Disease

The association between high dietary fat intake, particularly saturated fat, and the risk for developing CHD has been well researched.[7,8] This association is presumed to reflect the increased serum cholesterol and low-density-lipoprotein cholesterol (LDL-C) levels that result from a high intake of saturated fat.[9] Large-scale clinical trials have shown conclusively that reducing serum LDL-C levels reduces the number of acute cardiac events and deaths from CHD both in patients with existing disease and those at-risk due to elevated lipids.[10–12] Angiographic studies have demonstrated that LDL-C reduction slows the progression of atherosclerosis in patients with known disease.[10] Atherosclerosis is now viewed not simply as the deposition of lipid in the artery, but as a complex inflammatory response to damage of the endothelial lining of arteries.[5]

Dietary Lipids

It is important for Nurse Practitioners to understand the basic biochemistry of fatty acids in order to address the role of dietary fat in the prevention and treatment of heart disease. Dietary fats are composed mainly of three fatty acids attached to a glycerol molecule.[13] All fats are a combination of saturated, monounsaturated, and polyunsaturated fatty acids.[14] Fat is the most calorically dense nutrient, supplying nine calories per gram. Therefore, a diet high in fat is also generally high in calories. Reducing total fat intake and adhering to an exercise program can help patients lose weight.[14,15]

Saturated Fats

Saturated fats are fatty acids with no double bonds. With the exception of palm and coconut oil, foods high in saturated fat are solid at room temperature and come primarily from animal sources. Major contributors of saturated fats are shown in Table 8-1. According to the NHANES data, approximately 11–12% of the calories in the American diet come from saturated fat while less than 7% is recommended.[9,16,17] Saturated fatty acids (in contrast to unsaturated fatty acids) decrease the synthesis and activity of LDL-C receptors, promoting an increase in serum LDL-C, thereby contributing to atherogenesis.[18] An increase of 1 mg/dL in serum LDL-C increases CHD risk by 1%.[5] A meta-analysis of dietary studies concluded that for every 1% increase in calories from saturated fat, serum LDL-C increases approximately 1%.[5]

Table 8-1 Dietary Sources of Saturated Fats

Meats/Poultry: brisket, regular ground beef, sausages, hot dogs, bacon, fatty luncheon meats (bologna, pastrami, corned beef, salami, tongue), pâté, spare ribs, lamb, lard, poultry skin, chicken fat, beef fat, and fried foods.

Dairy Foods: butter, whole milk, 2% milk, heavy cream, stick margarine, half-and-half, whipped cream, full-fat yogurt, whole milk cottage and ricotta cheeses, ice cream, hard cheeses, cream cheese, and sour cream.

Breads/Snacks: potato chips, croissants, butter or sweet rolls, quick breads, and biscuits.

Desserts/Sweets: donuts, cakes, candy, pies, pastries, and cookies.

Source: Lisa Hark, PhD, RD and Fran Burke, MS, RD, 2012. Used with permission.

Polyunsaturated Fats

The two major categories of polyunsaturated fatty acids (PUFA) are omega-6 and omega-3 fatty acids. Vegetable oils such as corn, canola, cottonseed, peanut, sunflower, safflower, and soybean contain omega-6 fatty acids.[19] Linoleic acid, an essential omega-6 fatty acid, cannot be synthesized by the body and is therefore required in the diet.[13] Arachidonic acid, which is synthesized from linoleic acid, is the major omega-6 fatty acid found in cell membranes and the precursor of prostaglandins. Substitution of PUFA for saturated fat in the diet lowers LDL-C and reduces risk for CHD.[21]

Omega-3 fatty acids include the very long chain eicosapentanoic acid (EPA) and docosahexenoic acid (DHA), as well as the 18-carbon alpha-linolenic acid, another essential fatty acid.[5] The highest concentrations of DHA are found in eye/brain tissue and depend on dietary intake. The long-chain fatty acids have been shown to decrease serum triglycerides, reduce platelet aggregation, lower blood pressure and inflammation, and improve endothelial cell function.[19,21] Dietary sources of omega-3 fatty acids are shown in Table 8-2. Epidemiologic studies suggest that healthy individuals who consume 7 oz of fish per week are 30–40% less likely to die from a cardiac event than those who do not regularly consume fish.[22,23]

On the basis of currently available evidence, the AHA has recommended that all adults eat fish (particularly fatty fish) at least twice a week and vegetables containing plant-derived omega-3 fatty acids (ALA) and that patients with documented coronary heart disease consume approximately 1 g of EPA and DHA per day (combined), from oily fish or fish-oil capsules (after consultation with a physician).[7,24,25] The AHA recommendations also state that EPA/DHA supplements may be useful in patients with severe hypertriglyceridemia (>500 mg/dL). Doses of 2–4 g of EPA/DHA per day may lower triglyceride levels by 20–40%.[26] The AHA advises caution with respect to environmental contaminants in fish noting that many species of fish are low in methyl-mercury and that fish-oil supplements are free of methyl-mercury.[27] Some clinical trials suggest that an intake of approximately 1 g/day of EPA/DHA can reduce deaths from cardiac events.[26,28]

Table 8-2 Types and Dietary Sources of Polyunsaturated Fats

Omega-6 fatty acids: (Linoleic acid)
Food Sources: vegetable oils: corn, canola, safflower, sunflower, soybean, cottonseed, and peanut.

Omega-3 fatty acids
Alpha linolenic acid (ALA) (18:3).
Food Sources: canola, flaxseed, soybean oil, and walnuts.
Eicosapentaenoic acid (EPA) (20:5) and Docosahezaenoic acid (DHA) (22:6).

Food Sources of EPA and DHA: fish (salmon, sardines, tuna, swordfish, herring), fortified foods (eggs, soy milk, yogurt), fish oil supplements, cod liver oil supplements.

Source: adapted from Superko.[20]

Other studies indicate a trend toward fewer restenoses after angioplasty for patients receiving omega-3 dietary supplements.[14]

The American Heart Association recommendations:[3,25]

- All adults without CHD: eat fish (fatty) at least two times a week; include oils and foods rich in ALA.
- All adults with CHD: consume approximately 1 g/day of EPA+DHA preferably from oily fish. EPA+DHA supplements could be considered in consultation with the physician.
- All adults with high triglycerides: consume 2–4 g/day EPA+DHA as capsules under a physician's care.

Monounsaturated Fats

Monounsaturated fatty acids (MUFA) contain one double bond; oleic acid is the most common dietary form.[9,29] Oils high in oleic acid include canola, peanut, and olive oil. Other sources of MUFA include avocados, almonds, walnuts, and pecans. Epidemiologic evidence from the Mediterranean region, where diets are rich in MUFA, have demonstrated a lower incidence of CHD and these findings have been corroborated by the Lyon Diet Heart Study.[30,31] Shorter-term clinical trials of a Mediterranean style diet have shown improvement in a number of risk factors, including lowering serum triglycerides and reducing of inflammatory markers, such as C-reactive protein.[31,32] Substitution of oleic acid for saturated fatty acids reduces LDL-C levels.[9] A diet high in MUFA lowers LDL-C and serum triglycerides without lowering HDL-C. Provision of some calories from MUFA, which might otherwise be provided from carbohydrate, can lower LDL-C without lowering HDL-C or raising triglyceride levels.[32] Figure 8-1 shows sources of dietary fats.

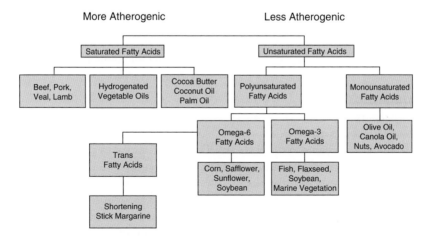

Figure 8-1 Sources of Dietary Fats
Source: Lisa Hark, PhD, RD and Linda VanHorn, PhD, RD, 2012. Used with permission.

Trans Fatty Acids

Hydrogenation, the addition of hydrogen atoms to an unsaturated fat, can change a fatty acid double bond from a *cis* to *trans* configuration.[33] The major source of dietary *trans* fatty acids is partially hydrogenated vegetable oils.[34] Food manufacturers have used this process to prolong the shelf-life of foods such as crackers, cookies, potato chips, and puddings. Randomized clinical trials indicate that *trans* fatty acids raise LDL-C and decrease HDL-C levels when compared with naturally occurring *cis* fatty acids.[9] The structural similarity of *trans* fat to saturated fat may explain the detrimental effects.[35] Numerous studies in men have shown that eating a diet high in *trans* fat increases the likelihood of having a heart attack.[28,33] Women with higher *trans* fat intake have 50% greater chance of having heart disease. Replacing *trans* fats with monounsaturated fat can lower LDL-C levels.[9]

Although margarines contain *trans* fatty acids, use of a soft or liquid margarine maintains a lower LDL-C than does a comparable diet containing butter (a source of saturated fat and cholesterol).[36] There are *trans*-free tub margarines available that may be recommended.[28] Since 2006, the Food and Drug Administration (FDA) has required food manufacturers to include *trans* fat information on food labels, and as a result, many food processors have substituted either a healthier vegetable oil, a specially produced inter-esterified fat that has less *trans* fat, or saturated fat blends (such as palm and canola oils). It is likely that these actions have reduced the *trans* fat intake in the US.

Dietary Cholesterol

Although saturated fat is the major dietary fat responsible for raising serum LDL-C levels, a high intake of dietary cholesterol can also increase serum LDL-C. Animal foods are sources of cholesterol, with the highest being egg yolks, shellfish, and organ meats. Meat and dairy sources of saturated fat, such as cheese, cream, and fatty meats, also contain substantial amounts of cholesterol. Two prospective cohort studies, The Nurses' Health Study and the Health Professionals Follow-up Study reported no significant association between egg consumption (up to 1 egg per day) and risk of CHD and stroke after adjusting for age, smoking, and other risk factors.[37] Since eggs are low in saturated fat and contain key nutrients such as vitamin A, D, folate, selenium, and zeaxanthin, they can be included in a heart healthy diet for adults and children.

Hyperlipidemia

Hyperlipidemia, the clinical term used to describe elevated cholesterol, or triglyceride levels, increases the risk of atherosclerosis.[5] When atherosclerosis proceeds to occlusion or rupture of a blood vessel, myocardial infarction, stroke, or peripheral vascular disease result (depending upon the affected site). Various lipoproteins transport cholesterol and triglycerides in the blood. The majority of cholesterol is carried in the blood by LDL-C and are the major atherogenic lipoproteins.[9] In contrast, cholesterol carried by HDL-C represents cholesterol being released by the cells. The majority of serum triglycerides are present in very low-density lipoproteins (VLDL). A fasting lipid profile of the patient's LDL-C, HDL-C, and triglyceride levels is now recommended by the National Cholesterol Education Program, Third Adult Treatment Panel (NCEP ATP III), rather than an earlier clinical approach of assessing total cholesterol.

Table 8-3 Target LDL-C Goals Based on Risk Category

Risk Category	LDL Goal	LDL Level to Initiate TLC Diet	LDL Level at Which to Consider Drug Therapy
CHD or CHD Risk Equivalents (10-year risk >20%)	<100 mg/dL	100 mg/dL	130 mg/dL (100–129 mg/dL: drug optional)
2+Risk Factors (10-year risk 20%)	<130 mg/dL	130 mg/dL	10-year risk 10–20%: 130 mg/dL 10-year risk <10%: 160 mg/dL
0–1 Risk Factor	<160 mg/dL	160 mg/dL	190 mg/dL (160–189 mg/dL: LDL-lowering drug optional)

Source: Gaziano.[38]

Target LDL-C Goals

The clinical approach to the hyperlipidemic patient is well outlined in the NCEP ATP III guidelines.[17] Key steps include the assessment of risk factors that allows determination of lipoprotein goals and delineation of the need for lifestyle change and, if needed, the addition of pharmacological treatment. Individuals with existing evidence of CHD or diabetes should aim for a goal LDL-C of 100 g/dL or less. Individuals without either diagnosis, but with two or more risk factors are further stratified as to their risk of a coronary event within the next 10 years based on Framingham data as shown in Table 8-3. This estimate of risk takes into account the patient's age, gender, total cholesterol, smoking history, HDL-C, and blood pressure.

Metabolic Syndrome

The association of obesity with the development of hypertension, type 2 diabetes, and consequent CVD further heightens the need for Nurse Practitioners to be educated in the role of nutrition in health promotion and disease prevention.[3] Recent attention regarding risk for CHD has focused on a constellation of characteristics termed metabolic syndrome. A series of simple measurements, shown in Table 8-4 provide the diagnostic criteria for metabolic syndrome. Patients with any three or

Table 8-4 Diagnostic Criteria for Metabolic Syndrome

Abdominal obesity	Waist circumference: Men >40 inches Women >35 inches
High blood pressure	BP≥130/85 mmHg or documented use of antihypertensive therapy
High fasting glucose	FBG≥100 mg/dL
High triglycerides	≥150 mg/dL
Low HDL-C	Men <40 mg/dL Women <50 mg/dL

Source: Gaziano.[38]

more of the five criteria can be diagnosed with metabolic syndrome, and nutrition therapy for each issue should be addressed.[5,6,39,40] The presence of abdominal obesity is a valuable clue to metabolic syndrome and can be easily identified by measuring the patient's waist circumference, as described in Chapters 2 and 6 and these cut-off points vary by different ethnic groups.

Nutrition Therapy for Hyperlipidemia and Metabolic Syndrome

Diet and exercise are the cornerstones of effective treatment for hyperlipidemia and each criteria of the metabolic syndrome.[5,16,17,39,40] The NCEP ATP III Guidelines include the Therapeutic Lifestyle Changes Diet (TLC) for achievement of LDL-C goals as shown in Table 8-5. Translating the TLC diet into food-based recommendations is shown in Table 8-6.

In patients with metabolic syndrome, a low-fat, high complex carbohydrate diet can raise post-prandial triglyceride levels. This can be prevented with the inclusion of omega-3 fats in the diet.[42] According to a consensus statement from the AHA, optimal fasting triglyceride levels should be defined as <100 mg/dL and considered a parameter of metabolic health. Since most patients are screened with a non-fasting blood test, non-fasting triglyceride levels of <200 mg/dL should be indicative of a normal (<150 mg/dL) or optimal (<100 mg/dL) fasting triglyceride level and requires no further testing.[43] Overall, the consensus statement supports the treatment of elevated triglyceride levels using the TLC diet. Increased exercise leading to weight loss of 5–10% will lower triglycerides by 20%.

Reducing calories from added sugars and fructose (carbohydrates), while increasing unsaturated fat intake, can reduce triglyceride levels by an additional 10–20%.[44] Restriction or elimination of saturated and *trans fats*, and increasing consumption of omega-3 unsaturated fats is also indicated.[30] Reductions of 50% or more in triglyceride levels are achievable through intensive therapeutic lifestyle change.[44] Therefore Nurse Practitioners should advise patients diagnosed with metabolic syndrome with

Table 8-5 Therapeutic Lifestyle Changes (TLC)

Nutrient Composition Nutrient	Recommended Intake
Saturated fat	Less than 7% of total calories
Polyunsaturated fat	Up to 10% of total calories
Monounsaturated fat	Up to 20% of total calories
Total fat	25–35% of total calories
Carbohydrate	50–60% of total calories
Dietary fiber	20–30 g per day
Protein	Approximately 15% of total calories
Cholesterol	Less than 200 mg/day
Total calories*	Maintain desirable body weight to prevent weight gain

*Total calories should be adjusted to maintain desirable body weight and prevent weight gain. Physical activity should include enough moderate exercise to expend at least 200 calories per day.
Source: ATP III Guidelines.[16]

Table 8.6 Food-Based Advice for Therapeutic Lifestyle Changes (TLC) Diet

Food Items to Choose More Often	Food Items to Choose Less Often
Breads and Cereals	
≥6 servings per day, adjusted to caloric needs	Bakery products, including doughnuts, cakes, biscuits, croissants, Danish, pies, muffins, cookies
Whole grain breads, cereals, pasta, brown rice, sweet potatoes, dry beans and peas, low-fat crackers	Potato chips, cheese puffs, snack mix, buttered popcorn
Vegetables and Fruits	
3–5 servings vegetables per day fresh, frozen, or canned, without added fat, sauce, or salt	Vegetables fried or prepared with butter, cheese, or cream sauce
2–4 servings fruits per day fresh, frozen, canned, dried	Fruits fried or served with butter or cream
Dairy Products	
2–3 servings per day fat-free, 1% milk, buttermilk, low-fat yogurt and cottage cheese, and fat-free or low-fat cheeses	Whole milk/2% milk, whole-milk yogurt, ice cream, cream, full-fat cheeses
Eggs	
≤2 egg yolks per week Egg whites or egg substitute	>3 egg yolks per week
Meat, Fish and Poultry	
≤5 oz per day Lean cuts: loin, leg, round, extra lean ground beef, cold cuts made with lean meat or soy protein, skinless poultry, all types of fish – broiled, baked, and grilled	High fat meat cuts: ribs, t-bone steak, regular hamburger, bacon, sausage; cold cuts: salami, bologna; hot dogs; organ meats: liver, brains, sweetbreads; poultry with skin; fried meat, fried poultry, fried fish
Fats and Oils	
Amount adjusted to caloric level: unsaturated oils, soft or liquid margarines and vegetable oil spreads, salad dressings, seeds, and nuts	Butter, shortening, stick margarine, chocolate

Source: Lisa Hark, PhD, RD, adapted from Mozaffarian.[41] Used with permission.

Table 8-7 Key Diet History Questions for Patients with Hyperlipidemia

How often do you eat fatty meats (hot dogs, bacon, sausage, salami, pastrami, corned beef)?
How often do you eat fish? How is it prepared?
What types of fats do you use in cooking and baking?
What do you spread on your bread?
What type of snacks and desserts do you eat?

Source: Lisa A. Hark, PhD, RD, 2012. Used with permission.

hypertriglyceridemia to include more fish in their diet, consider an omega-3 supplement, and follow a diet high in monounsaturated fats (Mediterranean). Key diet history questions to ask patients with hyperlipidemia are shown in Table 8-7. Nurse Practitioners need to collaborate with dietitians who routinely counsel patients with hyperlipidemia by supporting these recommendations and providing ongoing encouragement (Table 8-8).

Table 8-8 When To Refer to A Registered Dietitian

- A comprehensive assessment of nutritional status is required.
- Negotiated and tailored behavior change goals should be developed.
- Nutrition strategies to achieve these goals need to be established.
- Patient needs counseling to reduce portion sizes at home and eating out.
- Patient needs help with healthy food purchasing and preparation.
- Continued reinforcement and monitoring of diet and lifestyle will be helpful.

Source: Lisa Hark, PhD, RD and Fran Burke, MS, RD, 2012. Used with permission.

Case 1

Harry is a 52-year-old accountant and reports a high stress level both at work and at home. Over the past 2 years he has gained 12 lb. Harry attributes this to his sedentary, high-stress lifestyle, as well as to dining out with clients two to three nights per week. He does not smoke cigarettes and is not taking any medication. He drinks a 20 oz (600 mL) cup of coffee every morning and two alcoholic beverages every evening. Harry is married and has one daughter.

MEDICAL HISTORY: Harry's family history is positive for heart disease. His father died of a heart attack at age 54, and his father's brother had a heart attack at age 55. Harry's uncle is currently being treated for high cholesterol. There is no family history of high blood pressure, diabetes, or obesity. Harry has high normal blood pressure at 139/88 mmHg (pre-hypertensive). He is 5'10" and currently weighs 212 lb. BMI: 30.4. His weight 2 years ago was 200 lb (91 kg). His current waist circumference is 42 inches (107 cm) (<40 inches for men). Cholesterol: 260 mg/dL, fasting HDL-C: 32 mg/dL, LDL-C: 158 mg/dL, and triglycerides: 350 mg/dL. He does not exercise.

DIET HISTORY: For breakfast, Harry has a large bagel with 2 tablespoons of cream cheese and coffee with half-and-half cream. For lunch he eats two slices of pepperoni pizza or an Italian hoagie and a large 12 oz soda. He snacks on candy, cookies, donuts, or left over pizza. For dinner he usually orders prime rib or a sirloin steak, baked potato with sour cream and butter or French fries. He always has dessert, which is either a slice of cake, pie, or a bowl of ice cream. He drinks two bottles of beer with dinner.

LIFESTYLE CHANGES: Harry's modifiable risk factors for heart disease include obesity, high saturated fat diet, and sedentary lifestyle. Implementing a number of lifestyle and behavior changes could improve his risk profile significantly. Harry also has metabolic syndrome based on his elevated waist circumference, low HDL-C levels, and moderately high blood pressure.

ADVICE: The first lines of therapy for metabolic syndrome are weight reduction and increased physical activity. Treatment goals are to lower his cholesterol, LDL-C, and triglycerides, and raise HDL-C levels. He can achieve these goals by adhering to the TLC diet and reducing his total calories and saturated fat. Monounsaturated fat and omega-3 fatty acids should be substituted for saturated fat. Saturated fat is mostly coming from high fat dairy foods (half-and-half, cream cheese, mozzarella cheese), red meat, and ice cream. To lose weight, Harry can reduce his calories by cutting back on his portion sizes and increasing his exercise. Eating more fruits and vegetables (5–8 servings per day), whole grains, beans and legumes (7–8 servings per day), low fat or non-fat dairy products, white meat chicken without skin, fish, or lean meats will be beneficial. Harry should increase his intake of viscous (soluble) fiber (10–25 g/day) from oats, psyllium, dried beans and fruits. Margarine containing plant stanol/sterols (2 g /day) could be included to further lower LDL-C in place of other spreads. Harry may benefit from reducing his sodium intake.

For breakfast, he could have oatmeal with low-fat milk and an orange. For lunch, he could order a tuna or turkey sandwich without cheese. When he is out for dinner, he could order fish and chicken more often and limit the red meat to less than one time per week.

Other Nutritional Components
Stanol/Sterol Esters
Plant sterols and their chemically modified counterpart, plant stanols, have been esterified and incorporated into a growing number of products, such as margarine, milk, yogurt, and orange juice.[45] Clinical trials have shown up to 14% reduction in LDL-C levels in individuals consuming 2 g/day.[46] Consuming two tablespoons/day of sterol-fortified spread can provide 2–3 g of sterol/stanol esters per day and lower LDL-C levels by 7–15%.[36] In the gastrointestinal tract, sterol/stanol esters compete with cholesterol for incorporation into micelles and thus block the absorption of cholesterol. Two possible concerns regarding the use of plant sterol/stanol fortified margarines are: (1) if margarine use is increased, some caloric reduction is needed to maintain energy balance; (2) concurrent reduced absorption of dietary carotenoids requires the need to increase consumption of fruits and vegetables.[47]

Dietary Fiber
Inclusion of viscous or soluble dietary fiber can decrease LDL-C levels by forming a gel-like substance which binds and removes bile acids from the body through the stool preventing reabsorption. Based on evidence from a meta-analysis of over 50 clinical trials, ATP III recommends the inclusion of at least 5–10 g of viscous fiber daily, with the option of greater intakes in the range of 10–25 g daily.[5,7,16] The 5–10 g/day dose has been shown to reduce LDL-C by about 5%. Some of the best dietary sources of viscous fiber (providing 2–4 g per serving) include dried beans such as lima, pinto, and kidney beans, oatmeal, oat bran, citrus fruits, pears, and Brussels sprouts. Recommendations for increasing viscous dietary fiber are shown in Table 8-9.

Soy
In 1999, the FDA approved a health claim for soy foods: *25 g of soy protein per day, as part of a diet low in saturated fat and cholesterol, may reduce the risk of heart disease.*[48] Studies indicate small reductions in LDL-C (2–7%) with the ingestion of 50–55 g of soy protein daily.[49] The AHA has concluded that the major benefit of soy protein is its use as a substitute for less heart-healthy fatty animal products, rather than a substantial benefit inherent in the soy itself.[1,16,17]

Table 8-9 Recommendations for Increasing Viscous Fiber to the Diet

- Consume at least three servings of fruits and vegetables daily.
- Choose fresh fruits with pectin (apples, oranges, grapefruits).
- Eat skins of potatoes, apples, pears.
- Increase whole grain foods, especially whole oats.
- Use whole wheat pasta, whole grain breads, brown rice.
- Put oats in a blender and use as a filler in casseroles or in baked goods.
- Eat a high fiber cereal daily, including oatmeal.
- Increase intake of beans and legumes.
- Consider psyllium, guar gum, or glucomannen supplement.

Source: Lisa Hark, PhD, RD and Fran Burke, MS, RD, 2012. Used with permission.

Niacin

Niacin is a B vitamin which has been prescribed at pharmacological doses (2000–3000 mg/day) to patients with hyperlipidemia for several decades.[4] There are three different forms of niacin supplements: immediate-release (IR) nicotinic acid, sustained-release (SR) nicotinic acid, and extended-release (ER) nicotinic acid. Although all work in a similar manner to lower cholesterol, differences exist.[4,50] IR nicotinic acid is most commonly associated with the side effects of flushing, warmth, itching, headache, and nausea. SR nicotinic acid, also known as "timed-release" nicotinic acid, is associated with higher risk of liver toxicity. ER nicotinic acid, available only by prescription, and is associated with poor compliance does cause increased serum glucose levels and is not associated with liver toxicity. A recent randomized controlled clinical safety trial looking at the combination of ezetimibe and simvastatin (E/S) with ER niacin was done with 942 patients with type IIa/IIb hyperlipidemia.[50] Patients received either E/S (10/20 mg) with niacin (to 2 g), or E/S (10/20 mg) alone for 64 weeks, or niacin (to 2 g) for 24 weeks and then E/S (10/20 mg) with niacin (2 g) or E/S (10/20 mg) alone for an additional 40 weeks. The study showed that the combination of E/S with niacin was generally well tolerated and was more effective in improving HDL-C, triglyceride, and LDL-C levels compared with E/S alone.[50]

Supplemental Vitamins

Although supplementation with antioxidants, folate, and other B vitamins was tried in the 1990s as a strategy to reduce CHD risk, clinical trials have failed to demonstrate significant benefit in reducing cardiac events or mortality in patients receiving these supplements.[50–53] In fact, use of an antioxidant "cocktail" of vitamins C and E, beta-carotene, and selenium actually lowered the beneficial sub-fraction HDL-C$_2$ cholesterol in patients receiving simvastatin and niacin treatment and reduced the stenosis – the lowering effect of the medical treatment.[54,55] A recent meta-analysis reviewing 11 clinical trials evaluating all cause mortality associated with vitamin E supplementation (>400 IU/day) and CVD showed a statistically significant increase in all cause mortality in patients taking vitamin E in doses greater than 150 mg/day.[55] The conclusion derived from the analyzed data is that the use of vitamin E supplements does not help decrease CVD risk. Beyond using a daily multivitamin supplement, patients should be encouraged to obtain antioxidants and other vitamins from a diet rich in colorful fruits and vegetables and grains, rather than through supplements.[53,56]

Alcohol

Questions about alcohol consumption are often raised by patients with heart disease. A first step in advising patients regarding alcohol is to obtain an accurate alcohol intake history. Alcohol has both positive and negative effects in relation to heart disease.[57] Although light-to-moderate intake of alcohol has been shown to reduce the risk of CHD, intake over 30 g/day (more than two drinks) is associated with an increased mortality due to hypertension, pancreatitis, hypertriglyceridemia, gastrointestinal malignancies, stroke, cardiomyopathy, cirrhosis, accidents, and breast cancer.[58] Moderate alcohol intake is defined as no more than two drinks per day for men and one drink per day for women. A drink is defined as 5 oz of wine, 1.5 oz of 80-proof liquor, or 12 oz of beer.[4]

The beneficial cardioprotective effects of alcohol may be due to increasing HDL-C levels, reducing LDL-C oxidation via the antioxidant polyphenols (catechin, quercetin, resveratrol), and causing short-term vasodilatation.[57] A patient with CHD can continue to drink alcohol in moderation if free of other medical, psychiatric, or social problems. However, it is *not* appropriate to recommend alcohol intake to a non-drinker or an at-risk drinker for its cardioprotective effect, as there are many other effective non-pharmacological therapies.[59] Alcohol should also be avoided in patients diagnosed with hypertriglyceridemia.[32]

Weight Control to Reduce the Risk of CHD

Attention to calorie balance is important for most patients. The keys to weight maintenance and weight reduction are fostering control of calorie intake and encouraging physical activity. Weight reduction in overweight patients improves parameters associated with metabolic syndrome, including reducing LDL-C and triglycerides, increasing HDL-C, reducing blood pressure, and normalizing elevated serum glucose levels. In many cases, a 7–10% reduction in weight can eliminate the need for drug therapy in these clinical syndromes.[32] As shown in Table 8-10, weight loss is beneficial and a recommended therapy for the majority of risk factors for CVD.[3] Conversely, it is possible that initiation of a lipid-lowering medication prompts patients to feel attention to diet is no longer needed. Failure to follow appropriate diet with use of

Table 8-10 Summary of Dietary Recommendations Based on CVD Risk Factors

Risk Factor	Recommendation
Elevated LDL-C	↓ saturated fat, ↓ soluble fiber, weight loss, ↓ trans fat,
Low HDL-C	↑ exercise, weight loss, avoid smoking
Diabetes and insulin resistance	Weight Loss, ↓ blood pressure, ↓ carbohydrates
Elevated triglycerides	↓ Fish oils, weight loss, ↓ alcohol
Obesity (BMI > 30)	Weight loss, ↑ exercise, ↓ portion sizes
Hypertension	↓ blood pressure, ↓ alcohol, weight loss, ↑ exercise
Metabolic syndrome	Weight loss, ↑ exercise, customized recommendations for total fat, carbohydrate and calorie intake

Source: Lisa Hark, PhD, RD and Fran Burke, MS, RD, 2012. Used with permission.

drugs can necessitate higher doses of drugs, increasing the potential for side effects and limiting benefits. Therefore, Nurse Practitioners should continue to emphasize the underlying benefit of a calorically balanced, low saturated fat diet even when lipid-lowering drugs are necessary.

Hypertension

According to the Joint National Committee on Prevention, Detection, Evaluation, and Treatment of High Blood Pressure (JNC VII), hypertension affects over 50 million people in the US and is a major risk factor for the development of CHD, cardiomyopathy, and stroke.[60-62] Dietary lifestyle management is appropriate for all patients with hypertension, and has enormous potential for the prevention and treatment of hypertension and in some cases it can mitigate the need for drug therapy or lower the doses required.[63-65] This is particularly evident in patients with pre-hypertension (blood pressure: 120/80–139/89 mmHg) and, given the benefit of dietary therapy at these blood-pressure levels, patients should adopt the same dietary changes.[66] Therefore, Nurse Practitioners caring for patients with pre-hypertension or hypertension can utilize many of the following evidence-based dietary recommendations. Nutritional factors that may contribute to the development of essential hypertension include obesity, high sodium intake, low potassium and calcium intake, and excessive alcohol consumption.[67,68] The Dietary Approaches to Stop Hypertension (DASH) trial and the subsequent DASH-sodium trials and the PREMIER study have substantiated the benefit of a comprehensive dietary approach in the prevention and treatment of hypertension.[63,64,69,70]

The DASH diet, shown in Table 8-11, provides for a substantial intake of potassium and calcium mostly from fruits, vegetables, and low-fat dairy foods.[65] In addition, meat portions are limited and nuts are used to provide magnesium and additional fiber. The diet limits saturated fat and cholesterol intake comparable to the TLC diet. Clinical trials have demonstrated that the DASH diet reduced diastolic blood pressure by as much as 5 mmHg, regardless of age, gender, ethnicity, or pre-existing hypertension.[65,70] The DASH diet was more effective among African American and hypertensive individuals. For patients with Stage 1 hypertension (blood pressure: 140/90–159/99 mmHg) the diet's effectiveness in lowering blood pressure was similar to that of a single-agent anti-hypertensive medication.[63,70] After the original trial, the DASH-sodium trial investigated the effect of the DASH diet combined with three different levels of sodium (3300 mg, 2400 mg, and 1500 mg).[64,65] Reductions in blood pressure were proportional to the level of sodium restriction. Questions to ask patients with hypertension or pre-hypertension should include:

- Do you use a salt shaker at the table or in cooking?
- Do you read food labels for sodium content (<400 mg/serving permitted)?
- How often do you eat canned, smoked, frozen, or processed foods?

Obesity and Hypertension

Obesity is a major risk factor in the development of hypertension. It has been estimated that 60% of hypertensive patients are overweight.[71] A linear relationship exists between the degree of obesity and the severity of hypertension. The beneficial effect

Table 8-11 Dietary Approaches to Stop Hypertension (DASH Diet) Recommendations

Food Group	Daily Servings	Serving Sizes
Grains and grain products	7–8	1 slice bread 1 cup dry cereal 1/2 cup cooked rice, pasta, or cereal
Vegetables	4–5	1 cup raw leafy vegetable 1/2 cup cooked vegetable 6 oz vegetable juice
Fruits	4–5	6 oz fruit juice 1 medium fruit 1/4 cup dried fruit 1/2 cup fresh, frozen, or canned fruit
Low-fat or fat-free dairy foods	2–3	8 oz milk 1 cup yogurt 1 1/2 ounces cheese
Meats, poultry, and fish	2 or less	3 oz cooked meats, poultry, or fish
Nuts, seeds, and dry beans	4–5 per week	1/3 cup or 1 1/2 ounces nuts 2 tbsp or 1/2 ounces seeds 1/2 cup cooked dry beans
Fats and oils	2–3	1 tsp soft margarine 1 tbsp low fat mayonnaise 2 tbsp light salad dressing 1 tsp vegetable oil
Sweets	5 per week	1 tbsp sugar 1 tbsp jelly or jam 1/2 oz jelly beans 8 oz lemonade

This DASH eating plan is based on 2000 calories daily. The number of servings may vary from those listed depending on caloric needs. Serving sizes may vary between 1/2 and 1 1/4 cups. Fat content changes serving counts for fats and oils (1 tbsp of regular salad dressing equals 1/2 serving; 1 tbsp of fat-free dressing equals 0 servings). Source: National Heart, Lung, and Blood Institute.[70]

of weight reduction in hypertensive individuals has been clearly documented.[72] Controlled dietary intervention trials estimate that a mean reduction in body weight of 20 lb (9.2 kg) is associated with a 6.3 mmHg reduction in systolic blood pressure and a 3.1 mmHg reduction in diastolic blood pressure.[73] The exact mechanism of obesity-induced hypertension is unclear, but increased cardiac output, sodium retention, and increased sympathetic activity in response to elevated insulin levels are all thought to be significant contributors.[74] Weight reduction should be the primary goal for the overweight hypertensive patient, since even a 10% change in body weight is sufficient to reduce blood pressure.[62]

Dietary Sodium Intake and Hypertension

Population studies have repeatedly demonstrated a relationship between hypertension and a high sodium intake. However, not all individuals respond the same way to dietary sodium. Depletion and loading studies indicate that up to 50% of hypertensive patients are salt-sensitive.[75] Salt sensitivity appears to be associated with several demographic variables such as obesity, African American race, and older age. Unfortunately, there is no simple solution to determine salt sensitivity in the clinical setting.

The JNC-VII recommends limiting sodium to no more than 2400 mg daily for patients with hypertension. The 2010 *US Dietary Guidelines* now recommends 1500 mg sodium/day for adults age 51 and over and for individuals of any age who are African American or diagnosed with hypertension, diabetes, or chronic kidney disease. The typical American diet contains 4–8 g of sodium per day.[69] Table salt and foods high in sodium such as salted, smoked, canned, and highly processed foods should be limited. The use of convenience foods, fast foods, and eating out frequently all contribute to higher sodium intake among Americans. Low sodium foods are listed in Appendix X.

Dietary Potassium Intake and Hypertension

Epidemiologic and observational studies have reported an inverse correlation between potassium intake and blood pressure, especially among African Americans and individuals consuming a high sodium diet.[76] More recently, several small intervention studies have shown that potassium supplementation results in a modest hypotensive effect. Although the exact mechanism remains unclear, the effects of potassium supplementation include naturesis, inhibition of renin release, and decreased thromboxane production.[67] For practical purposes, increasing dietary intake of potassium may have a beneficial effect on blood pressure. Foods high in potassium include oranges, orange juice, potatoes (especially with the skins), and bananas. To maintain a high potassium intake, the DASH diet includes 8–10 servings of fruits and vegetables daily. Certain diuretic therapy, specifically loop diuretics, induce potassium wasting. Increasing dietary potassium intake in these patients may obviate the need for potassium supplements, which require close monitoring. Good sources of potassium are listed in Appendix J.

Dietary Calcium Intake and Hypertension

Calcium intake may be lower among those with hypertension compared with normotensive individuals. Increased dietary calcium intake may reduce the incidence of hypertension and calcium supplements may produce a hypotensive effect in some patients.[76] Although dietary calcium has been correlated with blood pressure, calcium supplementation has not been consistently shown significantly to lower blood pressure. Subsequently, the inclusion of low-fat dairy foods, within the framework of the DASH diet, did provide additional blood pressure lowering as shown in Table 8-11, which advises two to three servings per day of fat-free or low-fat dairy food. Dietary sources of calcium are listed in Appendices G and H.

Alcohol Intake and Hypertension

Individuals who drink three or more alcoholic beverages per day account for 5–7% of those diagnosed with hypertension. Evidence shows that two or more drinks per day can lead to an increase in blood pressure and the relationship is dependent on the amount of alcohol consumed, rather than the type of alcohol.[69] Although alcohol acts as a vasodilator, chronic alcohol ingestion is associated with increased formation of

Table 8-12 Lifestyle Modifications to Manage Hypertension (JNC 7)

Modification	Recommendations	Approximate Systolic BP Reduction
Weight reduction	Maintain normal body weight (BMI: 18.5–24.9)	5–20 mmHg for each 10 kg weight loss
Adopt DASH eating plan	Consume diet rich in fruits, vegetables, low-fat dairy foods and low saturated fat	8–14 mmHg
Dietary sodium reduction	Reduce sodium to no more than 2.4 g/day	2–8 mmHg
Increase physical activity	Engage in regular aerobic activity such as walking (30 min/day on most days)	4–9 mmHg
Moderate alcohol consumption	Limit alcohol to no more than 2 drinks/day for men and 1 drink/day for women	2–4 mmHg

Source: JNC VII.[69]

the vasoconstrictor, thromboxane. Chronically increased levels of this prostaglandin metabolite may be partially responsible for the hypertensive effect of chronic alcohol ingestion. In controlled studies, reducing alcohol consumption in this specific population has been associated with a modest reduction in blood pressure. Lifestyle modifications to manage hypertension are shown in Table 8-12.

Heart Failure

Heart failure (HF) is a leading cause of disability and death in the US affecting nearly 5 million adults.[77] Heart failure is characterized by decreased cardiac output, venous stasis, sodium and fluid retention, and malnutrition.[78] Reduced function of the left ventricle and accompanying neuro-hormonal changes promote accumulation of sodium and water. Shortness of breath, fatigue, and inactivity are all symptoms patients with heart failure are likely to experience which can affect their food intake.[79] Chronic heart failure (CHF) is increasingly recognized as a multisystem disease with several co-morbidities such as anemia, insulin resistance, autonomic disturbance, or cardiac cachexia.[77] Nurse Practitioners working with heart failure patients need to be aware of the most common nutritional issues, including malnutrition, cachexia, fluid overload, sodium retention, and vitamin/mineral deficiencies, which may contribute to disease progression. Nurse Practitioners can also minimize morbidity from nutrition impairment through appropriate monitoring and correction of baseline and medication-induced electrolyte imbalances in addition to vitamin and mineral supplementation when appropriate.[80] By working closely with registered dietitians in acute care settings and upon discharge, Nurse Practitioners can significantly impact patients' functional capacity, mortality, and quality of life.[79]

Nutritional Effects of Heart Failure
Cardiac Cachexia

Cardiac cachexia is a syndrome characterized by wasting and under-nutrition seen in patients with CHF. Elevated levels of pro-inflammatory cytokines may lead to the development of cardiac cachexia. As myocardial function progressively deteriorates, patients present with loss of adipose tissue, bone mineral density, and loss of lean body mass. Deficiencies in both macro- and micronutrients contribute to the progression of the disease, but rarely initiate the wasting process.[77,80,81] Upper-body and temporal wasting with lower-extremity edema are the hallmark features of this condition. New evidence suggests that patients with CHF also have alterations in intestinal morphology, permeability, and absorption function.[77] This intestinal dysfunction may lead to both the chronic inflammatory state and catabolic/anabolic imbalance seen in cardiac cachexia. The proposed mechanisms to explain cardiac cachexia include:

- Impaired cellular oxygen supply.
- Alterations of the gastrointestinal system and increased nutrient losses.
- Increased nutritional requirements.
- Decreased nutritional intake.

Impaired cellular oxygen supply: Decreased cardiac output reduces oxygen delivery to cells, resulting in inefficient substrate oxidation and inadequate synthesis of high-energy intermediary metabolites.

Gastrointestinal (GI) alterations and increased nutrient losses: Recent studies suggest that patients with CHF have alterations in their GI tract due to reductions in peripheral blood flow, non-occlusive mesenterial ischemia, and restricted intestinal microcirculation, leading to decreased nutrient absorption. Thickening of the bowel wall seen in patients with CHF compared with controls, results in nutrient malabsorption.[77] Hypoxemia and increased venous pressure may also cause bowel wall edema with subsequent fat and protein malabsorption. Decreased synthesis of hepatic bile salts and pancreatic enzymes caused by oxygen deprivation to the liver and pancreas may further contribute to this. Proteinuria is also a feature of heart failure (HF) secondary to the reduced renal blood flow characteristic of this disorder.

Increased nutritional requirements and inhibition of food intake: Patients with HF can be hypermetabolic and therefore have increased nutritional requirements. This hypermetabolic state is caused by the increased work required for breathing, the mechanical work of the heart and oxygen consumption, and activation of neuroendocrine factors and proinflammatory cytokines, such as tumor necrosis factor-alpha (TNF-alpha). These cytokines also appear to inhibit food intake in animal models.[77] In CHF, skeletal muscle insulin resistance occurs and contributes to impaired energy metabolism.[82] If additional calories are not ingested to meet these increased demands, weight loss ensues. Additional factors that may result in an inadequate food intake in patients with HF include:

- Hepatomegaly and ascites (reduce functional gastric volume causing early satiety).
- Dyspnea and fatigue induced by eating.
- Unpalatable low-sodium diets.
- Anorexia, nausea, or vomiting from medications used to treat CHF.

Nutrition Therapy for Heart Failure

Nutrition therapy for patients with HF should be aimed at controlling sodium and fluid retention, restoring and maintaining body weight, providing adequate energy, protein, vitamins, and minerals, and repletion of protein stores in patients who have lost lean body mass.[12,83] Patients with HF also have several co-morbidities, requiring certain dietary restrictions, which must be considered.

Dietary Sodium Intake

HF patients retain sodium and fluid and therefore dietary sodium restriction is a cornerstone of treatment. The level of sodium restriction may be individualized according to the severity of the HF. The Heart Failure Society of America's (HFSA) comprehensive practice guidelines recommend that patients with symptomatic HF reduce dietary sodium intake to 2–3 g (2000–3000 mg) per day.[84] The American Dietetic Association's Evidence Analysis Library reports fair evidence for restricting sodium intake to 2 g/day.[12] Sodium restriction supports the effectiveness of diuretic agents in achieving negative sodium balance. One-fourth or more of hospital re-admissions for patients with HF are due to non-compliance with dietary advice.[12] Patients need more than to be told "stay away from salt." They need to be able to understand their recommended level of dietary sodium, use values on the nutrition label to guide their intake, and distinguish between high and low sodium foods.

A recent study in an urban heart failure clinic linked knowledge of dietary sodium sources with consumption of fewer high sodium foods.[85] Another report indicated that one hour of education before hospital discharge decreased likelihood of re-hospitalization by 35% and saved $2823 per patient.[86] Whether the patient is seen in the acute care or ambulatory care setting, referral to the registered dietitian for assessment of their dietary intake and assistance in achieving the skills needed to manage a sodium-restricted diet at home is appropriate for cost-effective management of HF. Salt substitutes are available to flavor foods, but many of them substitute potassium for sodium. Patients with renal failure or those taking potassium-sparing diuretics should be instructed to avoid these products (see Appendix X for Low Sodium Foods).

Fluid Management

Heart failure associated with dilutional hyponatremia may require restricting fluid intake to 1500–2000 mL/day.[87] Fluid may be restricted slightly more in the hospital setting. Some suggest limiting daily fluid intake to an amount equal to the 24-hour urine output volume plus 500 mL. Traditional nutrition assessment parameters, such as actual body weight or weight change, may not accurately reflect nutritional status in HF patients. For example, cardiac cachexia may go undetected if body weight is normal or elevated because of sodium and water retention. In addition, serum protein levels, such as albumin, may be decreased secondary to either under-nutrition or artificially as a result of fluid overload. When HF appears well-controlled with no evidence of edema or ascites, and low serum BNP (B-type natriuretic peptide) levels, increase in weight is more likely actual dry weight gain.

Calories and Protein

The HFSA guidelines recommend that patients with HF consume a prudent diet which provides adequate protein, carbohydrate, and calories appropriate for their age, gender, and activity level.[84-86] If needed, daily caloric intake should be adequate to promote weight gain in underweight patients with HF. HF patients generally need higher calories compared with a healthy control subject, but more research is warranted to provide an accurate assessment of how many calories most HF patients need.[84-86] Some practitioners estimate dietary calories at 1.5 times the basal energy expenditure. Another set of recommendations suggests 28–30 kcal/kg of ideal body weight for weight maintenance and 32–35 kcal/kg of actual weight for the undernourished patient. Since disease states increase protein turnover and the body's demand for protein, patients with HF may benefit from higher protein intakes. Provision of 1.5 g/kg/day of protein can promote anabolism and achieve positive nitrogen balance in a patient with cardiac cachexia. High-protein, high-calorie supplements are often necessary to achieve this calorie requirement, especially when the patient has a poor appetite. Nutritional supplements, including both liquid and pudding forms, are available and provide a higher concentration of calories and protein in a relatively small volume. The sodium and fluid content of HF supplements must be considered in total daily sodium and fluid allowance. Small, frequent meals also may assist HF patients achieve an adequate dietary intake. Patients who cannot meet their caloric and protein require-ments orally may require enteral tube feeding (Chapter 13). Enteral feeding in a HF patient can be difficult as it can result in overfeeding, which will aggravate the primary condition. For some patients, obesity places additional strain on an already compro-mised heart. Thus, careful assessment of nutritional status and monitoring of dietary intake are valuable in providing for optimum nutritional support.

Other Nutrients and Supplements

The HFSA guidelines recommend a daily multivitamin and mineral supplement to offset the reduced nutrient absorption, loss of nutrients caused by diuretic therapy, and overall reduced food intake often seen in patients with HF. It is important, however, to ask patients about over-the counter-supplements to avoid the possibility of an adverse reaction from drug-nutrient interactions or megavitamin use. Thiamin deficiency has been noted more frequently among heart failure patients. It has been estimated that the incidence of thiamin deficiency in HF patients can range from 13 to 93%, suggesting that supplementation may be beneficial. Possible detrimental effects of thiamin defi-ciency on the heart include myocardial hypertrophy, myocardial failure, and sodium and water retention.[85,86] CHF patients often experience low vitamin D levels, which increases their risk for osteopenia and osteoporosis, especially with weight loss. Frequently prescribed loop diuretics can lead to calcium loss via the kidney.[77] Although a number of additional supplements have been studied in HF patients, there is limited evidence to support this practice.

Summary: Role of Nurse Practitioners

Nurse Practitioners need to be able to identify patients at risk for CHD using the NCEP and AHA guidelines and determine appropriate LDL-C goals. Recognition of the important role that nutrition plays in patients with CHD, HTN, and HF will help Nurse Practitioners gain knowledge and skills in this area and be able to provide appropriate nutritional guidance and evidence-based practice to their patients. Given a patient's medical, social, dietary history, and laboratory data Nurse Practitioners completing this chapter will be able to develop lifestyle goals with their patients to reduce risk for CHD and HTN.

References

1. American Heart Association Web Site. www.heart.org. Accessed 2012.
2. Centers for Disease Control and Prevention. National Center for Health Statistics, 2010.
3. Gidding SS, Lichtenstein AH, Faith MS, et al. Implementing American Heart Association Pediatric and Adult Nutrition Guidelines: A Scientific Statement from the American Heart Association Nutrition Committee of the Council on Nutrition, Physical Activity and Metabolism, Council on Cardiovascular Disease in the Young, Council on Arteriosclerosis, Thrombosis and Vascular Biology, Council on Cardiovascular Nursing, Council on Epidemiology and Prevention, and Council for High Blood Pressure Research. *Circulation* 2009;119:1161–1175.
4. Krauss RM, Eckel RH, Howard B, et al. AHA Dietary Guidelines: revision 2000: a statement for healthcare professionals from the Nutrition committee of the American Heart Association. *Circulation* 2000;102:2284–2299.
5. Grundy SM, Cleeman JI, Merz CN, et al. Implications of recent clinical trials for the National Cholesterol Education Program Adult Treatment Panel III guidelines. *Circulation* 2004;110: 227–239.
6. Eckel RH, Grundy SM, Zimmet PZ. The metabolic syndrome. *Lancet* 2005;365:1415–1428.
7. Lichtenstein AH, Appel LJ, Brands M, et al. Diet and Lifestyle Recommendations Revision 2006. A Scientific Statement from the American Heart Association Nutrition Committee. *Circulation* 2006;114:82–96.
8. Mente A, de Koning L, Shannon HS, et al. A systematic review of the evidence supporting a causal link between dietary factors and coronary heart disease. *Arch Intern Med* 2009;169: 659–669.
9. Judd JT, Baer DJ, Clevidence BA, et al. Dietary cis and trans monounsaturated and saturated FA and plasma lipids and lipoproteins in men. *Lipids* 2002;37:123–131.
10. Fletcher B, Berra K, Ades P, et al. AHA Scientific Statement. Managing abnormal blood lipids, a collaborative approach. *Circulation* 2005;112:3184–3209.
11. Mills EJ, O'Regan C, Eyawo O, et al. Intensive statin therapy compared with moderate dosing for prevention of cardiovascular events: a meta-analysis of>40 000 patients. *Eur Heart J* 2011;32:1409–1415.
12. American Dietetic Association. ADA Evidence Analysis Library. Disorders of lipid metabolism. Available at www.adaevidencelibrary.com. Accessed 2012.
13. Harper CR, Jacobson TA. The fats of life: the role of omega-3 fatty acids in the prevention of coronary heart disease. *Arch Intern Med* 2001;161:2185–2192.
14. Fernandez ML, West KL. Mechanisms by which dietary fatty acids modulate plasma lipids. *J Nutr* 2005;135:2075–2078.
15. van Horn L, McCoin M, Kris-Etherton PM, et al. Evidence base for dietary prevention and treatment of cardiovascular disease: a 21st century perspective. *J Am Diet Assoc* 2008;108:287–331.
16. Expert Panel on Detection, Evaluation, and Treatment of High Blood Cholesterol in Adults. Executive summary of the third report of the national cholesterol education program (NCEP) expert panel on detection, evaluation, and treatment of high blood cholesterol in adults (Adult Treatment Panel III). *JAMA* 2001;285:2486–2497.

17. National Heart, Lung, and Blood Institute *Third Report of the National Cholesterol Education Program Expert Panel on Detection, Evaluation, and Treatment of High Blood Cholesterol in Adults (Adult Treatment Panel III). Executive Summary.* National Institutes of Health, Bethesda, MD, 2001. NIH publication 01-3670. 2/3/2011.

18. Parikh P, McDaniel MC, Ashen MD, et al. Diets and cardiovascular disease. *J Am Coll Cardiol* 2005;45:1379–1387.

19. Albert C, Hennekens C, O'Donnell C, et al. Fish consumption and risk of sudden cardiac death. *JAMA* 1998;279:23–28.

20. Superko RH. Advanced lipoprotein testing and subfractionation are clinically useful. *Circulation* 2009;119:2383–2395.

21. Balk EM, Lichtenstein AH, Chung M, et al. Effects of omega-3 fatty acids on coronary restenosis, intima-media thickness, and exercise tolerance: a systematic review. *Atherosclerosis.* 2006;184:237–246.

22. Hu FB, Bronner L, Willett WC, et al. Fish and omega-3 fatty acid intake and risk of coronary heart disease in women. *JAMA* 2002;287:1815–1821.

23. Hu FB, Willett WC. Optimal diets for prevention of coronary heart disease. *JAMA* 2002;288:2569–2578.

24. American Dietetic Association. ADA Evidence Analysis Library. Heart Failure. Available at www.adaevidencelibrary.com. Accessed 2012.

25. Kris-Etherton PM, Harris WS, Appel LJ. American Heart Association Nutrition Committee. Fish consumption, fish oil, omega-3 fatty acids, and cardiovascular disease. *Circulation* 2002;106:2747–2757.

26. Wang C, Harris WS, Chung M, et al. N-3 fatty acids from fish or fish-oil supplements, but not alpha-linolenic acid, benefit cardiovascular disease outcomes in primary-and secondary-prevention studies: a systematic review. *Am J Clin Nutr* 2006;85:5–17.

27. De Caterina R. n–3 fatty acids in cardiovascular disease. *N Engl J Med* 2011;364:2439–2450.

28. Oomen CM, Ocké AC, Feskens EJ, et al. Association between trans fatty acid intake and 10-year risk of coronary heart disease in the Zutphen Elderly Study: a prospective population-based study. *Lancet* 2001.357:746–751.

29. de Lorgeril M, Renaud S, Mamelle N, et al. Mediterranean alpha-linolenic acid-rich diet in secondary prevention of coronary heart disease. *Lancet* 1994;343:1454–1459.

30. de Lorgeril M, Salen P, Martin JL, et al. Mediterranean diet, traditional risk factors and the rate of cardiovascular complications after myocardial infarction. Final report of the Lyon Diet Heart Study. *Circulation* 1999;99:779–785.

31. Jenkins DJ, Kendall CW, Marchie A, et al. Direct comparison of a dietary portfolio of cholesterol-lowering foods with a statin in hypercholesterolemic participants. *Am J Clin Nutr* 2005;81:380–387.

32. Williams MA, Haskell WL, Ades PA, et al. American Heart Association Council on Clinical Cardiology; American Heart Association Council on Nutrition, Physical Activity, and Metabolism. Resistance exercise in individuals with and without cardiovascular disease: 2007 update. A scientific statement from the American Heart Association Council on Clinical Cardiology and Council on Nutrition, Physical Activity, and Metabolism. *Circulation* 2007;116:572–584.

33. Baylin A, Kabagambe EK, Ascherio A, et al. High 18:2 trans-fatty acids in adipose tissue are associated with increased risk of nonfatal acute myocardial infarction in Costa Rican adults. *J Nutr* 2003;133:1186–1191.

34. Eckel RH, Borra S, Lichtenstein AH, et al. Understanding the complexity of trans fatty acid reduction in the American diet: American heart association Trans Fat Conference 2006: report of the Trans Fat Conference Planning Group. *Circulation* 2007;115:2231–2246.

35. Mozaffarian D, Katan MB, Ascherio A, et al. Trans fatty acids and cardiovascular disease. *N Engl J Med* 2006;354:1601–1613.

36. Denke MA, Adams-Huet B, Nguyen AT. Individual cholesterol variation in response to a margarine- or butter-based diet. *JAMA* 2000;284:2740–2747.
37. Hu FB, Stampfer MJ, Rimm EB, et al. A prospective study of egg consumption and risk of cardiovascular disease in men and women. *JAMA* 1999;281:1387–1394.
38. Gaziano JM, Ridker PM, Libby P. Primary and secondary prevention of coronary heart disease. In: Bonow RO, Mann DL, Zipes DP, Libby P (Eds), *Braunwald's Heart Disease: A Textbook of Cardiovascular Medicine*, 9th edition. Saunders, Philadelphia, PA, 2011.
39. Deen D. Metabolic syndrome: what is it and what can I do about it? *Am Fam Physician* 2004;69:2887–2888.
40. Deen D. Metabolic syndrome: time for action. *Am Fam Physician* 2004;69:2875–2882.
41. Mozaffarian D. Nutrition and cardiovascular disease. In: Bonow RO, Mann DL, Zipes DP, Libby P (Eds), *Braunwald's Heart Disease: A Textbook of Cardiovascular Medicine*, 9th edition. Saunders, Philadelphia, PA, 2011.
42. Jiménez-Gómez 2010. A low-fat, high-complex carbohydrate diet supplemented with long-chain (n-3) fatty acids alters the postprandial lipoprotein profile in patients with metabolic syndrome. *J Nutr* 2010;140:1595–1601.
43. An American Heart Association/National Heart, Lung, and Blood Institute Scientific Statement: Executive Summary. Diagnosis and Management of the Metabolic Syndrome. *Circulation* 2005; *112: e285–e290*.
44. Miller M, et al. Triglycerides and cardiovascular disease: a scientific statement from the American Heart Association. *Circulation* 2011;123:2292–2333.
45. Blair SN, Capuzzi DM, Gottlieb SO, et al. Incremental reduction of serum total cholesterol and low-density lipoprotein cholesterol with the addition of plant stanol ester-containingspread to statin therapy. *Am J Cardiol* 2000;86:46–52.
46. Miettinen TA, Puska P, Gylling H, et al. Reduction of serum cholesterol with sitonstanol-ester margarine in a mildly hypercholesterolemic population. *N Engl J Med* 1995;333:1308–1312.
47. Hallikainen MA, Sarkkinen ES, Uusitupa MI. Plant stanol esters affect serum cholesterol concentrations of hypercholesterolemic men and women in a dose-dependent manner. *J Nutr* 2000;130:767–776.
48. Stein K. FDA approves health claim labeling for foods containing soy protein. *J Am Diet Assoc* 2000;3:292.
49. Sacks FM, Lichtenstein A, van Horn L, Harris W, Kris-Etherton P, Winston M for the American Heart Association Nutrition Committee. Soy protein, isoflavones, and cardiovascular health. *Circulation* 2006;113:1034–1044.
50. Fazio S, Guyton JR, Polis AB, et al. Long-term safety and efficacy of triple combination ezetimibe/simvastatin plus extended-release niacin in patients with hyperlipidemia. *Am J Cardiol* 2010;105:487–494.
51. Davey SG, Ebrahim S. Folate supplementation and cardiovascular disease. *Lancet* 2005;366:1679–1681.
52. Bleys J, Miller ER, Pastor-Barriuso R, et al. Vitamin-mineral supplementation and the progression of atherosclerosis: a meta-analysis of randomized controlled trials. *Am J Clin Nutr* 2006;84:880–887.
53. Lichtenstein AH. Nutrient supplements and cardiovascular disease: a heartbreaking story. *J Lipid Res* 2009;50:S429–S433.
54. Sesso HD, Buring JE, Christen WG, et al. Vitamins E and C in the prevention of cardiovascular disease in men. *JAMA* 2008;300:2123–2133.
55. Miller ER, Pastor-Barriuso R, Dalal D, et al. Meta-analysis: high dose vitamin E supplementation may increase all cause mortality. *Ann Intern Med* 2005;142:37–46.
56. Kris-Etherton PM, Lichtenstein AH, Howard BV, et al. Antioxidant vitamin supplements and cardiovascular disease. *Circulation* 2004;110:637–641.

57. Costanzo S, Di Castelnuovo A, Benedetta Donati M, et al. Cardiovascular and overall mortality risk in relation to alcohol consumption in patients with cardiovascular disease. *Circulation* 2010;121:951–959.

58. Goldberg IJ, Mosca L, Piano MR, Fisher EA. AHA Science Advisory. Wine and your heart: a science advisory for healthcare professionals from the Nutrition Committee, Council on Epidemiology and Prevention, and Council on Cardiovascular Nursing of the American Heart Association. *Stroke* 2001;32:591–594.

59. De Oliveira e Silva ER, Foster D, et al. Alcohol consumption raises HDL cholesterol levels by increasing the transport rate of apolipoproteins A-I and A-II. *Circulation* 2000;102:2347–2352.

60. Ong KL, Cheung BM, Man YB, et al. Prevalence, awareness, treatment, and control of hypertension among United States Adults 1999–2004. *Hypertension* 2007;49:69–75.

61. Kotchen TA. Hypertension control: trends, approaches, and goals. *Hypertension* 2007;49:19–20.

62. The Seventh Report of the Joint National Committee on Prevention, Detection, Evaluation, and Treatment of High Blood Pressure. *JAMA* 2003;289:2083–2093.

63. Appel LJ, Moore TJ, Obarzanek E, et al. A clinical trial of the effects of dietary patterns on blood pressure. DASH Collaborative Research Group. *N Engl J Med* 1997;336:1117–1124.

64. Appel LJ, Champagne CM, Harsha DW, et al. Effects of comprehensive lifestyle modification on blood pressure control: main results of the PREMIER clinical trial. *JAMA* 2003;289:2083–2093.

65. Appel LJ, Brands MW, Daniels SR, et al. Dietary approaches to prevent and treat hypertension. *Hypertension* 2006;47:296–308.

66. Sacks FM, Campos H. Dietary therapy in hypertension. *N Engl J Med* 2010;362:2102–2112.

67. Adrogu´e HJ, Madias NE. Sodium and potassium in the pathogenesis of hypertension. *N Engl J Med* 2007;356:1966–1978.

68. Bosworth HB, Olsen MK, Neary A, et al. Take Control of Your Blood pressure (TCYB) study: A multifactorial tailored behavioral and educational intervention for achieving blood pressure control. *Patient Educ Couns* 2008;70:338–347.

69. Chobanian AV, Bakris GL, Black HR, et al., for The National High Blood Pressure Education Program Coordinating Committee. The seventh report of the Joint National Committee on Prevention, Detection, Evaluation, and Treatment of High Blood Pressure: the JNC 7 Report. *JAMA* 2003;289:2560–2572.

70. Sacks FM, Svetkey LP, Vollmer WM, et al. Effects on blood pressure of reduced dietary sodium and the Dietary Approaches to Stop Hypertension (DASH) diet. DASH-Sodium Collaborative Research Group. *N Engl J Med* 2001;344:3–10.

71. Mitka M. DASH dietary plan could benefit many, but few hypertensive patients follow it. *JAMA* 2007;298:164–165.

72. Mellen PB, Gao SK, Vitolins MZ, et al. Deteriorating dietary habits among adults with hypertension: DASH dietary accordance, NHANES 1988–1994 and 1999–2004. *Arch Intern Med* 2008;168:308–314.

73. Elmer PJ, Obarzanek E, Vollmer WM, et al. for PREMIER Collaborative Research Group. Effects of comprehensive lifestyle modification on diet, weight, physical fitness and blood pressure control: 18-month results of a randomized trial. *Ann Intern Med* 2006;144: 485–495.

74. Lin PH, Appel LJ, Fun K, et al. The PREMIER intervention helps participants follow the dietary approaches to stop hypertension dietary pattern and the current dietary reference intake recommendations. *J Am Diet Assoc* 2007;107:1541–1551.

75. Dickinson BD, Havas S. Reducing the population burden of cardiovascular disease by reducing sodium intake. *Arch Intern Med* 2007;167:1460–1468.

76. Beyer FR, Dickinson HO, Nicolson DJ, et al. Combined calcium, magnesium, and potassium supplementation for the management of primary hypertension in adults. *Cochrane Database of Systematic Reviews.* 2006, Issue 3. Art No.:CD004805. DOI:10.1002/14651858.CD004805.pub2.

77. Sandek A, Doehner W, Anker S, et al. Nutrition in heart failure: an update. *Curr Opin Clin Nutri Met Care* 2009;12:384–391.
78. Hunt SA, Abraham WT, Chin MH, et al. ACC/AHA guideline update for the diagnosis and management of chronic heart failure in the adult: summary article. *Circulation* 2005;112:1825–1852.
79. Koelling TM, Johnson ML, Cody RJ, et al. Discharge education improves clinical outcomes in patients with chronic heart failure. *Circulation* 2005;111:179–185.
80. Dunn SP, Bleske B, Dorsch M, et al. Nutrition and heart failure: impact of drug therapies and management strategies. *Nutr Clin Pract* 2009;24:60–75.
81. Anker SD, Sharma R. The syndrome of cardiac cachexia. *Int J Cardiol* 2002;85:51–66.
82. Doehner W, Rauchhaus M, Ponikowski P, et al. Impaired insulin sensitivity as an independent risk factor for mortality in patients with stable chronic heart failure. *J Am Coll Cardiol* 2005; 46:1019–1026.
83. Azhar G, Wei JY. Nutrition and cardiac cachexia. *Curr Opin Clin Nutr Metab Care* 2006;9:18–23.
84. Heart Failure Society of America, Lindenfeld J, Albert NM, Boehmer JP, et al. HFSA 2010 Comprehensive Heart Failure Practice Guideline. *J Card Fail* 2010;16:e1–194.
85. Francis GS, Greenberg BH, Hsu, et al. ACCF/AHA/ACP Task Force. ACCF/AHA/ACP/HFSA/ISHLT 2010 clinical competence statement on management of patients with advanced heart failure and cardiac transplant: a report of the ACCF/AHA/ACP Task Force on Clinical Competence and Training. *J Am Coll Cardiol* 2010;56:424–453.
86. Francis GS, Greenberg BH, Hsu DT, et al. ACCF/AHA/ACP/HFSA/ISHLT 2010 clinical competence statement on management of patients with advanced heart failure and cardiac transplant: a report of the ACCF/AHA/ACP Task Force on Clinical Competence and Training. *Circulation* 2010;122:644–672.
87. Payne-Emerson H, Lennie TA. Nutritional Considerations in Heart Failure. *Nurs Clin N Am* 2008;43:117–132.
88. Hanninen SA, Darling PB, Sole MJ, et al. The prevalence of thiamin deficiency in hospitalized patients with congestive heart failure. *J Am Coll Cardiol* 2006;47:354–361.

9 Endocrinology Care of the Diabetic Patient

Neva White, DNP, MSN, CRNP, CDE
Rickie Brawer, PhD, MPH, CHES
Cheryl Marco, RD, LDN, CDE

OBJECTIVES

- Describe the most common macrovascular and microvascular complications associated with diabetes mellitus.
- Describe the role of glycemic control, nutrition therapy, and physical activity in reducing diabetic complications.
- Describe all of the components of a comprehensive assessment for patients with diabetes.
- Develop an individualized problem list based on the comprehensive assessment.
- Describe how physical activity and optimal nutrition contribute to the health of diabetic patients.
- Describe strategies that may enhance the patients' self-management of diabetes.

Introduction

According to the *Healthy People 2020* goals, diabetes mellitus is an increasingly prevalent disorder predicted to cause a significant economic burden in the near future.[1,2] Nurse Practitioners in every specialty area will treat patients with diabetes and this chapter will provide evidence-based guidance on the promotion of self-management for diabetes. The goal of self-management is to achieve glycemic control in order to minimize acute complications (hypoglycemia and hyperglycemia with or without acidosis), and microvascular and macrovascular complications. The chapter will also discuss weight control goals and management of dyslipidemia in patients with diabetes.

Diabetes is a group of disorders which results from inadequate insulin effects on the tissues of the body. This may result from an underproduction of insulin by the pancreas, resistance to the effects of insulin by the tissues, or a combination of both factors.[4] In addition to type 1 and type 2 diabetes, other clinical presentations resulting in hyperglycemia include gestational diabetes, diabetes linked to genetic defects of

---

The Nurse Practitioner's Guide to Nutrition, Second Edition. Edited by Lisa Hark, Kathleen Ashton and Darwin Deen.
© 2012 John Wiley & Sons, Inc. Published 2012 by John Wiley & Sons, Inc.

beta-cell function or insulin action, diseases of the pancreas (e.g. alcoholic pancreatitis), and diabetes that is drug or chemically induced.[3] The goal of diabetes management is to initiate early and effective therapy that promotes glycemic control as close to normal as possible, while simultaneously avoiding adverse outcomes associated with hypoglycemia.[3-5] Complications associated with diabetes include:[3]

1. *Acute Life-threatening Consequences of Uncontrolled Hyperglycemia*
   - Diabetic ketoacidosis (DKA)
   - Hyperosmolar hyperglycemic syndrome (HHS)
2. *Microvascular Complications of Diabetes*
   - Diabetic nephropathy
   - Diabetic peripheral and autonomic neuropathy
   - Diabetic retinopathy
3. *Macrovascular Complications of Diabetes*
   - Atherosclerosis
   - Cardiovascular disease
   - Cerebrovascular disease
   - Periperheral vascular disease
4. *Other Complications of Diabetes*
   - Depression
   - Acanthosis nigrican
   - Dental disease (gum disease, infections, changes in saliva, tooth decay)

Prevalence of Diabetes

Diabetes affects approximately 25.8 million people of all ages in the US; however, up to 7 million individuals with diabetes are unaware of their condition.[2] While type 1 diabetes most typically presents in childhood or early adolescence, it can develop at any age and is not generally correlated with the presence of obesity. The development of type 2 diabetes on the other hand, correlates with the presence of obesity and generally increases with age.[2] Patients with either of these conditions are also at high risk for cardiovascular disease if lifestyle prevention strategies are not implemented (see Chapter 8).

Diagnosis of Diabetes Mellitus and Pre-diabetes

Of the four different methods available to diagnose diabetes (Table 9-1), each should be repeated on a subsequent day to confirm the diagnosis unless classic symptoms of hyperglycemia are exhibited. Symptoms of hyperglycemia include the following (however, the patient may also be asymptomatic): [3-5]

- Polyuria: excessive excretion of urine.
- Polydipsia: excessive thirst.
- Polyphagia: frequent hunger.
- Unexplained weight loss.

In type 2 diabetes, patients may also present with extreme fatigue, blurred vision, sexual dysfunction, slow healing wounds, recurrent bladder, skin, and gum infections.[3-5]

Table 9-1 Clinical Guidelines for the Diagnosis of Diabetes, Pre-Diabetes, and Gestational Diabetes

	Clinical Guidelines
Diagnosis of Diabetes Hemoglobin A1C	A1C ≥ 6.5%
Fasting plasma glucose (FPG)	≥ 126 mg/dL (7.0 mmol/L)
Random plasma glucose	> 200 mg/dL (11.1 mmol/L) with classic symptoms of polyuria, polydipsia, and unexplained weight loss
2-hour plasma glucose	≥ 200 mg/dL (11.1 mmol/L) during an oral glucose tolerance test (OGTT) using a glucose load containing the equivalent of 75 g of anhydrous glucose dissolved in water
Diagnosis of Pre-diabetes Hemoglobin A1C	5.7–6.4%
Fasting plasma glucose	100 mg/dL (5.6 mmol/L) to 125 mg/dL (6.9 mmol/lL)
2 hour plasma glucose	140–199 mg/dL mg/dL (11.1 mmol/L) during an oral glucose tolerance test (OGTT) using a glucose load containing the equivalent of 75 g of anhydrous glucose dissolved in water

Diagnosis of Gestational Diabetes
The ADA recommends that all pregnant women with no history of diabetes be screened at 24–26 weeks, using a 75 g oral glucose tolerance test (GTT)
Plasma glucose measurement:
    Fasting ≥ 92 mg/dL (5.1 mmol/L)
    1 hour after the administration of a 75 g oral glcouse tolerance test (OGTT) ≥ 180 mg/dL
    (10.0 mmol/l)
    2 hours ≥ 153 mg/dL (8.5 mmol/L)

Source: Adapted from ADA.[3]

Pathophysiology of Diabetes

Pre-diabetes

Hyperglycemia that does not meet diagnostic criteria for diabetes is categorized as either impaired fasting glucose (IFG) or impaired glucose tolerance (IGT). Both IFG and IGT are considered pre-diabetes and are risk factors for the development of diabetes and cardiovascular disease.[3,6,7] Hemoglobin A1C levels between 5.7 and 6.4% may reflect pre-diabetes.[7] Guidelines for screening for pre-diabetes and type 2 diabetes in asymptomatic adults should be considered when risk factors shown in Table 9-2 are present. Current recommendations for seeing patients without risk factors suggest beginning at age 45[4] and if screening results are normal, they should be repeated at 3 year intervals.[3] Guidelines for screening children and youth at increased risk for type 2 diabetes recommend starting at age 10 or at the onset of puberty if risk factors are present. If tests are normal, repeat every 3 years.[3,4,8]

Table 9-2 Guidelines for Screening Asymptomatic Adults for Diabetes

- BMI >25 kg/m²
- Physical inactivity
- Family history of diabetes (first degree relative)
- Member of a high risk race/ethnicity (e.g. Latino, African American, Native American, Asian American, Pacific Islander)
- History of gestational diabetes
- Hypertension (sustained blood pressure greater than 135/80)
- History of cardiovascular disease
- Women with history of polycystic ovarian syndrome (POS)
- History of pre-diabetes
- HDL-C level <35 mg/dL
- Triglyceride level >250 mg/dL

Source: Adapted from American Diabetes Association.[3]

Clinical Presentation and Diagnosis of Type 1 and Type 2 Diabetes

Type 1 diabetes accounts for 5–10% of all diagnosed cases of diabetes. The primary defect is pancreatic beta-cell destruction leading to absolute insulin deficiency (insulinopenia), and resulting in hyperglycemia, polyuria, polydipsia, unexplained weight loss, dehydration, electrolyte disturbance, and ketoacidosis.[3] The capacity of a healthy pancreas to secrete insulin is far in excess of what is needed normally. Therefore, the clinical onset of diabetes may be preceded by an extensive asymptomatic period (months to years), during which beta-cells are undergoing gradual destruction. Patients with type 1 diabetes are dependent on exogenous insulin to prevent ketoacidosis and death.[3,4] Although type 1 diabetes can occur at any age, most cases are diagnosed in patients younger than 30 years of age, with peak incidence between 10 and 12 years in girls and 12 and 14 years in boys.[3–5]

Type 1 diabetes is a result of a genetic predisposition combined with autoimmune destruction of the pancreatic beta-cells. At diagnosis, 85–90% of patients with type 1 diabetes have one or more circulating auto-antibodies, the measurement of which can assist in the diagnosis. Antibodies identified as contributing to the destruction of beta-cells are: (1) islet cell auto-antibodies (ICAs); (2) insulin auto-antibodies (IAAs) which may occur in patients who have never received insulin therapy; (3) auto-antibodies to glutamic acid decarboxylase (GAD65), a protein on the surface of beta-cells (GAD auto-antibodies appear to provoke an attack by the T-cells [killer T lymphocytes], which may be what destroys the beta-cells in diabetes); and (4) auto-antibodies to the tyrosine phosphatases IA-2 and IA-2β.[4] Frequently, after diagnosis and the correction of hyperglycemia, metabolic acidosis, and ketoacidosis, endogenous insulin secretion recovers. During this "honeymoon phase", exogenous insulin requirements decrease dramatically. However, the need for exogenous insulin is inevitable, and within 8–10 years after clinical onset, beta-cell loss is complete and insulin deficiency is absolute.[3–5]

Type 2 diabetes accounts for 90–95% of all diagnosed cases of diabetes and is a progressive disease that is often present long before it is diagnosed. Although approximately 50% of men and 70% of women are obese at the time of diagnosis, type

2 diabetes can occur in non-obese patients, especially in elderly patients.[3] An affected patient may or may not experience the classic symptoms of uncontrolled diabetes, although they are not prone to develop ketoacidosis. Insulin resistance begins and progresses for many years before the development of diabetes, but impaired beta-cell insulin secretory function must be present before hyperglycemia is seen. By the time diabetes is diagnosed, the patient has lost as much as 50% of beta-cell function.[3,9]

In type 2 diabetes, the normal biphasic insulin response to glucose is altered, resulting in post-prandial hyperglycemia. The inadequate first-phase insulin response is also unable to suppress pancreatic alpha-cell glucagon secretion, resulting in glucagon hypersecretion, which leads to an increase in hepatic glucose production and fasting hyperglycemia. The second major metabolic abnormality is a decrease in the ability of insulin to act on target tissues, specifically the muscles, liver, and fat cells. Compounding the problem is glucotoxicity, the impact of elevated glucose levels on both insulin sensitivity and insulin secretion, hence the importance of achieving near-euglycemia in patients with type 2 diabetes.[3] Insulin resistance is also demonstrated in adipocytes, leading to lipolysis and an elevation in circulating free fatty acids. These increased free fatty acids cause a further decrease in insulin sensitivity at the cellular level, impair insulin secretion, and augment hepatic glucose production (lipotoxicity).[9] All of these defects (cellular, hepatic, and beta-cell) contribute to the development and progression of type 2 diabetes.[4] As type 2 diabetes progresses, insulin production progressively declines. Therefore, patients with diabetes usually require more medication(s) over time and eventually exogenous insulin will be required. This is not due to a diet or medication failure, but rather represents a continued decline in beta-cell function.

Gestational Diabetes (see Chapter 4)

Gestational diabetes (GDM) is glucose intolerance that is experienced or recognized for the first time during pregnancy and includes those cases of diabetes diagnosed at the time of pregnancy (Table 9-1).[10] Pregnant women are targets for glycemic control and insulin is currently the agent of choice due to potential teratogenic effects of oral agents. It is important that Nurse Practitioners conduct a risk assessment for GDM at the first prenatal visit. Women at high risk or with a strong family history of diabetes should be tested as soon as possible to avoid complications of pregnancy caused by hyperglycemia. The American Diabetes Association (ADA) recommends that all pregnant women with risk factors but no history of diabetes be tested for GDM as early as possible and retested again at 24–28 weeks if the first test is normal.[4] Those without risk factors should be screened initially at 24–28 weeks. Most cases of GDM resolve after delivery. However, diabetes persists in some women, and those who have experienced GDM have an increased risk for the development of diabetes in the future.[10] Clinical guidelines for the diagnosis of diabetes, pre-diabetes and gestational diabetes are shown in Table 9-1.

Clinical Management of Diabetes

In the clinical management of diabetes, Nurse Practitioners should utilize a multidisciplinary team approach. Management includes appropriate nutrition therapy, regular physical activity, self-management education, and medication. Providing the

Table 9-3 Glycemic Control Treatment Goals

Hemoglobin A1C	<7.0%
Pre-prandial plasma glucose	90–130 mg/dL (5.0–7.2 mmol/L)
Post-prandial plasma glucose	<180 mg/dL (<10.0 mmol/L)
Blood pressure	<130/80 mmHg
LDL-cholesterol	<100 mg/dL (<2.6 mmol/L)
HDL-cholesterol	>40 mg/dL (>1.1 mmol/L)
Triglycerides	<150 mg/dL (<1.7 mmol/L)

Source: Adapted from ADA.[3]

patient with the necessary tools to achieve the best possible control of blood glucose, lipids, and blood pressure will prevent, delay, or arrest the microvascular and macro-vascular complications of diabetes while minimizing hypoglycemia and excess weight gain. Glycemic control treatment goals are shown in Table 9-3.

Two large, long-term studies have demonstrated a clear link between glycemic control and the development of microvascular complications in patients with type 1 and type 2 diabetes.[11-13] They also provide strong evidence for the role of nutrition therapy in the management of diabetes. The Diabetes Control and Complications Trial (DCCT), a long-term, randomized-controlled, multi-center trial, studied approximately 1441 young adults (aged 13–39 years) with type 1 diabetes. These subjects were treated with either intensive therapy (multiple injections of insulin or use of insulin pumps guided by blood glucose monitoring data) or conventional therapy (one or two insulin injections per day). Both groups received nutrition counseling by a nursing professional. The DCCT clearly showed that even small improvements in glucose control reduced the rate of microvascular complications. Patients in the intensive treatment group showed a 50–75% reduction in the risk of progression to retinopathy, nephropathy, and neuropathy. Subjects in the intensive therapy group who reported following their meal plan greater than 90% of the time had hemoglobin A1C levels that were 1% lower than those who reported following their meal plan only 40% of the time.[11]

In a 17-year follow-up study of DCCT patients, intensive treatment during the trial reduced the risk of any cardiovascular event by 42% and the risk of non-fatal myocardial infarction, stroke, or death from cardiovascular disease (CVD) by 57% compared with conventional therapy.[12] These findings support the importance of early intensive therapy to reduce the risk of diabetes complications.

The United Kingdom Prospective Diabetes Study (UKPDS) demonstrated that reduction of elevated blood glucose levels reduced microvascular complications in type 2 diabetes but the reduction in all-cause mortality did not reach statistical significance (a 7% reduction in mortality for every percentage point decrease in hemoglobin A1C).[13] The 5102 newly diagnosed patients with type 2 diabetes were randomized into a group treated conventionally and an intensively treated group. The intensively treated group experienced a 25% reduction in the rate of retinopathy and nephropathy. Improved blood pressure control resulted in a 34% reduction in all macrovascular endpoints and a 37% reduction in all microvascular endpoints.

The UKPDS also illustrated the progressive nature of type 2 diabetes. At diagnosis and before randomization into intensive or conventional treatment, subjects received individualized intensive nutrition counseling for 3 months. During this period, A1C levels decreased by approximately 2% (from 9% to 7%) and patients lost an average of 3.5 kg (8 lb). Researchers concluded that a reduction of energy intake was at least as important, if not more important, than the actual weight lost in determining glucose improvements.[13] However, as the study progressed, nutrition counseling alone was not enough to keep the majority of the patients' A1C levels at 7%. Medication(s), and for many, insulin, needed to be combined with nutrition therapy. Researchers suggest it was not the "diet" failing, but instead it was the pancreas failing to secrete enough insulin to maintain adequate glucose control.

While these studies show that achieving an A1C less than 7% is beneficial, the risk of hypoglycemia and sudden coronary events increases especially in older adults.[14] Therefore, targeting less than 7% A1C levels in patients with diabetes should focus on younger individuals with a longer life expectancy and minimal complications. Appropriate A1C targets for older adults and those with significant complications, higher risk for hypoglycemia, and coronary events, A1C should be aimed at 7–8%.[14]

Diabetes Self-Management Education/Training

Diabetes self-management education/training (DSME/T) is an ongoing process to help facilitate the knowledge, skills, and resources necessary for patients with diabetes or at risk for diabetes to live with the day-to-day challenges of the disease.[15-16] The American Diabetes Association and American Association of Diabetes Educators (AADE) sponsor Diabetes Education Accreditation.

The goal of DSME/T is to promote behaviors that lead to lifestyle changes consistent with improved glycemic control.[15-16] DSME/T shifts the role of Nurse Practitioners from providing direct medical care to supporting self-management among patients with diabetes and their families. Many Nurse Practitioners choose to use a team approach to DSME/T with registered dietitians (as well as other team members) in their practice setting or delegating the educational and skill-building components to an outside diabetes educator. Nurse Practitioners need to be aware of and have access to resources available for DSME/T within the practice, the nearest hospital, and other community-based settings.

It is essential that DSME/T be a collaborative process focused on behavior modification and guided by goal-setting to achieve better glycemic control.[15] The AADE has identified seven specific self-care behaviors that meet National Standards for DSME and can assist Nurse Practitioners in documenting patient outcomes and establishing measures of success. The seven AADE self-care behaviors provide common language for inter-professional coordination of care that is consistent with the Chronic Care Model.[17,18] These self-care behaviors include:

- Healthy Eating
- Being Active
- Taking Medication
- Monitoring
- Healthy Coping
- Problem Solving
- Reducing Risks

The Health Belief Model, as discussed in Chapter 3, suggests that patients who hold the following two important beliefs are more likely to engage in self-management behaviors compared with those who do not hold these beliefs: (1) consider diabetes to be serious and (2) believe that their own actions make a difference.[19] A patient's self-efficacy and self-confidence in making and maintaining a change are significant predictors of later adherence. A simple, but effective role that all Nurse Practitioners can provide is to endorse and support lifestyle changes and to express confidence in their patient's ability to make behavior changes. Patients may need support coping with the increased demands of caring for a chronic medical condition and they may present with numerous and uncertainties about treatment. For example, there are often numerous concerns about administering daily insulin injections and monitoring blood glucose levels.

Monitoring of Metabolic Outcomes

The goal of monitoring is to achieve individualized glycemic goals while minimizing the frequency and severity of episodes of hypoglycemia. Patients may assess day-to-day glycemic control by self-monitoring blood glucose levels (SMBG). Patients with diabetes can use SMBG to determine the impact that food choices and physical activities have on blood glucose levels and make adjustments in lifestyle and medications required to achieve glycemic goals. SMBG should be done three or more times daily by patients using multiple insulin injections or insulin pump therapy.[4] For patients on non-insulin therapy, SMBG should be done often to facilitate reaching glucose goals.[20,21] To achieve post-prandial glucose goals, post-prandial SMBG is also helpful. The accuracy of SMBG depends on the instrument and the user, and monitoring techniques must be evaluated on a regular basis. Patients also should be taught how to use the data to adjust food intake, exercise level, and medications to achieve glycemic goals. Negotiating shared goals, using the techniques discussed in Chapter 3, such as Motivational Interviewing, can be very helpful.[20–22]

Continuous glucose monitoring (CGM) measures interstitial fluid glucose (which correlates with blood glucose) in a continuous and minimally invasive manner.[22] Continuous glucose sensors have optional user-established alarms for hypo-and hyperglycemia and small studies have shown that CGM decreases the average time patients spend in hypo-and hyperglycemic ranges. Currently, its use is recommended as a supplement to SMBG for selected patients with type 1 diabetes.[23]

Complementing day-to-day testing are measurements of hemoglobin A1C that reflect a weighted average of plasma glucose measurements over the preceding 6–8 weeks, and long-term glycemic control.[24] When hemoglobin and other proteins are exposed to glucose, the glucose becomes attached to the protein in a slow, non-enzymatic, and concentration-dependent manner. In non-diabetic patients, A1C values are 4–6%, which correspond to an estimated average glucose up to 126 mg/dL as shown in Table 9-4.[25] A1C measurements should be taken approximately every 3 months to determine whether a patient's glycemic goals have been reached and maintained. Lowering A1C to an average of approximately 7% has clearly been shown to reduce complications of diabetes; however, some epidemiologic

Table 9-4 Comparison of A1C Percentages and
Estimated Average Blood Sugar Levels

A1C Reading (%)	Average Blood Glucose Level (mg/dL)
5	97
6	126
7	154
8	183
9	212
10	240
11	260
12	298

Adapted from ADA[4] and Handelsman.[5]

studies have reported benefit to lowering A1C into the normal range (<6.5%).[11–13] Since atherosclerosis is the primary cause of mortality in patients with diabetes, lipid levels, and blood pressure should be closely monitored. Lipids should be measured annually and blood pressure checked at every visit.[26]

Glucose-Lowering Medications to Treat Diabetes

If metabolic goals are not being met in patients with type 2 diabetes, there are various classes of oral medications as well as injectable medications, including insulin, that can be prescribed in combination with nutrition therapy and exercise. These provide numerous options for achieving euglycemia in patients with type 2 diabetes. Many patients benefit from taking two or more medications since each medication may address a different problem. Such combination therapy is so common that a number of combination pills have been made available as shown in Table 9-5. However, because of the progressive nature of type 2 diabetes, many patients will eventually require insulin injections to achieve glycemic control.

Insulin

All patients with type 1 diabetes and many patients with type 2 diabetes who no longer produce adequate endogenous insulin need replacement of insulin that mimics normal insulin release patterns (Table 9-6). After eating, plasma glucose and insulin concentrations increase rapidly, peak in 30–60 minutes, and return to basal concentrations within 2–3 hours in non-diabetics. To mimic this, rapid-acting insulin, such as lispro, aspart, or glulisine, is given at mealtime with doses adjusted based on the amount of carbohydrate in the meal.[28]

Basal or background insulin, such as determir, glargine, or NPH, is required in the post-absorptive state to restrain endogenous glucose output primarily from the liver and to limit lipolysis and excess flux of free fatty acids to the liver.[29] Glargine and detemir are 24-hour duration insulin analogs with virtually no peak

Table 9-5 Type 2 Diabetes Medications

Class and Generic Names	Mechanism of Action
DPP-4 Inhibitors Januvia (Stagliptin) Onglyza (Saxagliptin) Trajenta (Linagliptin)	Enhances glucose-dependent insulin secretions
Sulfonylureas (Second generation) Glipizide (Glucotrol) Glipizide, long-acting (Glucotrol XL) Glyburide, micronized (Glynase Prestabs) Glimepiride (Amaryl)	Stimulates insulin secretion from the beta cells
Meglitinide Repaglinide (Prandin), Nateglinide (Starlix)	Stimulates insulin secretion from beta cells
Biguanide Metformin (Glucophage) Metformin Extended Release (Glucophage XR) Metformin, liquid (Riomet)	Decreases hepatic glucose production
Thiazolidinediones Pioglitazone (Actos)	Improves peripheral insulin sensitivity
Alpha Glucosidase Inhibitors Acarbose (Precose), Miglitol (Glyset) Victoza (Litaglutide)	Delays carbohydrate absorption
Incretin Mimetics Exenatide (Byetta)	Enhances glucose-dependent insulin secretion and suppresses glucagon secretion
Amylinominetic Pramlintide (Smylin)	Decreases glucagon production which decreases mealtime hepatic glucose release and prevents postprandial hyperglycemia
Combination Drugs Metformin/glyburide (Glucovance) Metformin/poiglitazone (ActosPlus) Metformin/sitagliptin (Janumet) Metformin/glipizide (Metaglip)	Combined action of each medication

Source: Adapted from ADA[4] and Mensing.[27]

action time. They can be injected any time during the day, as long as they are taken around the same time each day, but cannot be mixed with other insulins.[30] NPH is also occasionally used as background insulin and can be administered with short-acting insulin, but usually has to be given twice daily. The type and timing of insulin regimens should be individualized based on eating and exercise habits and blood glucose concentrations.

There are also pre-mixed insulins that may be used in patients with type 2 diabetes, often when insulin is initiated (Table 9-6). Many patients find insulin pens to be a convenient way to inject their insulin doses. Insulin pens are available containing regular, NPH, lispro, aspart, glulisine, or 70/30 or 75/25 pre-mixed insulin.[32] Insulin

Table 9-6 Insulin Therapy

Type of Insulin	Onset of Action	Peak Action	Usual Effective Duration	Monitor Effect After
Bolus insulin (mealtime)				
Rapid-acting	<15 min	1–2 h	3–4 h	2 h
Insulin lispro (Humalog)				
Insulin aspart (Novolog)				
Insulin glulisine (Apidra)				
Short-acting	0.5–1 h	2–3 h	3–6 h	4 h
Regular				(next meal)
Basal insulin (background)				
Long-acting				
Insulin glargine (Lantus)	<1 h	Peakless	20–24 h	10–12 h
Insulin determir (Levemir)	1–2 h	5–14 h	14–3 h	10–12 h
Intermediate-acting				
NPH	2–4 h	6–10 h	10–16 h	8–12 h
Mixtures				
70/30 (70% NPH, 30%	0.5–1 h	Dual	10–16 h	
regular)	<15 min	Dual	10–16 h	
Humalog Mix 75/25				
(75% neutral protamine	<15 min	Dual	10–16 h	
lispro [NPL], 25% lispro)				
Novolog Mix 70/30 (70%				
neutral protamine aspart				
[NPA], 30% aspart)				

Source: Adapted from ADA[4] and Rodbarg.[31]

pump therapy delivers insulin in two ways: in a steady, measured, and continuous dose (the basal insulin), and as a surge (bolus) dose at mealtime. Insulin pumps can also deliver precise insulin doses for different times of day, which may be necessary to correct for situations such as the dawn phenomenon (increase in blood glucose level that occurs in the hours before and after waking). Pump therapy requires a committed and motivated patient who is willing to test their blood glucose levels at least four times per day, keep blood glucose logs and food records, and learn the technical features of pump usage.[33]

Nutrition and Diabetes

Patients with diabetes have multiple defects in the metabolism of carbohydrates, proteins, and fats. Nurse Practitioners should be knowledgeable about evidence-based diabetes nutrition recommendations. Healthy eating messages can be reinforced to promote lifestyle modifications. The ADA recommends that each patient be given a nutrition prescription based on treatment goals, the patient's metabolic profile, known strategies that would assist the patient in meeting these treatment goals, and most importantly, tailored messages based on changes the patient is willing and able to make.[34,35]

Nutrition Therapy

The primary goal of nutrition therapy for patients with diabetes mellitus is to attain and maintain optimal metabolic outcomes.[35–37] This includes:

- Blood glucose levels in the normal range to the greatest extent possible to prevent the complications of diabetes.
- A lipid and lipoprotein profile that reduces the risk for cardiovascular diseases.
- A blood pressure level that reduces the risk for vascular diseases.

Nutrition therapy for diabetes is guided by evidence-based recommendations based on the best available scientific evidence while taking into account patient circumstances, cultural and ethnic concerns, and involving the patient in decision-making.[36,38,39] Understanding the expected outcomes from nutrition therapy as well as evaluating the best implementation approach can assist Nurse Practitioners in the clinical decision-making process. If treatment goals are not being achieved by life-style interventions (nutrition therapy and physical activity), changes in medication(s) are required.

Clinical trials and outcome studies support nutrition therapy as an effective method to reach diabetes treatment goals.[35,36] The American Dietetic Association Evidence-Based Nutrition Practice Guidelines (EBNPG) documented decreases in A1C of 1–2% (range: −0.5% to −2.6%) with nutrition therapy depending on the type and duration of diabetes.[36,40] These outcomes are similar to those from glucose-lowering medications.[34,36] Nutrition therapy includes various types of nutrition interventions and requires multiple encounters in order to provide education and counseling on an ongoing basis.[34,36–38] Nurse Practitioners play a key role by obtaining a baseline diet history from all patients during the comprehensive diabetes assessment to determine what nutritional needs are present, and when appropriate, to refer to a registered dietitian. Table 9-7 highlights important diet history questions to include in the comprehensive diabetes assessment.

Nutrition and Insulin Therapy

The primary goal of dietary management in patients using insulin is to provide optimal nutrient intake while maintaining target glycemic goals and minimizing the occurrence of hypoglycemia. It is important for Nurse Practitioners to assist patients requiring insulin therapy to integrate an insulin regimen into their lifestyle. After the initial food/meal plan is determined by the registered dietitian (with the patient's input), it should be reviewed with the Nurse Practitioner in order to plan the insulin regimen. Today, the many insulin options available make it easier to select an insulin regimen that will conform to the patient's preferred meal times and food choices. Flexible insulin regimens using basal (background) insulin and bolus (mealtime) insulin or insulin pumps give patients freedom in the timing and composition of meals and are the preferred mode of therapy to maximize blood glucose control and minimize complications.[41]

The total amount of carbohydrate in the meal (and snacks, if desired) is the major determinant of the bolus rapid-acting insulin dose and post-prandial glucose response. After determining the amount of insulin required to manage the

Table 9-7 Nurse Practitioner Comprehensive Diabetes Assessment

---

Medical History
- History of diabetes (type, years of duration).
- History of diabetes-related complications (retinopathy, nephropathy, neuropathy, sexual dysfunction, gastric disorders, cardiovascular disease, cerebrovascular disease, and peripheral vascular disease).
- For females: history of polycystic ovarian syndrome, and gestational diabetes.
- History of diabetes emergency hospitalizations (severe hypoglycemia, DKA, HHS).
- Diabetes self-management education.
- History of mental disorders (major depression, etc.).
- All medications.

Nutrition History
- Height, weight, calculate BMI.
- Physical activity.
- Alcohol consumption.
- Smoking history.
- History of eating disorders.

Key Nutrition Assessment Questions
- At what times do you take your diabetes medications (including insulin)?
- At what times do you eat your meals and snacks?
- Do you ever skip meals during the day?
- How many servings of starchy foods such as breads, cereals, rice, pasta, corn, peas, or beans do you eat during a typical day?

Physical Examination
- Vital signs.
- Fundoscopic examination.
- Thyroid palpation.
- Skin examination (insulin injection sites, diabetic blisters, acanthois nigrican, itchy skin, etc.).
- Comprehensive foot exam.

Laboratory Evaluation
- Hemoglobin A1C.
- Lipid profile (HDL, LDL, triglycerides).
- Liver function tests.
- Kidney function tests (microalbuminemia and serum creatinine).

Source: Neva White, DNP, MSN, CRNP, CDE and Lisa Hark PhD, RD, 2012. Used with permission.

When to Refer to a Registered Dietitian

- Newly diagnosed patient with pre-diabetes or diabetes.
- Weight management concerns are present.
- There is a need to learn basic or advanced carbohydrate counting.
- The patient is requesting comprehensive nutrition education.

---

patient's usual meal carbohydrate intake, patients can be taught how to adjust bolus insulin doses based on the amount of carbohydrate they are planning to eat (insulin-to-carbohydrate ratio).[42,43] Consistency of day-to-day carbohydrate amount at meals is important for patients receiving fixed insulin regimens and for those not adjusting mealtime insulin doses.

Case 1

Deiana is a 64-year-old African American female who has had type 2 diabetes for 7 years. She retired last year from teaching high school for 30 years. She has experienced a difficult past 3 months with the death of her husband of 40 years. She presents at the clinic with an A1C of 9.2%. She is very unhappy because her A1C has been under 7% in the past. She is asking for menus, shopping lists, and any other help she can get to improve her eating habits.

APPROACH: Advise Deiana to complete a 3-day food and beverage diary to assess her eating patterns and work collaboratively with you to develop a plan for healthy eating. Refer Deiana to a diabetes self-management education class. Consider referring Deiana to a dietitian for a comprehensive nutrition assessment and follow-up counseling as indicated. If these interventions are not successful, carbohydrate counting may be an option.

Nutrition treatment guidelines for type 2 diabetes are often based on glycemic control as lifestyle modifications have an immediate impact on glucose concentrations. However, control of lipid levels and blood pressure goals are equally important (Chapter 8).[34] As patients move from being insulin resistant to insulin deficient, the goal of nutrition therapy shifts from weight loss to control of glucose, lipid, and blood pressure levels. Although moderate weight loss may be beneficial for some insulin resistant patients, for those with significant loss of beta-cell function, weight loss alone will not improve hyperglycemia.[36] The progressive nature of type 2 diabetes demands ongoing changes in both medication(s) and nutrition therapy. The two primary metabolic abnormalities in type 2 diabetes are insulin resistance (deficient response to insulin) and beta-cell failure (impairment in insulin secretion).[3,9]

Several strategies have been shown to improve health outcomes in patients with diabetes: teaching patients how to make appropriate food choices, often through the use of carbohydrate counting; increased physical activity; and using data from SMBG to evaluate glycemic control. These strategies should be implemented as soon as the diagnosis of diabetes is made. Some studies demonstrate that a modest amount of weight loss decreases metabolic abnormalities in some patients.[36] Weight loss, especially of intra-abdominal fat, reduces insulin resistance and helps correct dyslipidemias in the short-term (in weight loss studies involving subjects with type 2 diabetes). However, weight loss appears to plateau at 6 months and may be more difficult for patients with diabetes.[38] Furthermore, the American Dietetic Association's Evidence-Based Nutrition Practice Guidelines for diabetes indicates decreasing energy intake may improve glycemic control, though it is unclear whether weight loss alone will improve glycemic control, as sustained weight loss interventions lasting one year or longer report inconsistent effects on A1C. Therefore, it is recommended that if weight loss is a goal for patients with diabetes who are overweight or obese, glycemic control should be the primary focus.[36]

Carbohydrate Counting

Teaching patients with diabetes how to make appropriate food choices (usually by means of carbohydrate counting) and using data from blood glucose monitoring to evaluate short-term effectiveness are important components of successful nutrition therapy for type 2 diabetes (Table 9-8). Carbohydrate counting is useful in the management of all types of diabetes. However, instead of grouping foods into six lists as in the exchange system, it groups foods into three categories: carbohydrate, meat and meat substitutes, and fat. The carbohydrate list is composed of starches, starchy vegetables, fruits, milk, and sweets; one serving is the amount of food that contains 15 g of carbohydrate.[43] Learning how to read and understand nutrient facts on food labels is also useful. Additional recommendations for management of carbohydrate intake are shown in Table 9-9.

Many patients with type 2 diabetes also have dyslipidemia and hypertension, so decreasing intake of saturated fat, cholesterol, and sodium should also be a priority.

Table 9-8 Carbohydrate Counting (One Serving Contains 15 g of Carbohydrate)

Starch	Milk
1 slice of toast (1 oz)	1 cup low-fat milk
1/3 cup cooked pasta or rice	2/3 cup "lite" fruited yogurt (sweetened with non-nutritive sweetener) (6 oz)
4–6 crackers	
3/4 cup dry cereal	
1/2 small sweet potato with skin	
3/4 oz chips (unsalted)	
Fruit	**Sweets and desserts**
1 small fresh fruit (4 oz)	2 small cookies
1/2 banana	1 tablespoon jam, honey, syrup, table sugar
1/2 cup fruit juice (orange, apple)	1/2 cup ice cream, frozen yogurt, or sherbet

Source: Lisa Hark PhD, RD, 2012. Used with permission.

Table 9-9 Additional Recommendations for Management of Carbohydrate Intake

- In patients on nutrition therapy alone or when combined with glucose-lowering medications or fixed insulin doses, meal (and snack) carbohydrates should be kept consistent on a day-to-day basis, as consistency in carbohydrate intake has been shown to result in improved glycemic control. In patients with type 1 or type 2 diabetes who adjust their mealtime insulin or who are on insulin pump therapy, insulin doses should be adjusted to match carbohydrate intake.
- Recommendations for fiber intake are similar to recommendations for the general public (DRI: 14 g/1000 kcal per day). Diets containing 44–50 g of fiber per day are reported to improve glycemic control; however, more typical fiber intakes (up to 24 g/day) have not shown beneficial effects on glycemia. Diets high in total and soluble fiber, as part of cardioprotective nutrition therapy, have been shown to reduce total cholesterol by 2–3% and LDL-C up to 7%.
- If patients with diabetes choose to eat foods containing sucrose, the sucrose-containing foods should be substituted for other carbohydrate foods. Sucrose intakes of 10–35% of total energy intake do not have a negative effect on glycemic or lipid responses when substituted for isocaloric amounts of starch.
- Non-nutritive sweeteners and sugar alcohols are safe when consumed within the accepted daily intake levels established by the Food and Drug Administration. Some of these products, however, may contain energy and carbohydrate from other sources.
- Eating a minimum of five servings of vegetables and fruits daily is recommended for both prevention and treatment of high blood pressure.

Source: Bantle[34] Wheeler,[42] Franz.[36]

Case 2

Carlos is a 25-year-old, single, Hispanic male with type 1 diabetes. He is taking a 75/25 pre-mixed insulin dose in the morning and evening. He is currently struggling with late morning and overnight hypoglycemic episodes. He is not sure why this is happening. He does report a change in his work schedule from an all day shift to working mostly evenings and night shift.

APPROACH: Consider a more individualized physiologic insulin regimen (basal bolus pattern) to avoid hypoglycemia. Ask Carlos to complete a 3-day food and beverage diary to assess his eating patterns and modify his eating habits as needed to avoid hypoglycemia. It is critical to incorporate lifestyle and eating pattern consideration in Carlos's plan of care to avoid hypoglycemia. Carlos will require basic carbohydrate counting training. Refer Carlos to a registered dietitian for a comprehensive nutrition assessment and follow-up counseling as indicated. Refer Carlos to a diabetes self-management education class.

The sooner lifestyle strategies are implemented after diabetes is diagnosed, the greater the opportunity to prevent the chronic complications of the disorder.[34,36-39,44]

Researchers followed 37,083 men in the Health Professionals Follow-Up Study, 79,570 women in the Nurses' Health Study, and 87, 504 women in the Nurses' Health Study II over 10 or more years. After all collected data was analyzed with adjustments for age, body mass index (BMI), and other lifestyle and dietary risk factors, researchers found that consumption of a 50 g daily serving of processed meat (equivalent to one hot dog or two strips of bacon) was associated with 51% increase in diabetes incidence. They also found that protein from other sources such as nuts, seeds and whole grains will have the reverse effect.[45] In another study conducted at St Michael's Hospital and the University of Toronto, researchers reported that the daily consumption of 2 oz of nuts helped to control patients' type 2 diabetes via glycemic and serum lipid control and reduction of LDL-cholesterol. Patients measuring their blood glucose levels with the A1C test found a two-thirds reduction in their A1C when replacing some carbohydrates in their diet with nuts. Expected outcomes with effective nutrition therapy is shown in Table 9-10.

Nutrition Fact Label

Understanding food labels is essential to practical meal planning. Nurse Practitioners can provide the patient with a basic overview of the food label with a particular focus on serving size, total calories, and carbohydrates. Referral to a registered dietitian is useful to provide more comprehensive instruction when needed.

My Plate

Nurse Practitioners may advise patients to incorporate the use of a divided plate to aid in portion size control. The plate is divided into four sections: vegetables, proteins, grains, and fruit (Figure 9-1). One half of the plate is used for non-starch vegetables, one quarter for starches and starchy vegetables and the remaining one quarter for lean meat or protein.[46]

Table 9-10 Effectiveness of Nutrition Therapy

Endpoint	Expected Outcome	When to Evaluate
A1C	1–2% decrease	6 weeks to 3 months
Plasma fasting Glucose	50–100 mg/dL (2.78–5.56 mmol/L) decrease	
Lipids		
Total cholesterol	24–32 mg/dL (0.62–0.82 mmol/L) decrease	6 weeks; if goals are not achieved, intensify nutrition therapy and evaluate again in 6 weeks
LDL-C	19–25 mg/L (0.46–0.65 mmol/L) decrease	
Triglycerides	15–17 mg/dL (0.17–0.19 mmol/L) decrease	
HDL-C	With no exercise: no change With exercise: 7% increase	
Blood pressure	5 mmHg decrease in systolic 2 mmHg decrease in diastolic	Measure at every visit

Source: CDC.[2]

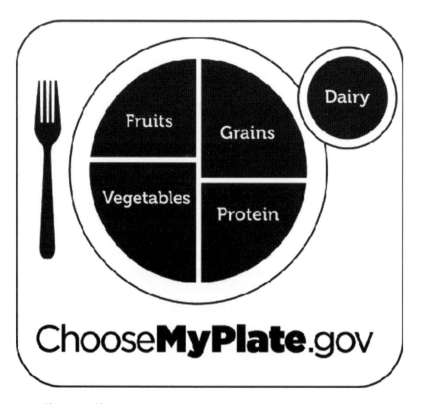

Figure 9-1 Choose My Plate
Source: http://choosemyplate.gov 2012[46]

Alcohol

Recommendations for alcohol intake among patients with well-controlled diabetes are similar to those for the general public. If patients choose to drink, alcoholic beverage consumption should be limited to no more than two drinks per day for men and no more than one drink per day for women.[34] One drink is defined as 12 oz of beer, 5 oz of wine, or 1.5 oz of distilled spirits, each of which contains approximately 15 g of alcohol.[36] For patients using insulin or insulin secretagogues, alcohol should be consumed with food to reduce the risk of hypoglycemia. Occasional use of alcoholic beverages should be considered an addition to the regular meal plan, and no food should be omitted.[34]

Moderate amounts of alcohol, when ingested with food, have minimal acute effects on glucose and insulin concentrations and light to moderate alcohol intake (one to two drinks per day) is associated with a decreased risk of CVD. The type of alcohol-containing beverage does not make a difference. On the other hand, excessive amounts of alcohol (three or more drinks per day), on a consistent basis, contribute to hyperglycemia, hypertension, and other medical conditions, as well as increase the risk of episodes of hypoglycemia due to changes in caloric intake patterns and diminished glycogen storage by the liver.[36]

Treatment of Hypoglycemia

Any available carbohydrate-containing food will raise glucose levels, including glucose tablets, sucrose, juice, non-diet soda, and syrup. Glucose is the preferred treatment, and commercially available glucose tablets have the advantage of being pre-measured to help prevent over-treatment. Treatment begins with 15–20 g of carbohydrate and an initial response should be seen in approximately 10–20 minutes.[41] Blood glucose should be evaluated again in approximately 60 minutes as additional treatment may be necessary. Adding protein has no benefit in treatment or preventing subsequent hypoglycemia.[36] Severe hypoglycemia (the patient is unable to ingest oral carbohydrate) requires intravenous glucose or the administration of glucagon. For insulin users, prevention of hypoglycemia is a critical component of diabetes management. Not all patients are equally aware of these hypoglycemic episodes. This variability in awareness impacts glycemic target goals, patient education, and management strategies.[47]

Health Maintenance Recommendations

- A1C every 6 months in well-controlled diabetes; every 3–4 months in patients not meeting treatment goals.
- Annual lipid panel.
- Blood pressure (at each office visit).
- Annual dilated eye examination.
- Annual kidney function test.
- Anti-platelet therapy as recommended.
- Dental examination every 6 months.
- Annual comprehensive foot examination.
- Annual vaccine (influenza, pneumoccocal as indicated).
- Smoking cessation.
- Depression screening.

Physical Activity

Regular physical activity improves blood glucose control and insulin sensitivity independent of weight loss.[9,36,38] In addition, physical activity reduces CVD risk factors, improves well-being, and is important for long-term weight maintenance.[38] Physical activity should be an integral part of the treatment plan for patients with diabetes. Exercise helps improve insulin sensitivity, reduce cardiovascular risk factors, control weight, and improve well-being. Patients with diabetes can exercise safely, but since diabetics are at significant risk for underlying CVD, consideration should be given to assessing exercise tolerance in this population. The exercise plan will vary depending on age, general health, and level of physical fitness. As demonstrated in the Diabetes Prevention Program (DPP), a minimum of 150 min/week of moderate intensity aerobic physical activity (50–70% of heart rate) is advised.[36] In the absence of contraindications, resistance training three times per week should be encouraged. Patients taking insulin or insulin secretagogues should monitor their blood glucose and take appropriate precautions to avoid hypoglycemia. Carbohydrates should be eaten if pre-exercise glucose levels are less than 100 mg/dL (5.6 mmol/L).[48,49] Based on the evidence, structured programs are recommended that emphasize lifestyle changes including education, reduced fat and calorie intake, regular physical activity, and regular participant contact. Such programs can produce long-term weight loss of 5–7% of baseline weight and reduce the risk of developing diabetes.[49-53]

Nutrition Recommendations for the Prevention of Diabetes

The increase in diabetes worldwide has made prevention of type 2 diabetes a high priority. Patients with pre-diabetes (A1C: 5.7–6.4%) are at risk for the development of diabetes and cardiovascular disease. The Finnish Diabetes Prevention Study and the Diabetes Prevention Program in the United States investigated the effects of lifestyle interventions on the prevention of diabetes in those at high-risk (impaired glucose tolerance).[49,50] In both studies, the incidence of diabetes was reduced by 58% in the intensive lifestyle intervention group. In a 7-year follow-up of participants in the Finnish Diabetes Study, after the first four years of an active lifestyle intervention, those still undiagnosed with diabetes reported continuing lifestyle changes and experienced a 43% lower diabetes risk.[49]

The DPP demonstrated that patients at high-risk for diabetes could delay or avoid developing type 2 diabetes through lifestyle interventions that included regular physical activity and eating a diet low in fat and calories that resulted in weight loss.[50] Both men and women benefited from the lifestyle interventions. Lifestyle modifications were most beneficial for participants age 60 and over. An estimated 5% of participants in the intervention group developed diabetes compared with 11% in the placebo group. Moderate physical activity of 150 minutes per week was the goal.

Several trials have tested how efficacious specific drugs (i.e. metformin, acarbose, orlistat, rosiglitazone) would be in the prevention of diabetes.[49-51] Each decreased the incidence of diabetes by various degrees. Based on cost and side effects, the ADA recommends that only metformin in combination with lifestyle counseling be considered in those who are at very high risk (combined IFG and IGT plus other risk factors) and who are obese and under 60 years of age.

Community Efforts

Managing chronic diseases such as diabetes requires a comprehensive approach that extends beyond traditional primary care. The focus must include community resources and attention to policies that support prevention, education, and patient motivation.[54] Socio-ecological models provide a framework for managing chronic diseases and focus on patient needs, such as community systems and policies that support healthy lifestyles.[55,56] Quality long-term diabetes management requires an integrated, comprehensive, whole system approach to care that serves the needs of both patients and health care professionals. The Chronic Care Model (CCM) for Obesity (Chapter 7) is geared to clinically oriented systems and is difficult to use for population disease prevention and health promotion efforts. The Expanded Chronic Care Model has been developed to integrate prevention and health promotion into the CCM. This model includes the six basic components of the CCM (community resources, health organization, self-management support, delivery system design, decision support, and clinical information systems) and integrates population health prevention efforts, social determinants of health, and community participation as factors that need to be considered by health systems in order to comprehensively address prevention and management of diabetes and its related co-morbidities.[57]

Diabetes management requires an integrated whole system approach designed to promote collaborative interactions and patient self-efficacy through education, motivation, and support. Nurse Practitioners must be aware of, promote, and partici-pate in community efforts as well as practice-based programs and interventions that address diabetes prevention and management.

Key Community Resources

Whole system approaches to care include input from the patient, provider, health care system, and other stakeholders that exist within the community. It is important that the Nurse Practitioner link patients to needed community resources, that may include:

- Access to quality, affordable, and healthy food.
- Safe and convenient places to walk.
- Adequate and accessible transportation.
- Affordable exercise programs.
- Access to affordable medication and diabetes care supplies.

Patient Education Resources

www.diabetes.org (American Diabetes Association)
www.americanheart.org (American Heart Association)
www.dLife.com (Diabetes Life)
www.eatright.org (American Dietetic Association)
www.ndep.nih.gov (National Diabetes Education Program)
www.platemethod.com
www.diabeteseducator.org (American Association of Diabetes Educators)
http://nnlm.gov/outreach/consumer/hlthlit.html (National Network of Libraries of Medicine)
www.divabetic.org

Key Resources for Nurse Practitioners

The following list of guidelines can assist Nurse Practitioners in the management of patients with diabetes:

- ADA Standards of Medical Care in Diabetes
- American Association of Clinical Endocrinologists (AACE) medical guidelines for clinical practices for developing a diabetes mellitus comprehensive care plan
- Veterans Health Administration/US Department of Defense (VA/DOD)
- American Association of Diabetes Educators (www.diabeteseducator.org)

References

1. US Department of Health and Human Services. *Healthy People 2020.* http://healthypeople.gov/
2. Centers for Disease Control and Prevention. *National Diabetes Fact Sheet: General Information and Nations Estimates of Diabetes in the United States, 2011.* Department of Health and Human Services, Atlanta, GA.
3. American Diabetes Association. Diagnosis and classification of diabetes mellitus (Position Statement). *Diabetes Care* 2011;34:S62–S69.
4. American Diabetes Association. Standards of medical care in diabetes–2010 (Position Statement). *Diabetes Care* 2012;35(Suppl 1):S11–S63.
5. Handelsman Y, Mechanick J, Blonde L, et al. American Association of Clinical Endocrinologists medical guidelines for clinical practice for developing a diabetes mellitus comprehensive care plan. *Endocr Pract* 2011;17(Suppl 2):1–53.
6. Nathan DM, Davidson MB, DeFronzo RA, et al. Impaired fasting glucose and impaired glucose tolerance: implications for care. *Diabetes Care* 2007;30:753–759.
7. Olson DE, Rhee MK, Herrick K, et al. Screening for diabetes and pre-diabetes with proposed A1C-based diagnostic criteria. *Diabetes Care* 2010;33:2184–2189.
8. The Writing Group for the Search for Diabetes in Youth Study Group. Incidence of diabetes in youth in the United States. *JAMA* 2007;297:2716–2724.
9. Kahn, S. The relative contributions of insulin resistance and beta-cell dysfunction to the pathophysiology of type 2 diabetes. *Diabetologia* 2003;46:3–19.
10. American Diabetes Association. Gestational Diabetes Mellitus. *Diabetes Care* 2004;27:S88–S90.
11. Diabetes Control and Complications Trial Research Group. The effect of intensive treatment of diabetes on the development and progression of long-term complications in insulin-dependent diabetes mellitus. *N Engl J Med* 1993;329:977–986.
12. The Diabetes Control and Complications Trial/Epidemiology of Diabetes Interventions and Complications (DCCT/EDIC) Study Research Group. Intensive diabetes treatment and cardiovascular disease in patients with type 1 diabetes. *N Engl J Med* 2005;353:2643–2653.
13. UK Prospective Diabetes Study Group: Tight blood pressure control and risk of macrovascular and microvascular complications in type 2 diabetes (UKPDS 38). *BMJ* 1998;317:703–713.
14. Donner T, Munoz M. Update on insulin therapy for Type 2 Diabetes. *J Clin Endocrin Met* 2012;97:1405–1413.
15. Funnel M, Brown T, Childs B, et al. National standards for diabetes self management education. *Diabetes Care* 2011:S89–S96.
16. Franz MJ. Lifestyle interventions across the continuum of type 2 diabetes: reducing the risks of diabetes. *Am J Lifestyle Med* 2007;1:327–334.
17. Siminerio L, Drab S, Gabbay R. AADE position statement: diabetes educators: implementing the chronic care model. *Diabetes Educ* 2008;34:451–456.

18. American Association of Diabetes Educators. AADE 7 self-care behaviors. *Diabetes Educator* 2008;34:445–449.
19. Becker M, Janz N. The health belief model applied to understanding diabetes regime compliance. *Diabetes Educ* 1985;11:41–47.
20. Rodbard HW, Jellinger PS, Davidson J, et al. American Association of Clinical Endocrinologists/American College of Endocrinology consensus panel on type 2 diabetes mellitus: an algorithm for glycemic control. *Endocrine Practice* 2009;15:540–559.
21. Polonsky W, Fisher L, Schikman C, et al. Structured self-monitoring of blood glucose significantly reduces A1C levels in poorly controlled, noninsulin-treated type 2 diabetes: results from the structured testing program study. *Diabetes Care* 2011;34:262–267.
22. Deiss D, Bolinder J, Riveline J. Improved glycemic control in poorly controlled patients with type 1 diabetes using real-time continous glucose monitoring. *Diabetes Care* 2006;29:2730–2732.
23. Halford J, Harris C. Determining clinical and psychological benefits and barriers with continuous glucose monitoring therapy. *Diab Tech Therapeutics* 2010;12:201–2.
24. Saudek C, Derr R, Kalvani R. Assessing glycemia in diabetes using self-monitoring blood glucose and hemoglobin A1c. *JAMA* 2006;295:1688–1697.
25. Nathan D, Kuenenm J, Borg R. Translating the A1C assay into estimated average glucose values. *Diabetes Care* 2008;31:1473–1478.
26. American Heart Association Scientific Statement. Managing abnormal blood lipids-a collaborative approach. *Circulation* 2005;112:3184–3209.
27. Mensing C. *The Art and Science of Diabetes Self-Management Education Desk Reference*, 2nd edition. American Association of Diabetes Educators, 2011.
28. American Diabetes Association. Insulin. *Diabetes Forecast 2010 Resource Guide* 2010;Jan:RG11-RG14.
29. Nathan D, Buse J, Davidson M, et al. American Diabetes Association, European Association for Study of Diabetes. Medical management of hyperglycemia in type 2 diabetes: a consensus algorithm for the initiation and adjustment of therapy: a consensus statement of the American Diabetes Association and the European for the Study of Diabetes. *Diabetes Care* 2009;32:193–203.
30. Fatourechi MM, Kudva YC, Murad MH, et al. Hypoglycemia with intensive insulin therapy: a systematic review and meta-analyses of randomized trials of continuous subcutaneous insulin infusion versus multiple daily injections. *J Clin Endocrinol Metab* 2009;94:729–740.
31. Rodbard D. Pharmacologic therapies: glucose management. In: Mensing C (Ed.), *The Art and Science of Diabetes: Self-Management Education Desk Reference*, 2nd Edition. American Association of Diabetes Educators, 2011.
32. Brunton S. Initiating insulin therapy in type 2 diabetes: benefits of insulin analogs and insulin pens. *Diab Tech Ther* 2008;10:247–256.
33. Pickup J, Renard E. Long-Acting insulin analogs versus insulin pump therapy for the treatment of type 1 and type 2 diabetes. *Diabetes Care* 2008;31:S140–S145.
34. Bantle JP, Wylie-Rosett J, Albright AL, et al. Nutrition recommendations and interventions for diabetes. A position statement of the American Diabetes Association. *Diabetes Care* 2008;31(Suppl 1):S61–S78.
35. Morris SF, Wylie-Rosett J. Medical nutrition therapy: a key to diabetes management and prevention. *Clinical Diabetes* 2010;28:12–18.
36. Franz MJ, Powers MA, Leontos C. The evidence for medical nutrition therapy for type 1 and type 2 diabetes in adults. *J Am Diet Assoc* 2010;110:1852–1889.
37. Franz MJ, Boucher JL, Green-Pastors J, Powers MA. Evidence-based nutrition practice guidelines for diabetes and scope and standards of practice. *J Am Diet Assoc* 2008;108(Suppl 1):S52–S58.

38. Franz MJ. The dilemma of weight loss in diabetes. *Diabetes Spectrum* 2007;20:133–136.
39. American Association of Diabetes Educators (AADE). Position statement: cultural sensitivity and diabetes education; recommendations for diabetes educators. *Diabetes Educ* 2007; 33:41–44.
40. American Dietetic Association Evidence Analysis Library Web site. Diabetes 1 and 2 Evidence Analysis Project: Available from https://www.adaevidencelibrary.com.
41. Samman A, Muhlhauser I, Bender R, Kloos C, Müller UA. Glycaemic control and severe hypoglycaemia following training in flexible, intensive insulin therapy to enable dietary freedom in patients with type 1 diabetes: a prospective implementation study. *Diabetologia* 2005; 48:1965–1970.
42. Kirk JK, Graves DE, Craven TE, et al. Restricted-carbohydrate diets in patients with type 2 diabetes: a meta-analysis. *J Am Diet Assoc* 2008;108:91–100.
43. Wheeler ML, Pi-Sunyer X. Carbohydrate issues: type and amount. *J Am Diet Assoc* 2008; 108(Suppl 1):S34–S39.
44. Pritchette L. Nutrition care process and model: ADA adopts roadmap to quality care and outcomes management. *J Am Diet Assoc* 2003;103:1061–1072.
45. Pan A, Sun Q, Berstein AM, et al. Red meat consumption and risk of type 2 diabetes: 3 cohorts of US adults and an updated meta-analysis. *Am J Clin Nutr* 2011 [Epub ahead of print].
46. US Department of Agriculture. *MyPlate*. http://www.choosemyplate.gov
47. Cox DJ, Gonder-Fredrick L, Ritterband L, Clarke W, Kovatchev BP. Prediction of severe hypoglycemia. *Diabetes Care* 2007;30:1370–1373.
48. Briscoe VJ, Tate DB, Davis SN. Type 1 diabetes: exercise and hypoglycemia. *Appl Physiol Nutr Metab* 2007;32:576–582.
49. Lindström J, Ilanne-Parikka P, Peltonen M, et al. on behalf of the Finnish Diabetes Prevention Study Group. Sustained reduction in the incidence of type 2 diabetes by lifestyle intervention: follow-up of the Finnish Diabetes Prevention Study. *Lancet* 2006;368:1673–1679.
50. Knowler WC, Barrett-Connor E, Fowler SE, et al. Diabetes Prevention Program Research Group. Reduction in the incidence of type 2 diabetes with lifestyle intervention or metformin. *N Engl J Med* 2002;346:393–403.
51. Knowler WC, Fowler SE, Hamman RF, et al. Diabetes Prevention Program Research Group. Ten-year follow-up of diabetes incidence and weight loss in the Diabetes Prevention Program Outcomes Study. *Lancet* 2009;374:1677–1686.
52. Look AHEAD Research Group. Reduction in weight and cardiovascular disease risk factors in patients with type 2 diabetes. *Diabetes Care* 2007;30:1374–1383.
53. Wadden TA, West DS, Neiberg RH, et al., the Look AHEAD Research Group. One-year weight losses in the Look AHEAD study: factors associated with success. *Obesity* 2009;17: 713–722.
54. Ratner R. Diabetes management in the age of national health reform. *Diabetes Care* 2011; 34:1054–1057.
55. Siminerio L, Piatt G, Zgibor J. Implementing the chronic care model for improvements in diabetes care and education in a rural primary care practice. *Diabetes Educ* 2005:225–234.
56. Funnell MM, Brown TL, Childs BP, et al. National standards for diabetes self-management education. *Diabetes Care* 2012;35: Suppl 1:S101–108.
57. Barr VJ, Robinson S, Marin-Link B, et al. The expanded chronic care model: an integration of concepts and strategies from population health promotion and the chronic care model, Vancouver health Authority. *Hosp Q* 2003;7:73–82.

10 Digestive Disorders and Gastrointestinal Care

Julie Vanderpool, RD, MPH, RN, MSN, ACNP
Beth-Ann Norton, MS, RN, ANP-BC

OBJECTIVES

- To increase the knowledge base of Nurse Practitioners on the role of nutrition in gastrointestinal diseases.

- To incorporate nutrition into the medical history, review of systems, and physical examination of patients with gastrointestinal diseases.

- To identify the causes of malnutrition in inflammatory bowel disease, liver diseases, and malabsorption syndrome.

- To describe why sodium and fluid restriction may be necessary for patients with liver disease.

- To explain the association between diet and lower esophageal sphincter pressure in patients with gastroesophageal reflux disease.

Introduction

Digestive disorders are often complex illnesses requiring a multi-faceted approach. Rarely is there one solution that will work for all patients. In addition to medical treatment of the underlying disease, nutrition therapy can improve gastrointestinal (GI) symptoms. The impact of dietary manipulations, such as dietary fiber in irritable bowel syndrome or a gluten-free diet in celiac disease, demonstrates the intricate role that nutrition therapy plays in the management of chronic digestive disorders. GI complaints, even seemingly mild, can negatively impact patients' quality of life. Nurse Practitioners often evaluate and treat digestive disorders, and patients seek care for various symptoms from food intolerances to chronic digestive diseases. Nurse Practitioners must determine whether symptoms such as abdominal pain, nausea, and altered bowel habits are caused by dietary intolerance, underlying GI pathology, or anxiety. The role of Nurse Practitioners is to differentiate between more benign versus potentially life-threatening GI symptoms. Once a diagnosis is found, the patient becomes a partner in the management of his/her GI problem. Management of these disorders frequently includes some degree of dietary manipulation. Some dietary guidelines, such as a diet rich in whole grain foods, can be useful across the

The Nurse Practitioner's Guide to Nutrition, Second Edition. Edited by Lisa Hark, Kathleen Ashton and Darwin Deen.
© 2012 John Wiley & Sons, Inc. Published 2012 by John Wiley & Sons, Inc.

spectrum of most GI symptoms, whereas certain disorders require specific nutritional modifications. Nurse Practitioners with a strong understanding of the role of nutrition in GI illnesses will be well suited to optimize disease management and improve patients' quality of life.

Digestion and Absorption

Nutrient digestion requires a controlled process of mechanical and chemical break-down, with subsequent enzymatic and secretory responses that facilitate nutrient absorption. Carbohydrate digestion requires adequate amylase to convert starches into disaccharides, which then undergo further hydrolysis into monosaccharides. Monosaccharides are absorbed through a process of either diffusion or active transport. Dietary fats require the action of lipase which results in the hydrolysis of free fatty acids from triglycerides. Once hydrolyzed, monoglycerides, glycerol, and fatty acids, as well as fat-soluble vitamins, undergo emulsification by bile acids in order to promote diffusion across the cell membrane of the enterocyte. Protein digestion requires adequate gastric acidity which activates pepsin and other proteases allowing breakdown of proteins into peptides and amino acids.[1] Defects in any of the mechanical, chemical, or secretory processes involved in digestion can result in nutrient maldigestion and malabsorption.

Malabsorption

Inadequate nutrient absorption can occur as a result of many diseases of the digestive system. In order effectively to treat the symptoms of malabsorption, one must first identify the cause, after which appropriate treatment can be implemented. The management of disorders of carbohydrate, protein, and fat malabsorption can often be improved with appropriate nutrition therapy.

Carbohydrate Malabsorption

Lactose intolerance is the most common form of carbohydrate malabsorption and has been estimated to affect approximately 70% of the world's population.[2] Lactose is a disaccharide sugar that requires hydrolysis by the enzyme lactase into glucose and galactose for absorption. Lactose malabsorption or intolerance is usually caused by sub-optimal activity or deficiency of lactase. Characteristic symptoms of lactose intolerance include bloating, abdominal pain, flatulence, borborygmi, nausea, or diarrhea after consumption of dairy foods. These symptoms are caused by the passage of undigested lactose into the colon where it is metabolized by colonic bacteria, producing excess fluid and gas in the bowel. In some cases, individuals will have delayed GI motility possibly due to the result of methane production. These patients will often present with consti-pation.[2] The diagnosis of lactose intolerance can frequently be made by improvement or resolution of symptoms after temporary avoidance of dairy foods. It is sometimes necessary to confirm the diagnosis with a lactose tolerance test or lactose hydrogen breath test if symptom etiology is present as other GI disorders, such as irritable bowel syndrome, inflammatory bowel disease, or celiac sprue may be suspected.[2]

Lactase production naturally declines as one ages. Lactose expression on the mucosal surface of the human enterocyte is at its peak at 34 weeks gestation, and begins to decline within the first few months of life.[2] Thus, while lactase deficiency may be pathological in infants, it is normal in most teens and adults. Secondary lactase deficiency can occur as a result of certain GI disorders including bacterial overgrowth, mucosal injury, or inflammatory bowel diseases. Effective treatment of these underlying disorders may improve lactose tolerance.[3]

The prevalence of lactase deficiency among populations suggests a certain genetic predisposition. Lactose malabsorption occurs in approximately 5–20% of Caucasians, but may be as high as 50–80% in Latinos, 60–80% among African Americans and Ashkenazi Jews, and nearly 100% among Asians and American Indians.[4] Despite the high prevalence of lactose malabsorption, lactose free dairy foods and lactase supplements allow individuals with lactose intolerance to consume adequate dietary calcium from dairy foods.[5] For patients with lactose intolerance, the severity of symptoms is often related to the quantity of lactose consumed. Given high calcium and vitamin D content in dairy foods, all individuals, regardless of lactose malabsorption, should be encouraged to include the three servings of low-fat dairy foods in their diet every day. Lactose hydrolyzed products can be well tolerated. In addition, fermented dairy foods such as yogurt, fermented cheese, and fermented milk contain lactic acid bacteria which improve tolerance and results in decreased symptoms related to lactose malabsorption. There may be some benefit from probiotics in patients with lactose malabsorption, possibly because microbial lactase is present within lactic acid bacteria in the probiotics themselves; however, research is ongoing in this area.[2] In addition, non-dairy milk enriched with calcium, including soy, hemp, almond, and rice milk are good options for patients who are lactose intolerant. The following ingredients may not be well tolerated by persons with lactose intolerance:

• Whey or lactose.
• Non-fat milk solids, buttermilk, or malted milk.
• Margarine or sweet or sour cream.

Lactose intolerant patients who are unable to tolerate adequate intake of dairy foods should be encouraged to consume calcium-fortified foods or take a 1000 mg calcium supplement once a day to ensure adequate recommended intake. The DRI for men and women aged 19–50 is 800 mg/day and 1000 mg/day for those over 51 years of age.[6] Appendix T identifies the recommended daily intake of calcium for all age groups. Food sources of calcium are shown in Appendices G and H.

Protein Malabsorption

Celiac disease, also termed gluten intolerance, is a small bowel absorption disorder characterized by chronic inflammation of small bowel mucosa, villous atrophy, and crypt hyperplasia. It is caused by intolerance to gliadin, the protein fraction of wheat, rye, and barley in genetically predisposed individuals.[7] The prevalence of celiac disease is approximately 1% in the general US population. However, the disorder remains largely under-diagnosed. Frequently there are delays in diagnosis even after a patient seeks medical care for symptoms. Currently the only treatment for celiac disease is a life-long adherence to a gluten-free diet.[8] Disease presentation is variable and onset of celiac disease can occur at any age. Presenting symptoms of celiac disease can be GI in nature (diarrhea, weight loss, vomiting, abdominal pain, bloating, distension, anorexia, and constipation) or may be less specific and include iron deficiency anemia, folic acid or vitamin B_{12} deficiency, osteoporosis or osteomalacia, infertility, or elevated transaminases.[7]. Neurological symptoms, such as ataxia, have also been traced to gluten sensitivity.[9] In recent years "silent" celiac disease or "non-celiac" gluten sensitivity has been described. Patients may present with non-specific symptoms such as those associated with irritable bowel syndrome or headaches.

Testing for celiac disease should be pursued in patients with persistent GI symptoms, such as chronic diarrhea, malabsorption, weight loss, or abdominal distension. Testing should also be considered in patients with unexplained iron deficiency anemia, vitamin deficiencies, infertility, or elevated transaminases.[7] Recent research suggests a higher prevalence of celiac disease among patients with osteoporosis but conflicting data have been presented.[10] High-risk populations for celiac disease include those with autoimmune endocrinopathies, especially type 1 diabetes mellitus, first and second-degree relatives of persons with celiac disease, and Turner syndrome.[7] The diagnostic evaluation of celiac disease should occur while the patient is on a gluten-containing diet and should include serologic testing followed by a small bowel biopsy if serologic testing is positive. The NIH consensus statement on celiac disease recommends the IgA antihuman tissue transglutaminase (TTG) and IgA endomysial antibody immunofluorescence (EMA) tests to avoid false negative results in IgA deficient patients.[11] Positive results warrant small bowel biopsies for histologic confirmation. Recommendations for people with celiac disease are shown in Table 10-1.

Table 10-1 Key Recommendations for Celiac Disease

- Consultation with a registered dietitian specializing in celiac disease.
- Education about the disease.
- Lifelong adherence to a gluten-free diet.
- Identification and treatment of nutritional deficiencies.
- Access to an advocacy group.
- Continuous follow-up by a multidisciplinary team.

Clinical evaluation should include an assessment for vitamin and mineral deficiencies. Initial blood work should include liver function tests, serum iron or ferritin, serum or red blood cell folate, vitamin B_{12}, calcium, and vitamin D. A DEXA scan should also be considered in patients diagnosed with celiac disease to screen for osteoporosis. In addition, serum albumin levels should be tested, as low levels may reflect small bowel protein loss. Serum albumin can also serve as one component of the overall assessment of nutritional status and be used as a baseline to monitor improvement as treatment progresses.[12] Identified deficiencies should be replenished, but long-term supplementation is likely not required once the disease is under control. Annual evaluation of vitamin status should be done as deficiencies of folate and vitamin B_6 have been documented in patients on long-term gluten-free diets.[13]

The gluten-free diet excludes all foods containing wheat, rye, and barley. Recent evidence suggests that patients can safely consume small amounts of oat-containing foods and gluten-free labeled oatmeal; however, questions about safety remain with an oat-containing gluten-free diet.[14] Some patients report worsened GI symptoms

Table 10-2 Gluten-Free Diet Guidelines

Celiac disease, sometimes called gluten intolerance, is a disorder that prevents wheat products from being properly digested. Gluten is found in most grain products, including wheat, barley, and rye. The list below provides basic guidelines for a gluten-free diet. It is important to get additional education from a nutrition professional who specializes in celiac disease.

Allowed Foods:
- Grains/flours: rice, corn, soy, potato, tapioca, beans, garfava, sorghum, quinoa, millet, buckwheat, arrowroot, amaranth, tef, nut flours, pure uncontaminated oats, and flax.
- Plain meat, chicken, fish, fruits and vegetables do not contain gluten and can be safely consumed.

Foods NOT ALLOWED:
- Grains/flours: wheat (including durum, semolina, kamut, spelt), rye, barley, triticale in any form, graham, farina, matzoh, couscous, commercial oats are not recommended.
- Foods that often contain gluten: breading and coating mixes, broth or soup bases, communion wafers, croutons, imitation bacon or seafood, marinades or sauces, salad dressings, processed meats, self-basting poultry, soy sauce, stuffings, thickeners.

Additional Recommendation:
- Read ingredient lists on all food labels. The following list includes ingredients which may contain gluten: brown rice syrup, caramel color, dextrin, flour or cereal products, malt or malt flavoring, malt vinegar, modified food starch, soy sauce or soy sauce solids.
- Check with your pharmacist about gluten content of vitamins, medications and toothpaste.

Source: The Celiac Disease Foundation and the Gluten Intolerance Group.[16]

when including oats in the diet, although mucosal integrity is maintained.[14,15] Table 10-2 describes the principles of a gluten-free diet. Patients should be advised to look for the many "gluten-free" products which are increasingly available in supermarkets and natural foods stores.

After diagnosis, patients should always be referred to a registered dietitian for assessment of nutritional deficits, degree of malnutrition, and education on a gluten-free diet. In addition, information on patient resources and support groups should be provided, as listed in Table 10-3. Whole grains that can be safely included possibly in a gluten-free diet include rice, corn, buckwheat, millet, amaranth, quinoa, and gluten-free oats. A recent study examining the nutritional quality of gluten-free diets demonstrated that despite adherence to dietary restrictions, diet quality was poor. The majority of women in the study consumed suboptimal intakes of whole grain foods, fiber, calcium, and iron. While men were more likely to consume adequate amounts of fiber and iron, diet choices remained low in calcium and whole grain foods.[17] It should be noted that while most wheat-based products in the US are fortified with vitamins and minerals, gluten-free products are usually not.[18] To improve diet quality, patients with celiac disease should be encouraged to consume 6–11 servings of whole grain or enriched gluten-free grains and three servings of gluten-free dairy foods per day. In addition, gluten-free vitamins are commercially available, and these may aid those with celiac disease in meeting daily vitamin and mineral requirements. Nurse Practitioners, in partnership with gastroenterologists and dietitians, should reinforce the need for life-long diet adherence to the gluten-free diet, particularly after symptom resolution.

Table 10-3 Patient Resources for Celiac Disease

- Celiac Sprue Association: www.csaceliacs.org or 1-877-CSA-4CSA. Non-profit organization that provides patient advocacy, gluten-free diet education, and links to national and local chapters/support groups.
- Celiac Disease Foundation: www.celiac.org. Nonprofit organization focusing on awareness, education, and advocacy about celiac disease.
- Gluten Intolerance Group of North America: www.gluten.net or 206-246-6652. Provides up-to-date information, education and support for patients and health care professionals.
- American Dietetic Association: www.eatright.org or 1-800-877-1600. National organization of registered dietitians and nutrition professionals.
- Celiac.com: www.celiac.com. Patient information website; includes gluten-free on-line store.
- Book: *Celiac Disease: A Hidden Epidemic* by Peter Green, MD and Rory Jones. Harper Collins Publishers, 2006.
- Book: *Celiac Disease Nutrition Guide* by Trisha Thompson, MS, RD. American Dietetic Association: 2nd edition, 2006.

Fat Malabsorption

Fat malabsorption is associated with many GI disorders and frequently presents with symptoms of steatorrhea. Fat malabsorption may occur in cases of impaired luminal transport of products of digestion, and is often seen in disorders causing widespread mucosal injury, such as celiac disease, inflammatory bowel disease, and bacterial overgrowth. In such cases, management of the underlying mucosal disorder is the treatment of choice. Steatorrhea can also be caused by maldigestion of fats, due to lipase deficiency or a lack of emulsification, as seen in chronic pancreatitis, cystic fibrosis, and bile salt deficiencies.[19] In addition, fat malabsorption can be seen in wasting syndromes, such as HIV wasting, or can be iatrogenic in nature, such as post-gastric bypass or extensive resection of the small bowel, particularly the terminal ileum.[20,21] Untreated fat malabsorption may result in weight loss, failure to thrive, osteomalacia, bone pain, infertility, dysmenorrhea, and amenorrhea. In addition, fat-soluble vitamin deficiencies (A, D, E, and K) may occur.

Adoption of a low-fat diet may aid in symptom management. Patients following a low-fat diet may have difficulty consuming adequate calories to maintain weight. Additional calories can be added to the diet with the use of medium chain triglycerides (MCT). These provide 115 calories per tablespoon. MCT oil is rapidly hydrolyzed and absorbed directly into portal circulation and therefore does not require bile salts or micelle formation for digestion. Factors limiting the use of MCT oil include poor palatability and possible side effects such as nausea and vomiting; therefore patients are typically unable to consume more than 3–4 tablespoons per day. Oral nutrition supplements with added MCT oil are commercially available and may provide some benefit. Unfortunately, these products tend to be very expensive and they are often not covered by medical insurance. For patients with pancreatic exocrine insufficiency, supplemental pancreatic enzymes may be necessary. Recent evidence suggests that patients with chronic pancreatitis may benefit from early screening for fat malabsorption. These patients may present with post-prandial abdominal pain resulting in reduced caloric intake even in the absence of clinically significant steatorrhea.[22] Conjugated bile acids may improve digestion of fat in patients with a history of ileal resection.

Fat malabsorption places patients at risk for vitamin and mineral deficiencies, specifically fat-soluble vitamins (vitamins A, D, E, and K). Monitoring for fat-soluble vitamin deficiencies should occur on an annual basis, with aggressive repletion as needed. Provision of fat-soluble vitamins in a water-miscible form may allow patients to have better vitamin absorption. Deficiencies of calcium, magnesium, zinc, and iron may also be present due to impaired absorption and increased intestinal losses and should be aggressively repleted.

Gastric Disorders

Gastroesophageal Reflux Disease (GERD)

Gastroesophageal reflux disease (GERD) is characterized by a burning sensation in the substernal area caused by abnormal reflux of acidic gastric contents into the esophagus. This condition has been reported to affect up to 20% of the population.[23] As many as one in seven persons may suffer from daily symptoms of "heartburn", which can negatively affect patients' quality of life.[24] Although the underlying causes of GERD are not known, the pathogenesis has been related to altered and intermittent relaxation of the lower esophageal sphincter. Over the long-term this can result in esophageal mucosal damage and erosion, and may increase risk of complications, such as peptic stricture, chronic esophagitis, Barrett's esophagus, and development of esophageal adenocarcinoma.[25]

Obesity is also considered a significant risk factor for development of GERD.[26] Increasing abdominal circumference is associated with increased intra-abdominal pressure and lower esophageal sphincter relaxation, which may contribute to the development of GERD.[25] The risk of GERD increases with increasing BMI.[24] Dietary factors have been evaluated as a cause of reflux disease. Although limited data are available, spicy foods, acidic foods, high-fat foods, chocolate, mint, alcohol, and caffeine (coffee, tea, cola) have been associated with GERD symptoms. High-fat intake, particularly saturated fat, has also been found to increase the risk of GERD.[27] High-fat foods or large meals delay gastric emptying time, which can lead to increased reflux of gastric contents.[28] There is some evidence that increasing dietary fiber may have a protective effect against reflux.[29] The mechanism is unclear, but may be related to fiber's role as a nitrite scavenger in the gut as nitrites have been implicated in contributing to a decrease in lower esophageal sphincter tone.[30]

Nutrition therapy for patients with GERD should be focused on minimizing reflux symptoms. Patients may have varying degrees of sensitivity to different high-risk foods. The goals of therapy should be to prevent relaxation of the lower esophageal sphincter, reduce volume of gastric acid, and prevent esophageal irritation. In addition, encouraging patients to increase gradually their intake of whole grain foods may reduce their reflux symptoms. Table 10-4 lists dietary recommendations for patients with GERD.

Peptic Ulcer Disease

The management of peptic ulcer disease (PUD) has changed significantly in recent decades. Early treatment of PUD included a bland diet as a mainstay of treatment. It is now understood that most gastric and duodenal ulcers are caused by damage to the

Table 10-4 Key Nutrition Recommendations for Gastroesophageal Reflux Disease

- Limit intake of high fat, high calorie meals.
- Avoid large meals during a single sitting.
- Eat smaller meals more frequently during the day.
- Drink most fluids between meals rather than with meals.
- Increase intake of high fiber foods (fruits, vegetables, and whole grains).
- Sit up or take a walk after eating rather than lying down.
- Avoid eating at least 2 hours before bedtime if possible.
- Limit foods that worsen symptoms, such as alcohol, chocolate, coffee, or caffeine-containing beverages, mints, citrus fruits, tomato products, spicy foods, or carbonated beverages.

Source: Lisa Hark, PhD, RD and Darwin Deen, MD, MS, 2012. Used with permission.

gastric mucosa, and the most common causative agents are *Helicobacter Pylori* and non-steroidal anti-inflammatory drugs (NSAIDS).[31] Treatment of the underlying cause of PUD may result in resolution of symptoms of PUD.

Gastric acid secretion occurs as a result of vagal stimulation of the parietal cells by the sight or taste of food. Although gastric acid is no longer thought to be responsible for ulcer development, reduction in gastric acid may facilitate healing and decrease abdominal discomfort. Certain foods are known to increase gastric acid secretions, including coffee, tea, colas, and alcohol. No difference has been found in randomized controlled trials that compared restricted diets with unrestricted diets in the resolution of ulcers. The focus of nutrition therapy should be based on individual tolerance and patients should be encouraged to avoid their individual triggers. Foods that are often poorly tolerated include coffee, orange juice, fried foods, spicy foods, and fruits. After treatment of *H. pylori*, improved tolerance of these trigger foods has been demonstrated.[32] Table 10-5 outlines key dietary recommendations for symptom management of PUD.

Table 10-5 Key Nutrition Recommendations for Peptic Ulcer Disease

- Limit intake of caffeine-containing beverages and foods including coffee, tea, iced tea, colas, and chocolate.
- Avoid alcohol, especially on an empty stomach.
- Don't skip meals.
- Avoid eating spicy foods, fried foods, and citrus fruits as these foods may worsen symptoms.
- Avoid other foods or drinks that cause discomfort.

Source: Lisa Hark, PhD, RD and Darwin Deen, MD, MS, 2012. Used with permission.

Small and Large Bowel Disorders
Diarrhea

Diarrhea is characterized by increased frequency of loose or watery stools, and may be acute or chronic in nature most often due to self-limited viral or bacterial infections. Acute diarrhea often resolves on its own, whereas chronic diarrhea lasts for more than 4 weeks. Up to 5% of the population may suffer from chronic diarrhea.[33] Chronic diarrhea occurs in many underlying GI illnesses, and therefore appropriate evaluation of symptoms is vital. Malabsorptive disorders, such as lactose intolerance, celiac disease, or inflammatory bowel disease may result in chronic diarrhea. Assessment should identify the frequency of stools, duration of symptoms, and potential weight loss. Stool characteristics (i.e. watery, mucousal, or fatty) can aid in further evaluation of the pathogenesis of diarrhea. Secretory diarrhea occurs as a result of a disruption in electrolyte transport within the epithelium. It may be caused by enterotoxins, intestinal resections or mucosal disease, or mesenteric ischemia due to atherosclerosis. Osmotic diarrhea occurs after ingestion of poorly absorbed cations and anions, such as sorbitol or sugar alcohols, magnesium, sulfate, or phosphate. Osmotic diarrhea may also be related to deficiencies of disaccharidases, as in lactase deficiency.[34]

In patients with chronic diarrhea, a comprehensive evaluation is necessary to determine the underlying cause. Management of diarrhea to prevent electrolyte abnormalities and potential weight loss is vital. Adequate fluids are also necessary to prevent dehydration. While diarrhea may be worsened by the intake of insoluble dietary fibers, soluble fibers may aid in improvement as they form a gel within the intestinal lumen, thus slowing intestinal transit. Table 10-6 reviews sources of soluble and insoluble dietary fiber. After diarrhea resolves, patients may tolerate gradual reintroduction of insoluble dietary fiber, such as whole grain breads and cereals. Other foods that may worsen diarrhea, such as lactose-containing foods or high-fat foods, should be avoided until diarrhea begins to resolve. Evidence suggests that incorporating functional foods containing live, active bacterial cultures such as yogurt or probiotic supplements may be helpful in treating diarrhea associated with antibiotic use, acute infectious diarrhea, travelers' diarrhea, and diarrhea-predominant irritable bowel syndrome. The most studied probiotic strains are *Lactobacillus*, *Bifidobacterium*, and *Saccharomyces*.[34] However, recent studies have shown adverse outcomes associated with administration of probiotics to critically-ill hospitalized patients. The use of probiotic supplementation in this population is not recommended.[35]

A thorough medication history can identify potential drugs that may exacerbate diarrhea. Sorbitol or lactose-containing medications should be adjusted if possible.

Table 10-6 Dietary Sources of Soluble and Insoluble Fiber

Soluble Fiber	Insoluble Fiber
Apples	Whole wheat flour
Citrus fruits	Bran
Strawberries	Vegetables
Carrots	Whole grains
Oats	Wheat
Beans	Fruits with edible seeds (strawberries, blueberries, etc.)
Legumes	
Barley	
Fiber supplements:	
Psyllium (Metamucil)	
Guar gum (Benefiber)	

Source: Lisa Hark, PhD, RD and Darwin Deen, MD, MS, 2012. Used with permission.

Significant amounts of sorbitol and other sugar alcohols found in low carbohydrate or sugar-free foods can also play a role. Patients should be encouraged to eliminate these foods temporarily and assess for symptom resolution.

Constipation

Constipation is a common complaint with prevalence estimates of 12–19% in North America. Risk factors for constipation include advancing age and female gender, with women being twice as likely as men to report symptoms.[36] Constipation is defined as less than two to three bowel movements per week and can be classified as primary constipation, which is caused by disordered movement of stool in the colon, or secondary constipation, which is caused by various systemic disorders or medications.[12] Because the causes of constipation are varied, it is important to rule out structural causes of constipation as well as organic disease.

Nutrition therapy for constipation focuses on increasing fluid intake, gradually increasing fiber intake, and increasing physical activity. It is important that patients are instructed to make gradual dietary changes, as rapid fluctuations in dietary fiber can worsen symptoms of constipation and abdominal discomfort. Dietary fiber intake should be increased as tolerated to approximately 25–35 g/day by including fruits, vegetables, whole grains, legumes, and nuts. *The Dietary Guidelines for Americans* recommend at least 2 cups or 3–4 servings of fruits and 2½ cups or 4–5 servings of vegetables every day. Population-based studies have demonstrated that women who are physically active on a daily basis and consumed approximately 20 g of fiber per day had a threefold lower prevalence of constipation.[37] Treating constipation in the elderly, another high-risk group, should also involve dietary management that promotes appropriate increases in fluid and fiber intake. Assessment for other contributing factors including co-morbid conditions, decreased mobility, and inability to sit on the toilet should be considered (in the case of bed-bound patients) and should be evaluated by Nurse Practitioners[12] (Appendix O for High Fiber Foods).

Inflammatory Bowel Disease

Inflammatory bowel disease (IBD), Crohn's disease, and ulcerative colitis are idiopathic, chronic, inflammatory conditions affecting the GI tract. Crohn's disease can involve any part of the digestive tract, while ulcerative colitis is limited to the colon. Because of the chronic involvement of the GI tract, most patients with IBD, particularly those with Crohn's disease, have some form of nutritional deficiency. Therefore, careful attention to diet and appropriate referral to a registered dietitian are important in order to prevent nutritional deficiencies. Dietary interventions in IBD should focus on maintaining or improving nutritional status through adequate intake, and avoiding foods that worsen symptoms.[38] Table 10-7 outlines when to refer patients with IBD to a registered dietitian.

Protein-calorie malnutrition is common among patients with IBD and correlates with disease activity which may be mediated by pro-inflammatory cytokines such as IL-1, IL-6, and tumor necrosis factor alpha.[38,39] Nutrition assessment is essential because of the severe consequences of malnutrition, including growth failure and developmental impairment in children and teenagers, impaired healing of the

Table 10-7 When to Refer a Patient with IBD to a Registered Dietitian

- Risk of failure to thrive (children, older adults).
- Child/teen with growth and development failure.
- Pregnant women not gaining weight appropriately.
- Following low-residue diet for more than 6 weeks.
- Evidence of fat malabsorption.
- Presence of comorbidities (diabetes, celiac, CAD, liver disease).
- Suspected or confirmed eating disorder.
- Needs motivation to eat well.
- Needs help with meal planning.
- Has or is at risk for nutrient-deficiencies due to malabsorption, restriction of a specific food group, or medication (e.g. prednisone, proton pump inihibitor).
- Experienced excessive weight gain secondary to medication (prednisone).
- Experienced unintentional weight loss (>5% in 1 month; >7.5% in previous 3 months; >10% in previous 6 months).

Source: Beth-Ann Norton, MS, RN, ANP-BC, 2012. Used with permission.

inflamed bowel, weight loss with loss of muscle mass, metabolic bone disease, and increased susceptibility to infection in children and adults.[38] In addition, a malnourished patient with IBD may present with defects in GI function that further limit the absorption and utilization of nutrients.

Causes of Malnutrition

Malnutrition occurs in patients suffering from IBD as a consequence of decreased dietary intake, increased nutrient losses, and increased nutrient requirements.

Decreased Dietary Intake

Inadequate dietary intake and poor appetite are the most important factors contributing to poor nutritional status in patients with IBD. GI symptoms such as nausea, diarrhea, and recurrent abdominal pain at mealtimes often decrease patients' appetites and food intakes. Fear of eating, oral aphthous ulcerations, and anorexia also contribute to decreased intake. Certain foods may increase the likelihood of symptoms or complications of IBD. For example, patients with Crohn's disease, where the lumen of the small bowel may be narrowed, may experience impaction of high-fiber foods in an inflamed or fibrotic section of bowel, which can precipitate an obstruction. High-fat foods or spicy foods may worsen diarrhea. Some medications that may be used to treat IBD such as metronidazole, methotrexate, or sulfasalazine may decrease appetite. To maximize nutrient intake, unwarranted dietary restrictions should be avoided.

Increased Nutrient Losses

In patients with Crohn's disease, small and large bowel inflammation and/or multiple bowel resections can decrease the absorptive surface area of both the small and large intestine and cause malabsorption of essential nutrients. Resections of the ileum can cause bile salt deficiency, resulting in steatorrhea or fat malabsorption and subsequent deficiency of fat-soluble vitamins A, D, E, and K. Bacterial overgrowth may also interfere with nutrient utilization.[40]

Vitamin B_{12} is coupled with intrinsic factor which is secreted by the parietal cells of the stomach. Because the vitamin B_{12}-intrinsic factor complex is absorbed in the terminal ileum, complete ileal resection or prolonged inflammation of the terminal ileum results in a vitamin B_{12} deficiency that requires treatment via subcutaneous or intramuscular injections, nasal spray, or sublingual vitamin B_{12}.

IBD also can result in a protein-losing enteropathy, through excessive intestinal transudate (movement of protein-rich fluids through the inflamed bowel wall). In the case of Crohn's disease, protein-rich fluid is lost through fistulas, particularly high-output fistulas. Severe diarrhea causes depletion of electrolytes, minerals, and trace elements, such as zinc. GI bleeding can also contribute to iron deficiency anemia. Prednisone, which is frequently used during IBD flares, reduces calcium absorption and increases protein breakdown.[40]

Increased Nutrient Requirements

The inflammatory process of IBD may increase resting energy expenditure, thereby contributing to weight loss and depletion of fat stores that occur when patients do not consume adequate calories and protein. Patients with fever, infection, sepsis, and those undergoing surgery also have greater requirements for protein, calories, and other nutrients compared with patients who are less severely ill. Increased intestinal cell turnover can also raise nutrient requirements in patients with IBD.

Nutrition Therapy for IBD

No specific diet has been shown to prevent or treat IBD. However, some diet strategies help control symptoms. Nutritional recommendations must take into account the patient's digestive and absorptive capabilities. They also depend on whether the patient is hospitalized in an acute flare-up or asymptomatic. Therefore, goals of nutrition therapy for patients with IBD are shown in Table 10-8.

Oral nutritional repletion may be difficult to achieve during symptomatic flares of active IBD since most patients' symptoms worsen both during and following meals. To decrease both the symptoms associated with eating and bowel activity during the healing process, patients hospitalized for IBD are sometimes placed on bowel rest. Prolonged bowel rest without nutrition support can lead to nutritional depletion. Any hospitalized patient on bowel rest for 7–14 days who is not anticipated to resume oral repletion should be considered for total parenteral nutrition (TPN) (Chapter 13).[41]

Table 10-8 Nutrition Therapy Goals for Patients with IBD

- To prevent symptoms associated with malabsorption, such as diarrhea.
- To correct and prevent nutritional deficiencies.
- To promote healing of the intestinal mucosa.
- To minimize stress on inflamed and often narrowed segments of the bowel (Crohn's disease).
- To promote normal growth and development in children and teenagers.

Source: DeLegge.[38]

Table 10-9 Key Recommendations for Patients with Active IBD

- Eat small meals/snacks often throughout the day (6 small meals or eat every 3–4 hours).
- Increase fluid intake to a minimum of eight 8 oz glasses (2000 ml) per day if loose stools persist. Include rehydration beverages.
- Incorporate a chewable multivitamin and mineral supplement daily.
- Eat foods high in potassium.
- Eat foods high in probiotics and prebiotics.
- Avoid lactose. Add milk back slowly to monitor tolerance when bowel movements normalize and when the patient is feeling better. Low-fat yogurt and cheese are better tolerated than milk.
- Avoid fried and high-fat meats, highly marbled or tough meats. Try lean meat such as skinless poultry, baked or broiled fish.
- Limit high fiber grains such as whole grain breads/cereals/pasta with greater than 2 g of dietary fiber per serving.
- Avoid raw vegetables. Try well-cooked, skinless vegetables.
- Avoid dry fruit and raw fruit with peels or skins. Try juice, bananas, melon, and canned fruits. Dilute juice with water if they are not tolerated at full strength.
- Limit fats and oils to 40 ml per day.
- Avoid caffeine (coffee, tea, cola, chocolate).
- Avoid alcohol.
- Avoid artificial sweeteners (sorbitol, mannitol, xylitol).
- Avoid concentrated sweets.

Source: Brown.[40]

An oral diet may be tolerated when active IBD is less severe. To control diarrhea and malabsorption, a low-fat, low-fiber, low-lactose diet is often prescribed. Small, frequent feedings may help to limit GI secretions as well as reduce the volume of food that the damaged bowel must handle at any one time. During a flare, the diet should be individualized according to the patient's clinical condition and food tolerances. Many patients with IBD believe that diet plays a role in the development of a flare, though there are no data to support this. While certain foods have been associated with causing increased GI pain or other symptoms, they are not believed to cause disease relapses. Restriction of diet when individuals do not have active IBD is not encouraged because it can further limit nutrient intake unnecessarily (unless there are fixed narrowings in the lumen of the GI tract). Key dietary recommendations for patients with IBD are listed in Table 10-9.

Patients should be advised to eat foods based on tolerance; however, there are certain foods that can be discouraged because they offer few redeeming nutritional qualities and have been associated with intestinal distress (e.g. popcorn, seeds). This can also allow patients to feel they have more control over their disease. For those who are symptomatic, the goal is to liberalize the diet as much as possible after symptoms have subsided, under the guidelines of a dietitian and Nurse Practitioner team.

Alcohol and caffeine can trigger diarrhea because they stimulate the GI tract; many times this can occur within 30 minutes of consumption. Similarly, diet foods and beverages containing sugar alcohols, such as sorbitol, xylitol, and mannitol can also cause intestinal discomfort and diarrhea, and patients should be encouraged to read labels and avoid these items. Though controversial, heavily spiced foods, fried foods, and concentrated sweets have also been associated with inducing diarrhea. Individuals who experience intense GI pain after eating benefit from keeping a food diary to determine if any specific foods or beverages they consume may act as a GI irritant. A food diary is essential for patients to gain a better understanding of what foods they can or cannot tolerate. Food diaries can be simple and could include columns in a notebook for:

- Type of food or beverage consumed.
- Amount of the food or beverage consumed.
- Where it was consumed (home, car, restaurant).
- Time of day.
- Symptoms.

Calories

In adults, ingested calories should be provided in amounts sufficient to maintain or restore bodyweight. In children, the amount of ingested calories should be adequate to support growth and development, as measured on the pediatric growth charts. Active disease and complications, such as fevers, infection, sepsis, and high output fistulas may increase caloric requirements in adults to as high as 35–45 kcal/kg/day, or approximately 1.5–1.7 times the basal energy expenditure. For example, a female patient with moderate to severe disease activity weighing 110 lb (50 kg) may require 1750–2250 kcal/day to maintain her weight. If a patient is severely malnourished and his or her calorie intake is low, the patient should be assessed by a registered dietitian to help determine the most appropriate feeding plan. Usually 20–25 kcal/kg/day may be initially prescribed to help avoid complications of refeeding syndrome. Supplemental calories can be given in the form of whole protein, elemental or semi-elemental products, and easy to metabolize MCT oils that do not require bile salts for digestion.

Protein

Protein needs are often increased in patients with IBD due to intestinal inflammatory complications of IBD, such as abscesses in Crohn's disease patients. The majority of IBD patients have daily protein needs of 1–1.5 g/kg ideal body weight. Therefore, a male weighing 155 lb (70.5 kg), without kidney disease, but with actively flaring IBD should consume approximately 70–105 g of protein each day. For weight gain and to restore loss of lean body mass greater than 10% after an acute flare, protein needs may be increased up to 3.0 g/kg.[38,42] Protein needs are also increased if the patient is taking prednisone.

Vitamins and Minerals

Patients with IBD are at higher risk for vitamin, mineral, and trace element deficiencies. Higher doses of specific nutrients are indicated if clinical or laboratory evidence identifies a deficiency due to possible poor absorption or increased requirements. Vitamin and mineral requirements for patients with IBD are described below and summarized in Table 10-10.

- Patients with Crohn's disease who have extensive damage due to prolonged inflammation and/or have undergone resection of the terminal ileum are likely to suffer from inadequate vitamin B_{12} absorption and thus require supplementation with intramuscular, sublingual sources or an intranasal spray of vitamin B_{12}.

Table 10-10 Vitamin and Mineral Requirements for Patients with IBD

Nutrient	Recommended Daily Requirements	Recommended Replacement for Deficiency (oral dose)
Zinc	15 mg	50 mg elemental/day
Iron	10–15 mg	300 mg 3×/day
Vitamin B$_{12}$	3 µg	1000 µg /day
Calcium	800–1500 mg	150–200 mg/day
Magnesium	400 mg	150 mg elemental 4×/day
Vitamin D	1000 IU	50 000 IU once weekly × 8 weeks

Source: adapted from Eiden.[43]

- IBD patients with persistent, watery diarrhea may have difficulty maintaining adequate zinc, potassium, and magnesium levels and require supplementation.
- Chronic blood loss and altered iron absorption, frequently observed in patients with IBD, can cause iron deficiency anemia. However, oral iron supplements in full therapeutic doses may exacerbate "GI distress." In particular, oral iron may cause symptoms of nausea, constipation, and abdominal cramping. Slower iron supplementation, along with ascorbic acid may be more effective, because ascorbic acid enhances the absorption of iron by converting the ferric ions to the ferrous form. Only 25–50 mg of ascorbic acid is needed daily to enhance the absorption of iron. If oral iron cannot be tolerated and/or ferritin levels are markedly low, intravenous iron should be considered.
- Though corticosteroids are not recommended as maintenance medication in IBD, long-term treatment with corticosteroids requires calcium and vitamin D supplementation because corticosteroids decrease calcium absorption and increase calcium excretion.
- Patients treated with sulfasalazine (Azulfidine) should receive oral folate supplements, 1 mg/day, because this medication inhibits folate absorption by competitive inhibition of the enzyme folate conjugase in the jejunum. Mexthotrexate also requires folate supplementation at 1 mg daily because it is a folate antagonist (it inhibits the enzyme dihydrofolate reductase) and folate deficiencies may lead to stomatitis and anemia.
- If a patient is taking cholestyramine, a bile salt sequestrant used to treat bile salt diarrhea, fat-soluble vitamins A, D, E, K can bind with the medication. Folate and magnesium absorption can also be impaired by cholestyramine.

Fiber

A low-fiber diet is often prescribed for patients with narrowed sections of bowel to decrease the possibility of intestinal obstruction, minimize physical irritation to the inflamed bowel, reduce stool weight and frequency, and slow the rate of intestinal transit. The diet consists of white bread and refined cereals and avoidance of high-fiber fresh fruits and vegetables, nuts, skins, and seeds. The benefit of a low-fiber diet in managing symptoms or affecting the course of IBD remains unclear. Diets should be recommended depending on a patient's individual tolerance and intolerance; intake of fiber-rich, nutrient-dense foods can generally be encouraged in the absence of bowel strictures and if there is no discomfort. A fiber-rich diet should not be prescribed in patients with strictures (Crohn's disease), as this could potentially contribute to a small bowel obstruction.

Lactose

Patients with IBD may have decreased lactose absorption because of the decline in brush border epithelial cell lactase activity and rapid intestinal transit. The enzyme lactase is most prevalent in the jejunum. Given that Crohn's disease is most prevalent in the ileocecal region it is not unexpected that the incidence of lactose intolerance among those suffering from Crohn's disease is similar to that of the general population. Lactose intolerance can also occur in patients with ulcerative colitis. Symptoms of lactose intolerance may include diarrhea, cramps, or gas. The symptoms of lactose intolerance can be minimized by avoiding dairy foods or by substituting lactose-reduced dairy foods.

Fat

Decreased fat intake may help control the symptoms of steatorrhea, especially in patients with Crohn's disease involving the small bowel. However, fats serve as a form of concentrated calories which are needed to promote weight gain in underweight or malnourished patients.[40] Dietary fats are also essential for the absorption of vitamins A, D, E, and K. In order to decrease bile salt diarrhea related to fat digestion, MCT oil can be substituted as it is more easily absorbed than other fats. MCT oil can be added to other foods, but this may change the palatability of the food. Doses should be given in less than 15 g amounts. Referral to a registered dietitian is essential for all patients requiring weight gain who present with fat malabsorption.

Inflammatory vs Anti-Inflammatory Fatty Acids

It has been demonstrated that gene mutations that affect the immune system, causing inflammation, are associated with IBD. Consequently, it has been hypothesized that the ratio of different polyunsaturated fats in the diet may play a role in helping to control inflammation. Current dietary intake of omega-6 fats (vegetable oils) is much greater than omega-3 fats. An increase in consumption of omega-3 fats and a decrease in omega-6 fats results in reduced arachidonic acid and it is hypothesized that reducing omega-6 fat sources and increasing omega-3 fatty acids results in a reduction of inflammation. However, there are insufficient data to recommend the use of omega-3 fatty acids to maintain remission and prevent flares in IBD.[44] While research has not demonstrated that supplementation with omega-3 is beneficial in helping to sustain remission, food sources of omega-3 fats pose little harm to IBD patients and should be encouraged, if tolerated. Dietary sources of omega-3 fats include fatty fish, walnuts, soy, flaxseed, canola oil, and in small amounts, certain leafy greens and are listed in Appendix M.

Oxalate

Calcium oxalate kidney stones are a common complication in patients with Crohn's disease who undergo intestinal surgeries such as ileal resection, or diverting ileostomy which can lead to malabsorption.[45] Dietary modification to prevent oxalate stones aim to increase intake of fluid, dietary calcium, potassium, and phytates while reducing intake of oxalate, animal protein, sucrose, fructose, sodium, supplemental calcium, and vitamin C. The role of vitamin D in stone formation remains unclear.[45] Drug therapy is indicated if the stone disease remains active (as evidenced by the formation of new stones, enlargement of old stones, or the passage of gravel) or if there is insufficient improvement in the urine chemistries despite attempted dietary modification over a 3–6 month period.[45]

Prebiotics and Probiotics

The intestinal tract is host to a vast ecology of microbes, which are necessary for health, but also have the potential to contribute to the development of disease by a variety of mechanisms.[46] Changes in intestinal epithelial barrier function or innate immune bacterial killing, for example, can lead to an inflammatory response caused by increased uptake of bacterial and food antigens that stimulate the mucosal immune system.[46] Research has been done that involves the deliberate manipulation of the intestinal bacteria with therapeutic intention.[46] There are three general methods by which intestinal microflora can be altered: administration of antibiotics, prebiotics (i.e. dietary components that promote the growth and metabolic activity of beneficial bacteria), or probiotics (i.e. beneficial bacteria).[46]

Probiotics — microorganisms thought to have a beneficial effect on gut health — may be beneficial to IBD patients. Dietary sources of probiotics, such as yogurt and kefir, contain probiotics, protein, and calcium and can be recommended. Patients should look for food labels of such sources that say "contains live and active cultures," indicating that the bacteria are viable. The bacteria studied in IBD include bifidobacterium, lactobacillus, and others. With regards to probiotic supplementation there are currently too few conclusive studies to be certain of the effect of probiotics in IBD.

Ulcerative colitis: Various probiotic species have shown promise in the treatment of ulcerative colitis in small studies, although a clear clinical benefit remains to be established, particularly for induction of remission. Prevention of relapse is better documented.[46]

Crohn's disease: Clinical trials of probiotics in Crohn's disease have shown mixed results. The reasons are unclear, but could be due to several factors such as the specific probiotics (and dosages) used, differences in study duration, characteristics of the included patients (e.g. location of disease), and endpoints that were measured.[46] Caution should be taken when prescribing probiotics to patients, as a few complications may result in patients who are immunocompromised, have short bowel of less than 150 cm, and are otherwise critically ill.

Prebiotics are non-digestible carbohydrates that upon reaching the colon undigested, may stimulate the growth of healthy bacteria found in the gut and may improve gut health. More studies are needed to support prebiotic supplementation in IBD patients. Prebiotic supplements such as fructooligosaccharides (FOS), an insulin-type probiotic, must initially be started in small amounts and slowly increased as they may cause significant gas production. Recommended maximum FOS intake is 15 g/day.[47]

Nutrition Support (Chapter 13)

Enteral nutrition support should be the primary source of nutrition if it is safe to provide and oral nutrition consumption is not an option. The liquid formula used to provide enteral nutrition support in patients with IBD should be low-fat, low-residue, and lactose-free. Elemental formulas (formulas that contain protein in the form of amino acids) for enteral tube feeding have been used successfully in this population. Because these formulas are completely absorbed in the upper small intestine and seem to be effective in reducing residue in the bowel, they are particularly appropriate for patients with Crohn's disease. Elemental formulas are also well tolerated because of their low-fat content.

Parenteral nutrition (PN) support is indicated only in severe cases of IBD when bowel rest is considered necessary and enteral nutrition (EN) support is not an option, as in cases of bowel obstruction or severe strictures, severe perianal or enterocutaneous fistulas that prohibit feeding, or with a length of less than 150 cm of functional small intestine (short bowel) remaining. Chapter 13 describes both EN and PN support regimens in detail.

Case 1

Laura is a 56-year-old Caucasian woman with a history of severe Crohn's ileitis, with three resections of the terminal ileum. She smokes one packet of cigarettes a day. She has been refractory to multiple medications and now has 12–15 watery stools per day accompanied by moderate post-prandial abdominal pain. She has a poor appetite and has lost 15 lb in 7 months (10% weight change). She is hypokalemic. (K: 4.8 mg/dL). She has bile salt diarrhea due to laxative effect of bile salts in the large intestine that have not been absorbed.

ADVICE: Laura is at risk for malnutrition and will likely require parenteral nutrition support if her weight loss continues. Another immunosuppressive medication should be prescribed to reduce her pain and control her diarrhea episodes. Quitting smoking will help to decrease the severity of her Crohn's disease.

Start her on an oral elemental diet and refer her to a registered dietitian. Laboratory work prior to that visit can include calcium, vitamin B_{12}, vitamin D, total protein, and albumin.

Consider oral repletion of her potassium with follow-up electrolytes, prescribe a bile salt sequestrant once daily to start that can be titrated to b.i.d. to t.i.d. dosing, and recommend a smoking cessation program.

Irritable Bowel Syndrome

Irritable bowel syndrome (IBS) is a functional GI disorder characterized by abdominal pain, altered bowel motility, and bloating or abdominal distension. The pathogenesis of IBS is not well understood; however, genetic and environmental factors are thought to play a role.[48] In addition, researchers have reported abnormal GI motility, visceral hypersensitivity, dietary intolerances, and psychological or emotional dysfunction in patients with IBS. No specific physiologic or psychologic abnormality has been shown to be absolutely indicative of this disorder.[48]

The abdominal pain associated with IBS is variable, and can be mild to severe. Diarrhea and constipation may occur in varying degrees, and despite extensive research, no one predominant pattern of small bowel or colonic dysmotility has been found.[19,48] IBS may present with diarrhea or constipation predominant symptoms; however, some patients have alternating diarrhea and constipation. An evaluation for organic causes of GI symptoms should be considered. Recent evidence suggests that carbohydrate malabsorption may precipitate symptoms of IBS.[49,50] Testing for lactose or fructose malabsorption should be considered in patients with symptoms consistent with IBS. Based on patient symptoms and physical exam, diagnostic tests such as motility studies and manometry may or may not be performed. If IBS is diagnosed, treatment should focus on management of symptoms.

Nutrition Therapy for IBS

Nutrition therapy for IBS is variable, as many patients have specific food intolerances. Following a lactose-restricted diet may improve symptoms for some patients with IBS, particularly those with diarrhea-predominant IBS. In addition, reducing the amount of dietary fructose, found in fruits, fruit juices, and foods prepared with high fructose corn syrup may be beneficial as fructose is not absorbed well by some individuals and can contribute to upset stomach and diarrhea. A high-fiber diet is often recommended, especially in patients with constipation-predominant IBS, as it aids in water absorption, promotes bulking of the stool, and can improve intestinal transit. Bijkerk and colleagues[51] examined the results of 17 clinical trials looking at the role of insoluble and soluble fiber in the treatment of IBS. Research results were inconsistent, with some studies showing only marginal improvement in global symptoms of IBS. Of note, some studies show that in patients with constipation-predominant symptoms, insoluble fiber caused their symptoms to worsen. This may be related to a functional decrease in small bowel or colonic motility seen in some patients with IBS.[52] These mixed results suggest individualized dietary counseling and recommendations for fiber intake are needed in patients with IBS.

Nurse Practitioners should consider the type of dietary fiber the patient is taking (soluble vs insoluble) and the amount. There has been some research to show that soluble fiber, such as guar gum, causes less abdominal pain and bloating than wheat bran; however, these studies show mixed results.[53] Research examining a role for probiotics in IBS is ongoing. It is thought that alterations of normal GI flora may play a role in symptom expression, and some studies have shown decreased levels of the healthy bacteria lactobacilli and bifidobacteria in patients with IBS.[54] It has been hypothesized that the restoration of normal gut flora may decrease abnormal gas production in some patients. In addition, it is thought that probiotics may decrease adherence of pathogenic bacteria to the GI mucosa, thereby decreasing symptoms of IBS.[54] Additional research is needed to determine the ideal balance between diet, fiber supplements, and probiotics in the management of IBS. Greater understanding can be expected from the continued study of their effects on enterocytes.[55]

Case 2

Melanie is a 35-year-old women diagnosed with IBS 5 years ago. She complains of crampy, abdominal pain that is relieved when she has a bowel movement. She often has loose stools or diarrhea followed by no bowel movement for several days. These irregular bowel movements worsen when she is under stress. Her weight has been stable and she does not have any fever or bleeding when she goes to the toilet.

LIFESTYLE: Melanie is a lawyer and is frequently under a lot of stress, especially when she is in court. Her symptoms seem to come several times a week and she says they are interfering with her ability to work. She eats two meals a day (lunch and dinner), frequently on the run, since she is so busy. Because she has diarrhea, she is not sure what to eat, but she drinks apple juice to prevent dehydration and replace potassium. She does not take a multivitamin supplement and does not exercise.

ADVICE: A combination of factors are most likely contributing to Melanie's current IBS problem. First, she is stressed and would benefit from stress reduction techniques, such as increasing her exercise and meditation. She also does not make the time for breakfast, which would help her bowels to be more regular from eating a high-fiber meal. She also may be experiencing cramping and gas from certain foods which produce gas, the most common being legumes, beans, onions, prunes, and cruciferous vegetables, such as cabbage, brussel sprouts, cauliflower, and broccoli. Melanie could try to systematically eliminate these foods to help to determine the relationship between the food and symptoms. Melanie could also temporarily eliminate dairy foods, since lactose intolerance is common and can cause symptoms similar to IBS or aggravate IBS. If this is helpful, she should take dietary calcium supplements to reach 1000 mg/day. Yogurt is often well-tolerated and is also a good source of calcium.

Increasing dietary fiber (either by adding certain foods to the diet or using fiber supplements) can also help to relieve Melanie's symptoms and help her to have regular bowel movements and improve the consistency of stools. It is often helpful to take a psyllium, guar, or methylcellulose dietary fiber supplement since it is difficult to consume enough fiber in the diet, particularly when avoiding foods known to increase intestinal gas. Dietary fiber supplements should be increased to the prescribed dose over several weeks to help reduce the symptoms of excessive intestinal gas, which can occur in some people when beginning fiber therapy. Alcohol, caffeine, sorbitol, and fructose have also been shown to aggravate symptoms in some people who have IBS. Melanie is drinking apple juice on a regular basis, which contains high amounts of fructose and could be contributing to her diarrhea. She should discontinue this and substitute water. Some diet drinks also contain sorbitol, so these should be discouraged as well.

Because symptoms are variable, encouraging patients with IBS to keep a food diary may allow them to determine specific dietary triggers, and the foods identified as triggers should be limited or avoided. In addition, a trial high-fiber diet may produce symptomatic improvement in some patients, especially if their dietary intake of fiber is less than the recommended 25–35 g/day. Nurse Practitioners should be aware of what type of fiber patients are consuming, and encourage them to experiment with more or less insoluble and soluble fibers depending on their symptoms. High-fiber

Table 10-11 Nutrition Recommendations to Decrease Gas and Bloating

---

Certain foods can produce excess gas during digestion and may worsen your symptoms of abdominal pain or bloating. Various foods affect people in different ways; avoid these foods if they cause discomfort.

Foods that may cause gas:
- Beans, cabbage, cauliflower, brussel sprouts, broccoli, asparagus, peppers, cucumbers, onions, garlic, radishes, sauerkraut.
- Raw apples, avocados, melon.
- Eggs, fried and fatty foods, spicy foods, carbonated beverages.

Swallowing air may also cause excess gas. To prevent this:
- Eat slowly.
- Avoid chewing gum, carbonated beverages, and smoking cigarettes.

Source: Lisa Hark, PhD, RD and Darwin Deen, MD, MS, 2012. Used with permission.

food sources are shown in Appendix O. Patients should be instructed to increase fiber intake gradually, and to increase fluid intake as fiber intake increases. Avoidance of lactose- or fructose-containing foods, as well as gas-producing foods may reduce episodes of bloating and abdominal pain. Key recommendations to reduce gas and bloating are listed in Table 10-11. Patients who avoid dairy foods due to symptoms of lactose intolerance should be encouraged to consume other calcium-rich foods or calcium supplements to meet the recommended daily intake of calcium as shown in Appendix T.

Diverticulosis

Diverticulosis is a disorder of the colon, most often the sigmoid colon, caused by multiple potential factors including age-related changes in the colonic wall, abnormal increases in colonic intraluminal pressure, and motor dysfunction. Inadequate fiber intake is thought to increase the risk for the development of diverticulosis.[56] The incidence of diverticulosis increases with age. The prevalence of diverticular disease has been reported at 10% of the population, most often occurring after age 40. It has been estimated that more than 30% of patients over age 60 and 50% of patients over age 80 have evidence of diverticulosis.[12]

Treatment of diverticulosis focuses on increasing dietary fiber intake via whole grain foods, fruits, and vegetables. Some studies have shown an improvement in symptoms of uncomplicated diverticular disease with a fiber intake of 25–30 g/day. The best results seemed to be obtained when a combination of soluble and insoluble fiber was included in the diet.[57] Appendix O lists high-fiber food choices. It may be necessary to increase fiber intake with the use of soluble fiber supplements, such as psyllium or guar gum. Early recommendations for diverticular disease encouraged the elimination of foods containing nuts and seeds due to concerns that these items could become lodged within the diverticuli. However, new evidence from large cohort studies suggest that nuts, corn, and popcorn are safe for most patients, and exclusion in the diet should be based on individual patient intolerance. The most current recommendations focus on increasing dietary fiber intake and do not recommend avoidance of nuts, seeds, and popcorn.[58] Vegetarians have been shown to be a third less likely to develop diverticular disease, possibly because of their high dietary fiber intake.[59] While seeds have not been specifically assessed for tolerance in clinical trials, blueberries and strawberries have been included in studies and have not been found to be associated with increased risk of diverticulitis.[60] It is important to advise patients to increase fluid intake as fiber intake is increased. Although no evidence is available to provide an exact recommendation for fluid intake, encouraging at least 64 oz of fluids daily is reasonable.

Diverticulitis

Diverticulitis occurs when there is inflammation or perforation at the site of a diverticuli. Management focuses on resolution of inflammation. Bowel rest is often indicated with gradual diet advancement. As eating resumes, patients should maintain a low-fiber intake until the inflammation is resolved. The diet should be advanced slowly as tolerance permits, and fiber intake should be gradually increased. Eventual return to a high-fiber diet should be encouraged, as well as consumption of adequate fluids.

Liver Disease

Fatty Liver

The development of fatty liver can occur as a result of chronic alcohol use or as a side effect of many medications. Recently, much emphasis has been focused on the development of non-alcoholic fatty liver disease (NAFLD). Two subsets of NAFLD include non-alcoholic steatohepatitis (NASH) and non-NASH fatty liver disease (NNFLD). NASH is characterized by steatosis with inflammation, cellular ballooning, and fibrosis.[61] Patients with NASH have the potential to progress to advanced cirrhosis and end stage liver disease. NNFLD is characterized by steatosis with minimal inflammation. These patients are at less risk for disease progression.[61]. The world-wide prevalence of NAFLD is increasing, and has been found to be associated with the increase in the prevalence of obesity and type 2 diabetes. Patients at risk for NAFLD are those with aspects of metabolic syndrome, including central obesity, elevated triglycerides, low HDL-cholesterol, hypertension, and insulin resistance.[62]

In patients who experience fatty liver as a result of alcohol use, abstinence from alcohol should be strongly encouraged. Nutrition therapy of NAFLD is aimed at a gradual weight loss of 1–2 lb/week. The ideal dietary composition for patients with NAFLD is unclear, but reduction in total calorie and fat intake and increased dietary fiber intake will likely aid in weight loss and improve other symptoms associated with metabolic syndrome.[63] Increased physical activity will aid the patient in weight loss maintenance. Patients may benefit from referral to a registered dietitian or weight loss programs that offer a support component, either through local hospitals or programs such as Weight Watchers. Chapter 7 describes weight reduction treatment recommendations and Chapter 9 describes treatment recommendations for metabolic syndrome.

Cirrhosis

Malnutrition and vitamin deficiencies are extremely prevalent in patients with cirrhosis because the diseased liver is no longer able to play a central role in the metabolism of carbohydrate, fat, and protein. It is estimated that protein calorie malnutrition affects anywhere from 10–100% of patients with liver disease and can occur throughout all stages of the disease. Protein calorie malnutrition is often considered a negative prognostic risk factor and is associated with poor outcomes and complications such as hepatorenal syndrome, refractory ascites, variceal hemorrhage, and spontaneous bacterial peritonitis.[64] Causes of malnutrition in this population vary. There is impaired nutrient metabolism, causing patients to move more rapidly from a fed state to a fasting state. Malabsorption may occur as a result of diminished bile acid production. Calorie requirements may be increased acutely during complications of ascites or spontaneous bacterial peritonitis. GI symptoms, such as anorexia, nausea, and early satiety may impact the intake of adequate nutrients.[65] In addition, highly restricted diets, lactulose therapy, frequent paracentesis, and diuresis are iatrogenic causes which may worsen malnutrition.[64]

Risk factors for development of cirrhosis include alcohol-related liver disease, hepatitis, non-alcoholic steatohepatitis (NASH), and cholestatic diseases. Nutrition therapy depends on the cause of the cirrhosis and the degree of decompensation. To prevent worsening of cirrhosis, patients who consume alcohol should be strongly encouraged to abstain. Nutrient deficiencies, particularly the B vitamins (thiamin, folate, B_{12}), are often seen in patients with alcoholic cirrhosis and supplementation may be necessary if they are diagnosed with anemia.[64]

The optimal macronutrient content of the diet in patients with cirrhosis has not been determined. Patients may suffer from insulin resistance, in which case intake of carbohydrates may need to be modified. Patients should be encouraged to increase consumption of whole grains and limit sweets. Fat intake should be adjusted based on symptoms of intolerance, particularly in cholestatic diseases. In patients with significant malnutrition and anorexia, increasing calorie intake by way of high-fat, energy-dense food choices may be helpful as long as they are not experiencing significant fat malabsorption. Protein restrictions have frequently been recommended in cirrhosis, especially with accompanying encephalopathy, often at levels of 40 g/day. However, it has been shown that excessive protein restriction can worsen outcomes in cirrhosis.[66] Protein restrictions should be limited to periods of acute encephalopathy, with gradual increases in protein intake after the resolution of encephalopathy. Protein restrictions instituted during periods of acute encepholapthy should be moderate and never less than 0.8 to 1.0 g/kg/day. Protein intake should provide an adequate substrate for energy synthesis and prevent muscle catabolism and release of amino acids, which can lead to increased levels of ammonia, and worsening of encephalopathy.[67] Cirrhosis is a catabolic illness, and evidence suggests that patients benefit from protein intake in a range of 1.0–1.5 g of protein/kg/day.[68] Protein requirements should be based on the estimated dry weight. Patients may have better tolerance to vegetable or dairy proteins rather than animal proteins as these foods are higher in branched-chain amino acids.[67] In addition, the increased fiber content of vegetable protein sources may facilitate desired nitrogenous losses in the stool. Avoidance of raw seafood and shellfish should be encouraged due to the risk of *Vibrio vulnificus* infections.[69]

Individuals with persistently inadequate oral intake may benefit from oral liquid nutrition supplements to increase calorie and protein intake. Oral supplements high in branched-chain amino acids (BCAA) have been developed specifically for patients with liver disease. Addition of BCAA to the diet is thought to improve hepatic encephalopathy by competing with aromatic amino acids for transport across the blood–brain barrier, and decreasing the synthesis of false neurotransmitters seen in acute encephalopathy. There is conflicting data on the benefits of BCAA supplementation in cirrhotic patients, and the formulations are expensive and often unpalatable. Therefore, there is limited use of these formulas in the clinical setting. However, current evidence supports the use of BCAA formulations for supplementation in decompensated cirrhosis.[64]

Many patients with cirrhosis will develop ascites, and therefore a low sodium diet is also indicated. Restriction of sodium to less than 2000 mg/day is often recommended. Further restrictions in sodium worsen the palability of the diet and increase the risk of inadequate nutrient intake. Fluid restriction may also be indicated. In patients with significant steatorrhea, it may be necessary to provide additional supplementation of the fat-soluble vitamins, preferably in a water-soluble form. Key nutrition recommendations for patients with cirrhosis and advanced liver disease have been recommended by the American Society of Parenteral and Enteral Nutrition.[70]

- Caloric intake goal of 30–35 kcal/kg dry body weight.
- 50–60% of calories from carbohydrate.
- 20–30% of calories from protein, or 1.0–1.5 g/kg/dry body weight.
- 10–20% of calories from fats.
- Avoid dietary restrictions if possible.
- Provide small, frequent meals throughout the day and small snacks.
- Screen for vitamin and mineral deficiencies, particularly fat-soluble vitamins (A, D, E, K), B vitamins (folate, B_{12}, thiamin), zinc, calcium.
- Avoid alcohol.

Gallbladder Disease: Cholelithiasis

Cholelithiasis is caused by a combination of lithogenic bile, cholesterol crystallization, and gallbladder stasis. The majority of cases of gallstone disease are related to cholesterol stones. Female gender, pregnancy, age, obesity, and certain ethnic backgrounds have higher rates of cholelithiasis. Rapid weight loss, family history, and certain medications may also increase the risk of developing gallstones. Although there are no specific diet recommendations for the management of gallstones, dietary factors may play a role in gallstone development. For example, excess energy intakes, as well as diets high in saturated fats and refined sugars, have been identified as risk factors for gallstone development.[71] The combination of dietary factors that predispose patients to weight gain and obesity also predispose them to gallstone disease. Recent evidence from long-term population studies suggest that high-fiber diets may reduce risk. In addition, there has been some evidence that diets high in poly and monounsaturated fats reduce the risk of cholelithiasis in both men and women.[72]

Patients who are at risk for the development of gallstone disease should be encouraged to adopt healthy lifestyle habits, including a diet low in saturated fats and refined sugars and high in dietary fiber. Increased consumption of high-fiber foods from whole grain breads and cereals, fruits, and vegetables reduce risk. If weight loss is indicated, patients should be encouraged to make gradual changes to support weight loss of no more than 1–2 lb/week. Rapid weight loss has been associated with gallstone formation.[71] In patients with current gallstone disease, a diet that restricts fat to 25–30% of total calories is indicated. Further restriction of fat should be avoided, as it may prevent adequate stimulation of gallbladder contraction. Food intolerances may be reported, specifically with foods that cause gas and bloating. Avoiding these foods may aid in symptom control. If steatorrhea is reported, supplementation of fat-soluble vitamins may be indicated.

Summary: Role of Nurse Practitioners

This chapter has provided general recommendations for nutritional management of GI disorders. Nurse Practitioners play a vital role in the diagnosis and treatment of a variety of GI disorders. The importance of a multidisciplinary team approach is required to care for GI patients appropriately and includes Nurse Practitioners, physicians, pharmacists, and dietitians. A dietitian should always be involved in the care of patients requiring complex dietary management, extensive dietary modifications, or for those patients who are at high risk for malnutrition, weight loss, or vitamin and mineral deficiencies.

References

1. Hark L, Morrison G. *Medical Nutrition and Disease: A Case-Based Approach*, 4th edition. Blackwell Publishing, Malden, MA, 2009.
2. Lomer MC, Parkes GC, Sandeson JD. Review article: lactose intolerance in clinical practice — myths and realities. *Ailment Pharmacol Ther* 2008;27:93–103.
3. Swagerty DL Jr, Walling AD, Klein RM. Lactose intolerance. *Am Fam Physician* 2002; 65: 1845–1850.
4. Sahi T. Genetics and epidemiology of adult-type hypolactasia. *Scand J Gastro Ent* 1994: 29:s202:7–20.
5. Suarez FL, Savaiano DA, Levitt MD. A comparison of symptoms after the consumption of milk or lactose-hydrolyzed milk by people with self-reported severe lactose intolerance. *N Engl J Med* 1995;333:1–4.
6. Food and Nutrition Board, Institute of Medicine. *Dietary Reference Intakes (DRI)* for energy, CHO, Fiber, Fat, Protein. National Academies Press, Washington, DC, 2011.
7. National Institutes of Health Consensus Development Conference Statement. Celiac Disease 2004. http://consensus.nih.gov/2004/2004CeliacDisease118html.htm. Accessed 2012.
8. Niewinksi M. Advances in celiac disease and gluten-free diet. *J Am Diet Assoc* 2008;108: 661–672.
9. Hadjivassilion M, Grunnewald RA, Davies-Jones GAB. Gluten sensitivity as a neurological illness. *J Neurosurg Psych* 2002;72:560–563.
10. Stenson WF, Newberry R, Lorenz R, Baldus C, Civitelli R. Increased prevalence of celiac disease and need for routine screening among patients with osteoporosis. *Arch Intern Med* 2005;165:393–399.

11. James SP. National Institutes of Health Consensus Development Conference Statement on Celiac Disease, 2004. *Gastroenterology* 2005;128:S1–S9.

12. McQuaid K. Gastrointestinal disorders. In: McPhee SJ, Papadakis MA (Eds), *Current Medical Diagnosis and Treatment*, 2010. McGraw-Hill Companies, New York, NY: 991–1078.

13. Hallert C, Grant C, Grehn S, et al. Evidence of poor vitamin status in celiac patients on a gluten-free diet for 10 years. *Aliment Pharmacol Ther* 2002;16:1333–1339.

14. Peraaho M, Kaukinen K, Mustalahti K, et al. Effect of an oats-containing gluten-free diet on symptoms and quality of life in celiac disease. *A randomized study. Scand J Gastroenterol* 2004;39:27–31.

15. Thompson T. Gluten contamination of commercial oat products in the United States. *N Engl J Med* 2004;351:2021–2022.

16. The Celiac Disease Foundation. www.celiac.org. Accessed 2012.

17. Thompson T, Dennis M, Higgins LA, Lee AR, Sharrett MK. Gluten-free diet survery: are Americans with celiac diease consuming recommended amounts of fiber, iron, calcium and grain foods? *J Hum Nutr Diet* 2005;18:163–169.

18. Niewinski MM. Advances in celiac disease and gluten-free diet. *J Am Diet Assoc* 2008; 108:661–672.

19. Feldman M, Friedman L, Sleisinger M. *Sleisinger and Fordtran. Gastrointestinal and Liver Disease*, Seventh edition. Elsevier, Philadelphia, PA, 2002.

20. Isaac R, Alex R, Knox R. Malabsorption in wasting HIV disease: diagnostic and management issues in poor resource settings. *Trop Doc* 2008;38:133–134.

21. Kumar R, Lieske JC, Collazo-Clavell ML et al. Fat malabsorption and increased intestinal oxalate absorption are common after roux-en-Y gastric bypass surgery. *Surgery*, 2011;154: 654–661.

22. Dumasy V, Delhaye M, Cotton F, Deviere J. Fat malabsorption screening in chronic pancreatitis. *Am J Gastroenterol* 2004;99:1350–1354.

23. Locke GR III, Talley NJ, Fett SL, Zinsmeister AR, Melton LJ III. Prevalence and clinical spectrum of gastroesophageal reflux: a population-based study in Olmsted County, Minnesota. *Gastroenterology* 1997;112:1448–1456.

24. Nandurkur S, Locke GR III, Fett S, Zinsmeister AR, Cameron AJ, Talley NJ. Relationship between body mass index, diet, exercise and gastro-oesophageal reflux symptoms in a community. *Aliment Pharmacol Ther* 2004;20:497–505.

25. Vermulapalli R. Diet and lifestyle modifications in the management of gastroesophageal reflux disease. *Nut Clinl Pract* 2008;23:293–298.

26. Nocon M, Labenz J, Jaspersen D, et al. Association of body mass index with heart burn, regurgitation and esophagitis: results of the Progression of Gastroesophageal Reflux Disease Study. *J Gastroenterol Hepatol* 2007;22:1728–1731.

27. El-Serag HB, Satia JA, Rabeneck L. Dietary intake and the risk of gastro-oesophageal reflux disease: a cross-sectional study in volunteers. *Gut* 2005;54:11–17.

28. Colombo P, Mangano M, Bianchi PA, Penagini R. Effect of calories and fat on postprandial gastro-oesophageal reflux. *Scand J Gastroenerol* 2002;37:3–5.

29. Nilsson M, Johnsen R, Ye W, Hveem K, Lagergren J. Lifestyle related risk factors in the aetiology of gastro-oesophageal reflux. *Gut* 2004;53:1730–1735.

30. Moller ME, Dahl R, Bockman OC. A possible role of the dietary fiber product, wheat bran, as a nitrite scavenger. *Food Chem Toxicol* 1988;26:841–845.

31. Sontag SJ. Guilty as charged: bugs and drugs in gastric ulcer. *Am J Gastroenterol.* 1997;92: 1255–1261.

32. Olafsson S, Berstad A. Changes in food tolerance and lifestyle after eradication of helicobacter pylori. *Scand J Gastroenterol* 2003;38:268–276.

33. Fine KD, Schiller LR. AGA technical review on the evaluation and management of chronic diarrhea. *Gastroenterology* 1999;116:1464.

34. Guarino A, Vecchio AL, Canani RB. Probiotics as prevention and treatment for diarrhea. *Curr Opin Gastroenterol* 2009;25:18–23.

35. Barraud D, Blard C, Hein F, et al. Probiotics in the critically ill patient: a double blind, randomized, placebo controlled trial. *Intensive Care Med* 2010;36:1540–1547.

36. Higgins PD, Johanson JF. Epidemiology of constipation in North America: a systematic review. *Am J Gastroenterol* 2004;99:750–759.

37. Dukas L, Willet WC, Giovannucci EL. Association between physical activity, fiber intake, and other lifestyle variables and constipation in a study of women. *Am J Gastroenterol* 2003;98:1790–1796.

38. DeLegge, M. Nutrition and dietary interventions in adults with inflammatory bowel disease. *UpToDate* 19.1, Feb, 2011.

39. Teitelbaum. J. Nutrient deficiencies in inflammatory bowel disease. *UpToDate* 19.1, Jan, 2011.

40. Brown AC, Rampertab SD, Mullin GE. Existing dietary guidelines for Crohn's disease and ulcerative colitis. *Expert Rev Gastroenterol Hepatol* 2011;5:411–425.

41. Hait E, *et al.* Overview of parenteral and enteral nutrition. *UpToDate* 12.3, Aug, 2004.

42. Milovic M, Grand R. Protein-losing gastroenteropathy. *UpToDate* 19.1, Jan, 2011.

43. Eiden K. Nutritional considerations in inflammatory bowel disease. *Pract Gastro* 2003; 27:33.

44. Turner D, Shah P, Steinhart, A, Zlotnik, S, Griffiths, A. Maintenance of remission in inflamma-tory bowel disease using omega-3 Fatty Acids (Fish Oil): a systematic review and meta-analyses. *Inflamm Bowel Dis* 2011;17:336–345.

45. Curhan G. Prevention of recurrent calcium stones in adults. *UpToDate* 19.1, Jan, 2011.

46. Sartor R. Probiotics for gastrointestinal diseases. *UpToDate* 19.1, Jan, 2011.

47. Benjamin J, et al. Randomised, double-blind, placebo-controlled trial of fructo-oligosaccharides in active Crohn's disease. *Gut* 2011;60:923–929.

48. Clark C, DeLegge M. Irritable bowel syndrome: a practical approach. *Nut Clin Pract* 2008; 23:263–267.

49. Vesa TH, Seppo LM, Marteau, PR, Sahi T, Korpela R. Role of irritable bowel syndrome in subjective lactose intolerance. *Am J Clin Nutr* 1998;67:710–715.

50. Choi YK, Johlin FC Jr, Summers RW, Jackson M, Rao SS. Fructose intolerance: an under-recognized problem. *Am J Gastroenterol* 2003;98:1348–1353.

51. Bijkerk CJ, Muris JW, Knotternerus JA, Hoes AW, de Wit NJ. Systematic review: the role of different types of fiber in the treatment of irritable bowel syndrome. *Ailment Pharmacol Ther* 2004;19:245–251.

52. Hebden JM, Blackshaw E, D'Amato M, Perkins AC, Spiller RC. Abnormalities of GI transit in bloated irritable bowel syndrome: effect of bran on transit and symptoms. *Am J Gastroenterol* 2002;97:2315–2320.

53. Parisi GC, Zill M, Miani MP, et al. High-fiber diet supplementation in patients with irritable bowel syndrome (IBS). A multicenter, randomized, open trial comparison between wheat bran diet and partially hydrolyzed guar gum (PHGG). *Dig Dis Sci* 2002;47:1697–1704.

54. Heitkemper MM, Jarrett ME. Update on irritable bowel syndrome and gender differences. *Nutr Clin Pract* 2008;23:275–283.

55. Aumugam M, *et al.* Enterotypes of the human gut microbiome. *Nature* 2010;473:174–180.

56. West B. The pathology of diverticulosis: classical concepts and mucosal changes in diverticula. *J Clinl Gastroenterol* 2006; 40:S126–S131.

57. Rocco A, Compare D, Caruso F, Nardone G. Treatment options for uncomplicated diverticular disease of the colon. *J Clin Gastroenterol* 2009;43:803–808.

58. Tarleton S, DiBaise JK. Low-residue diet in diverticular disease: putting and end to a myth. *Nut Clin Pract* 2011;26:137–142.

59. Crowe F, Appleby P, Allen A, et al. Diet and risk of diverticular disease in Oxford cohort of European Prospective Investigation into Cancer and Nutrition (EPIC): prospective study of British vegetarians and non-vegetarians. *BMJ* 2011;343.

60. Prasad S, Ewigman B, Hickner J. Let them eat nuts — this snack is safe for diverticulosis patients. *J Fam Pract* 2009;58:82–84.

61. Caldwell S, Argo C. The natural history of non-alcoholic fatty liver disease. *Dig Dis* 2010; 28:162–168.

62. Bellentaini S, Scaglioni F, Marino M, Bedogni G. Epidemiology of non-alcoholic fatty liver disease. *Dig Dis* 2010;28:155–161.

63. Solga S, Alkhuraishe AR, Clark JM, et al. Dietary composition and nonalcoholic fatty liver disease. *Dig Dis Sci* 2004;49:1578–1584.

64. Chadalavada R, Shekhar R, Biyyani S, Maxwell J, Mullen K. Nutrition in hepatic encephalopathy. *Nutr Clin Pract* 2010;25:257–264.

65. ASPEN Board of Directors and The Clinical Guidelines Task Force. Guidelines for the use of parenteral and enteral nutrition in adult and pediatric patients: liver disease. *JPEN* 2002; 26(1)Suppl:65SA–67SA.

66. Mullen KD, Dasarathy S. Protein restriction in hepatic encephalopathy, necessary evil or illogical dogma? *J Hepatol* 2004;41:147–148.

67. Cabral CM, Burns DL. Low protein diets for hepatic encephalopathy debunked: let them eat steak. *Nutr Clin Pract* 2011;26:155–159.

68. Plauth M, Merli M, Kondrup J, Weimann A, Ferenci P, Muller MJ. ESPEN guidelines for nutrition in liver disease and transplantation. *Clin Nutr* 1997;16:43–55.

69. Chen Y, Satoh T, Tokunya O. Vibrio vulnificus infection in patients with liver disease: reports of five autopsy cases. Virchows Archiv 2002;44:88–92.

70. *ASPEN Nutrition Support Practice Manual*, 2nd edition. American Society for Parenteral and Enteral Nutrition, Silver Spring. 2005.

71. Cuevas A, Miquel JF, Reyes MS, Zanlungo S, Nervi F. Diet as a risk factor for cholesterol gallstone disease. *J Am Coll Nutr* 2004;23:187–196.

72. Tsai CJ, Leitzman MF, Hu FB, Willett WC, Giovannucci EL. A prospective cohort study of nut consumption and the risk of gallstone disease in men. *Am J Epid* 2004;160:961–968.

11 Renal Care

Jean Stover, RD, LDN
Lauren Solomon, MSN, ANP-BC, GNP-BC

OBJECTIVES

- Explain the importance of regulating the intake of protein, calories, sodium, potassium, phosphorus, fluid, vitamins, and other minerals in patients with renal disease.
- Describe the specific nutrition therapy for acute kidney injury, chronic kidney disease, nephrotic syndrome, urinary tract infection, and nephrolithiasis.
- Describe the goals of nutrition therapy for patients on hemodialysis, peritoneal dialysis, and other forms of renal replacement therapy.
- Provide details on the nutrition goals after renal transplant.

Introduction

Nutrition therapy for patients with renal disease varies according to the type of disorder as well as the stage of disease. Variations in pathology, physiology, and disease presentation within the spectrum of renal disease require specific nutritional management and monitoring. Specific recommendations for fluid and mineral intake are required for patients with urinary tract infections and nephrolithiasis. Acute kidney injury, chronic kidney disease (CKD) (with or without dialysis), nephrotic syndrome, and renal transplant all focus on nutrition therapy regulating intake of protein, calories, sodium, potassium, phosphorus, fluid, specific vitamins, and other minerals.

Urinary Tract Infections

Urinary tract infections (UTI) are more common among women, but also occur in men. UTIs are also more common among patients with diabetes because the spillage of glucose into the urine provides a medium for bacterial growth. *Escherichia coli* (*E. coli*) is the most common causative pathogen in UTIs.[1] Empirical treatment should be offered to all individuals who present with UTI symptoms. Obtaining a urine dipstick to confirm pyuria will solidify the clinical picture, but the recommendation to make this routine practice varies by professional organization. It is not necessary

The Nurse Practitioner's Guide to Nutrition, Second Edition. Edited by Lisa Hark, Kathleen Ashton and Darwin Deen.
© 2012 John Wiley & Sons, Inc. Published 2012 by John Wiley & Sons, Inc.

to send urine for culture unless the initial antibiotic course fails.[2] Since antibiotic resistance is making the treatment of UTIs more difficult, it is important to decrease the frequency of UTI in at-risk individuals. UTI rates can be lowered by adopting certain dietary treatments. Adequate fluid intake, cranberry juice, and probiotics have all been reported to prevent incidence of UTIs and are described below.

Nutrition Therapy for Urinary Tract Infections
Cranberry Supplementation

Cranberry supplementation, in either juice or pill form, has been widely accepted and recommended to reduce the risk of UTIs.[3,4] Cranberry acidifies the urine, making a bacteriostatic environment. More recent studies have determined that the tannins in cranberries, or proanthocyanidins, prevent fimbriated *E. coli* from adhering to uroepithelial cells. The effect lasts for approximately 10 hours, so twice daily cranberry supplementation is most beneficial.[4] Cranberry tablets contain approximately 450 mg of cranberry concentrate, the equivalent of 2880 mL of cranberry concentrate juice.[5] In the case of diabetes or glucose intolerance, cranberry capsules or light, sugar-free, cranberry juice are suggested to decrease glucose load and are equally effective. Cranberry concentrate in high doses may inhibit warfarin metabolism and potentiate the anticoagulant effects of the drug.[6] Therefore, cranberry tablets are contraindicated for patients on warfarin therapy.

Probiotics

Probiotics have also demonstrated positive effects in reducing the risk of UTIs.[7] Probiotics are microorganisms administered at high doses to maintain or restore healthy internal gastroenteric and genitourinary flora. UTIs often occur from gut *E. coli* contaminating the genitourinary tract. Probiotics alter the p-fimbriae and type I attachment organelles on the *E. coli* cell to prevent adherence to the urogenital epithelial cells. Probiotics also act directly on promoting normal genitourinary flora, namely lactobacilli.[2] They are found in fermented dairy foods, such as yogurt, as well as in capsule or tablet form. *Lactobacillus bulgaricus* and *Streptococcus thermopiles* are found in all yogurts that meet the National Yogurt Association's (NYA) standard for live and active cultures.[8] Other commonly recommended probiotics are bifidus bacteria and acidophilus. For a yogurt manufacturer to obtain the NYA's probiotic approval seal, the product must contain at least 100 million cultures per gram at time of manufacturing. Frozen yogurt must contain 10 million cultures per gram. For patients with CKD who require potassium and phosphorus restrictions, probiotics are preferred instead of yogurt, which is high in both nutrients.

Fluids

Consuming increased volumes of fluid have long been suggested in the prevention of UTIs. It is thought that the fluids "flush" the genitourinary system and enhance bacterial eradification.[9] However, most of the literature on the subject is from the 1960s and 1970s, so there is no current clinical guideline. Advising patients to consume the recommended eight cups of fluid per day is appropriate, but has no proven benefit on incidence of UTIs. All fluids, including water, juice, tea, and coffee are considered part of this eight cups per day. However, caffeinated beverages are bladder irritants and could increase UTI symptoms until the infection resolves.[9]

Nephrolithiasis (Kidney Stones)

The goals of nutrition therapy for patients with kidney stones are to eliminate the diet-related risk factors for stone formation and prevent the growth of existing stones. The influence of fluids and specific nutrients such as calcium, oxalate, protein, and sodium on the risk for calcium stone formation is discussed in the following section.

Nutrition Therapy for Kidney Stones

Fluid

A high fluid intake is the most important and essential component of nutrition therapy for patients with kidney stones. An increase in urine volume to 2 L/day or more is needed to maintain dilute urine and reduce the concentration of stone-forming substances. Producing this volume of urine requires a fluid intake of approximately 2.5–3 L/day. Observational studies have suggested that coffee, tea, and wine may reduce the risk of stone formation while grapefruit juice and apple juice may increase the risk.[10] It is usually recommended, however, that most fluids be derived from water.

Calcium

Hypercalciuria (usually idiopathic) is one of the common urinary abnormalities seen in patients who form calcium stones. Although much attention is directed toward the effect of dietary calcium on urinary calcium excretion, in reality most cases of calcium urolithiasis are not attributed to high dietary calcium intake. In fact, a very low-calcium diet has been shown to increase the absorption and subsequent excretion of oxalate, which promotes formation of calcium oxalate stones in susceptible individuals. Large studies have also shown that the risk of forming stones is much lower when dietary calcium intake is greater than 1000 mg/day compared with those with dietary calcium intakes less than 600 mg/day.[11] In a large observational study however, the intake of calcium supplements increased the risk of kidney stone formation.[10] Therefore, dietary calcium, mainly coming from dairy foods and calcium-fortified foods, should be prescribed (three servings per day).

Oxalate

Changes in oxalate excretion are more important than calcium excretion in altering the probability of developing calcium oxalate stones. Oxalate has a greater relative effect than calcium on urine supersaturation of calcium oxalate. The role of dietary oxalate in the formation of calcium oxalate stones is not clear, and the proportion of urinary oxalate that comes from diet is controversial (estimated to range from 10 to 50%, but usually closer to 10%). The remainder of urinary oxalate is a product of endogenous metabolism.[10,11]

Gastrointestinal disorders that cause malabsorption are the most common cause of enteric hyperoxaluria. Oxalate absorption tends to be excessive when malabsorbed fat forms soaps and binds calcium in the gut. Free oxalate is then easily absorbed in the intraluminal intestine. Small increases in urinary oxalate concentration greatly increase the potential for crystal formation.[11] Hyperoxaluria has now been seen in an increasing number of patients who have undergone Roux-en-Y bariatric surgery.[12] Control of dietary oxalate therefore may benefit those susceptible to oxalate stones. Oxalate in the urine can be decreased by reducing oxalate in the diet while maintaining enough calcium to achieve a proper balance between these two elements. Vitamin C supplements should be discouraged since ascorbic acid breaks down to oxalic acid and is excreted in the kidney. Dietary sources of high oxalate foods are shown in Table 11-1.

Protein

Most studies have shown that animal proteins cause an unfavorable effect on stone formation because they increase calcium, phosphate, and uric acid excretion, while reducing citrate and urine pH. The increase in urinary phosphate and uric acid is due to the high purine and phosphorus content of animal proteins. The increase in urinary calcium and decrease in citrate and urine pH are due to the high content of sulphurated amino acids.[10] Limiting intake of foods such as meat, fish, poultry, and eggs, to achieve a total protein intake of 60–70 g/day, may be helpful for patients with kidney stones.[11]

Table 11-1 High-Oxalate Foods*

Apricots, dried	Figs
Barley, raw (1/2 cup)	Granola
Beans	Grits (white corn)
Chili	Kiwi
Black beans	Leeks
White beans	Lentil and potato soup
Great northern beans	Miso
Navy beans	Nuts, nut butters
Pink beans	Okra
Beets	Poppy seeds
Bran cereals, shredded wheat, cream of wheat	Potatoes, fried
Buckwheat flour	Raspberries (black)
Carob powder	Red currants
Chocolate/cocoa	Rhubarb
Cornmeal, yellow (1/2 cup)	Sesame seeds
Dark leafy greens	Soy products
Spinach	Sweet potatoes
Collards	Tumeric, ground
Swiss chard	Tomato, canned paste
Mustard	Wheat bran, crude (2T.)

*The oxalate content of foods is variable depending on climate, soil, portion of the plant analyzed, as well as method used for measurement. The above list is based on the "Very High" and "High" lists compiled from the website listed below. This list should only be used as a guide, as some of the "Medium" oxalate containing foods not listed may become high oxalate foods if eaten in significant amounts.
Source: The Oxalate Content of Food: http://www.ohf.org/docs/Oxalate2008.pdf

Sodium

A high sodium intake increases calcium excretion by expanding extracellular fluid volume, increasing the glomerular filtration rate, and decreasing renal tubular calcium reabsorption. These alterations result in an increased quantity of calcium-containing crystals in the urine. Therefore, a moderate reduction of high-sodium foods is recommended (2–4 g/day).[10, 11] High sodium foods are listed in Table 11-5.

Acute Kidney Injury

Acute renal failure (ARF) has recently been renamed and redefined as acute kidney injury (AKI).[13] Stages of AKI have been defined based on smaller changes in serum creatinine and decrease in urine output as shown in Table 11-2. Morbidity and mortality are highest as renal function declines, especially in the presence of sepsis, gastrointestinal dysfunction, or cardiorespiratory and/or hepatic failure.[14] In AKI precipitated by major trauma, critical illness, or sepsis, patients undergo metabolic stress that accelerates degradation of protein, resulting in the loss of lean body mass. With nutrition interventions, it is possible to improve wound healing, reduce infections, and lower mortality rates.[15]

Nutrition Therapy for Acute Kidney Injury

Since malnutrition is so often seen in patients with AKI and is known to be an independent risk factor for mortality, implementation of nutrition therapy is vital. Decisions on when to initiate nutrition therapy and how aggressive to be depend on the patient's current body weight loss compared with their ideal body weight and laboratory parameters such as blood urea nitrogen (BUN), serum albumin, total protein, lactate and carbon dioxide levels, brain natriuretic peptide (BNP), and electrolytes. It is also important to consider the stage of AKI, and plan for renal replacement therapy (RRT), defined as hemodialysis or peritoneal dialysis. Considering all of these variables, nutrition therapy for the patient with AKI is highly individualized. Goals are to preserve existing protein stores and maintain fluid, electrolyte, and acid-base homeostasis.

Table 11-2 Criteria for Stages of Acute Kidney Injury (AKI)

Stage	Creatinine	Urine Output
1	Serum creatinine increased by 0.3 mg/dL or 1.5–2x baseline value.	Less than 0.5 ml/kg/h for more than 6 h.
2	Serum creatinine increased 2–3x baseline value.	Less than 0.5 ml/kg/h for more than 12 h.
3	Serum creatinine increased more than 3x baseline value or serum creatinine more than or equal to 4.0 mg/dL with an acute increase of 0.5 mg/dL.	Less than 0.3 ml/kg/h for 24 h or anuria (no urine ouput) for 12 h.

Source: Gervasio and Cotton.[14]

Protein

The purpose of reducing protein intake in AKI is to limit uremic toxin formation. The degree of protein restriction depends on the stage of AKI, degree of catabolism, and need for RRT. Protein restriction less than or equal to 1.0 g/kg/day is indicated for patients with AKI when renal insufficiency is expected to be transient and for those who are not catabolic or receiving any form of RRT.[15] Since all forms of RRT result in protein loss, the recommended protein intake for patients who are receiving dialysis should be at least 1.2–1.5 g/kg/day. Severely catabolic patients with AKI may have even higher protein needs and require aggressive dialytic therapy or continuous renal replacement therapy (CRRT) to balance protein intake with uremic by-product removal.[15]

CRRT is used when the patient exhibits hemodynamic instability as it provides slower fluid and solute removal. With this therapy, a lower blood flow rate is utilized through a hemofilter in the extracorporeal circuit. It can rely on either arteriovenous (AV) access in which the patient's mean arterial pressure drives the process or veno-venous (VV) access which requires a pump-driven circuit providing a more constant and reliable blood flow rate and solute clearance.[16]

Energy

Caloric requirements for patients with AKI vary depending on the degree of hyper-metabolism. To determine caloric requirements accurately, indirect calorimetry is recommended. Using a calorimeter, the amount of heat generated in an oxidation reaction is determined by measuring the patient's consumption of oxygen (intake) and carbon dioxide production (release) or nitrogen. These quantities are then translated into a heat equivalent that reflects caloric consumption.[17]

Recommendations for caloric intake vary from 20–30 kcal/kg/day. Complications from slightly underfeeding are not as harmful as adverse effects from overfeeding, which can result in hyperglycemia and hypertriglyceridemia.[15] When peritoneal dialysis is utilized as RRT for AKI (though this is rare), calories from the dextrose in the dialysate solutions must be carefully monitored. A simple method for estimating calories absorbed is shown in Table 11-3.[18] This is only an estimate, as patients' peritoneal membrane characteristics are unique. Replacement fluids used with CRRT now contain only physiologic amounts of dextrose, and bicarbonate rather than lactate; therefore, they are generally not a significant source of calories.

Table 11-3 Caloric Absorption from Peritoneal Dialysate

Dextrose (%)	Dextrose (g/L)	Calories Available (3.4 g/L)
1.5	15	51
2.5	25	85
4.25	42.5	145

Approximately 60–76% of calories are estimated to be absorbed from longer dwell times with CAPD and 40–50% with shorter dwell times with CCPD.
Source: Burkhart.[18]

Patients who have adequate gastrointestinal (GI) tract function, but cannot tolerate food by mouth due to mechanical ventilation, altered mental status, anorexia, or nausea should receive nourishment by enteral tube feeding (Chapter 13). The specific formula used will depend on whether the patient is receiving RRT/CRRT and serum electrolyte levels, including calcium and phosphorus. A specialized renal product is not always necessary. Those without a functional GI tract require parenteral nutrition support (Chapter 13). The formulation of the parenteral nutrition will be determined by lab values and whether RRT or CRRT is being utilized. Peripheral insulin resistance may cause hyperglycemia in catabolic patients with AKI, therefore blood glucose levels should be closely monitored. Insulin may be required, especially with the use of parenteral nutrition. There may also be dysfunction of lipid metabolism.[15] Lipids are not precluded in parenteral feedings, but if lipids are added to parenteral nutrition, triglyceride levels must be monitored closely.

Sodium and Potassium

Electrolyte requirements for AKI vary by patient. For example, a patient with acute intrinsic renal failure, or acute tubular necrosis may experience dramatic sodium and water overload during the oliguric phase (< 400 mL urine output/day) and sodium and water depletion during the diuretic or recovery phase, when urine output can exceed 2–3 L/day. For this reason, serum electrolytes must be closely monitored in all patients with AKI. During the oliguric or anuric phase, patients require a sodium restriction of 2–3 g/day and a potassium restriction of 2–3 g/day. This may vary slightly depending on the type and frequency of RRT the patient is receiving.[15] As renal tubular function returns, sodium, potassium, and fluid may need to be replaced to replenish urinary losses.

Vitamins and Other Nutrients

Patients with AKI undergoing any form of RRT or CRRT should be prescribed a water-soluble vitamin supplement above the recommended dietary allowances (RDA) because these are depleted during these treatments. A regular multivitamin preparation is acceptable, as patients with AKI may have lower levels of vitamin A, E, and D.[15] Vitamin K levels may be normal or elevated. Also, with CRRT selenium loss is increased and replacement of this mineral has been shown to improve clinical outcomes in critically ill patients.[15] Phosphorus may actually need repletion if RRT/CRRT is being provided. Frequent monitoring of these levels, in addition to electrolyte levels is essential.

Fluid

Daily fluid intake for oliguric patients should equal urine output plus approximately 500 mL to replace insensible losses. Most anuric patients can tolerate approximately 1000 mL/day with hemodialysis three times per week. These restrictions may be liberalized for patients with fever, and for those receiving daily peritoneal dialysis, hemodialysis, or CRRT.

Chronic Kidney Disease (CKD)

In 2002, the National Kidney Foundation (NKF) published clinical care guidelines for patients with CKD.[19] These guidelines represent a consensus that established the stage of kidney disease based on degree of kidney damage and/or level of glomerular filtration rate (GFR) as shown in Table 11-4. Stage 1 includes kidney damage (e.g. proteinuria) with a normal GFR (90 mL/min/m² or above). Stage 2 represents mild kidney damage (GFR of 60–89). Stage 3 represents a moderate decrease in GFR (30–59). In Stage 4 the GFR is reduced to 15–29 and in Stage 5 the GFR is less than 15.[19]

Table 11-4 Stages of Chronic Kidney Disease

Stage of CKD	Level of Kidney Damage	GFR (mL/min)
1	Kidney damage (e.g. proteinuria)	Normal or ≥90
2	Mild kidney damage	60–89
3	Moderate decrease in GFR	30–59
4	More severe decrease in GFR	15–29
5	Severe decrease in GFR	<15

Adapted with permission from Table 10.1. Renal Disease. In: Hark L, Morrison G (Eds), *Medical Nutrition and Disease: A Case-based Approach*. Wiley-Blackwell, Malden, MA, 2009: 394–426. Original Source: National Kidney Foundation.

Nutrition Therapy for CKD

The goal of nutrition therapy for patients with CKD Stages 1 to 4 prior to dialysis or renal transplantation is to retard the progression of CKD while preventing or alleviating the symptoms of uremia, and restoring acid-base, calcium/phosphorus, vitamin, and iron balance. Treatment also aims to provide adequate calories to maintain or achieve ideal body weight.

Protein

As the GFR decreases, the excretion of nitrogenous wastes (byproducts of protein break-down) declines, producing azotemia and ultimately uremia. Protein restriction can minimize the symptoms of uremic toxicity by reducing the production of nitrogenous wastes in the blood. Evidence suggests that protein restriction early in the course of CKD may decrease glomerular stress and permeability and slow disease progression.[20] The generally accepted level of protein restriction for patients with CKD Stages 1–3 is 0.75 g/kg/day, which is approximately what the DRIs recommend for normal, healthy adults (but is significantly lower than the typical American diet). For Stages 4 and 5 (GFR <29 mL/minute), 0.6 g/kg/day (using an adjusted dry body weight) is advised.[19]

To ensure that essential amino acid requirements are met, it is recommended that approximately 50% of protein intake be from high biological value protein sources.[21] Such sources that contain all essential amino acids include eggs, meats, and other animal proteins. There is some evidence, however, that plant-based proteins may have less deleterious effect on GFR as compared with animal proteins.[21] Protein-restricted diets must be carefully balanced with an adequate caloric intake to prevent weight loss. A low-protein diet may not be appropriate for patients with CKD who are acutely ill and have a decreased oral intake.

Energy

To maintain body weight and allow for effective protein utilization, the recommended adequate energy intake for individuals with CKD not yet on dialysis has been estimated at 35 kcal/kg/day. It has been suggested that 30 kcal/kg/day may be a more appropriate guideline for those greater than 60 years of age assuming they lead a more sedentary lifestyle.[22]

Lipids

Recommendations for fat intake aim to balance adequate caloric intake with prevention of dyslipidemia. Recommendations are based on the KDOQI Clinical Guidelines for Diabetes and CKD and include less than 30% of total calories coming from fat, with 10% omega-3 fatty acids, 10% omega-9 fatty acids, 5% omega-6 fatty acids, and 5% saturated fatty acids.[23] Since dyslipidemia is prevalent in CKD, lipid levels should be monitored for all patients. Pharmacologic treatment, specifically statin therapy, has proven cardiovascular benefits in CKD Stage 2 and 3, but mixed outcome benefits in CKD Stage 4 and 5. For this reason, medical treatment of hyperlipidemia in the later stages of CKD will vary for each patient.[24]

Sodium

As renal failure progresses to a GFR of about 10–15 mL/min, renal sodium excretion decreases. Sodium intake must be limited to prevent sodium retention and subsequent increased thirst. Thirst will cause increased fluid intake which can lead to water retention, edema, hypertension, and/or chronic heart failure. *The NKF/KDOQI Clinical Practice Guidelines on Hypertension and Antihypertensives* recommend limiting sodium intake to less than 2.4 g/day unless a sodium wasting disease is present.[25] A low-sodium diet is difficult to maintain, but is a cornerstone of CKD management due to the strong link between sodium and hypertension.[25] Dietary sources of high sodium are shown Table 11-5.

Potassium

The kidneys regulate potassium efficiently until the GFR falls below 10 mL/min. Thus, a dietary potassium restriction may be necessary only during the later stages of CKD. Exceptions include renal diseases such as diabetic nephropathy, in which aldosterone deficiency develops and potassium excretion declines.[26] Hyperkalemia can be exacerbated by certain drugs, such as angiotensin-converting enzyme (ACE) inhibitors or potassium sparing diuretics (spironolactone). Contrarily, loop diuretics, such as furosemide, or torsemide increase potassium excretion and may cause hypokalemia, even in the presence of CKD. Serum potassium should be monitored more frequently in all the aforementioned cases.[6] When serum potassium levels are consistently greater than 5.0 mEq/L, a potassium-restricted diet of 2–3 g/day

Table 11-5 Foods With High Sodium Content

Bacon	Ham	Smoked meats or fish
Barbecue sauce	Hotdogs	Soy sauce
Bouillon cubes*	Meat tenderizers	Steak sauce
Canned seafood*	Nuts, salted*	Soups, canned* & dried mixes
Cheeses, processed	Olives	Tomato juice*
Chinese food	Packaged or prepared	Tomato sauce
Cold cuts	casserole dishes	Vegetable juice*
Corned beef	Popcorn	Worcestershire sauce
Corn chips	Pickles	
Crackers*	Pretzels*	
Dried beef	Relish	
"Fast Foods"	Salt pork	
Frozen dinners (unless of	Sauerkraut	
a healthy variety)	Sausages	
Gravy, canned or packaged	Scrapple	

Generally, any labeled snack food item with a sodium content ≤200 mg per serving is considered acceptable; some of the above foods may be acceptable if allowed in small servings. Whole dinners should be acceptable if ≤600 mg.
*These items may be purchased "salt-free" or "low sodium" in many grocery stores; check labels to be sure KCl is not added to replace NaCl (salt) if a potassium restriction is required.
Source: Jean Stover, RD, LDN 2012. Used with permission.

(51–77 mEq/day) should be initiated. Dietary sources of high and low potassium-containing foods are listed in Table 11-6.

Calcium, Phosphorus, Parathyroid Hormone and Vitamin D

CKD-Mineral bone disorder (MBD) refers to the clinical syndrome which results from the disturbances of mineral bone metabolism due to CKD. Renal osteodystrophy refers to only the bone disease associated with this disorder.[27] The three major types of renal osteodystrophy include adynamic bone disease, osteitis fibrosa, and osteomalacia. Bone biopsy is the only way to diagnose which type of bone disease a patient has, but the treatment, focused on controlling circulating parathyroid hormone (PTH), calcium, and phosphorus, is the same for all three disorders. MBD also refers to abnormal regulation of PTH, calcium, and phosphorus, which leads to increased vascular and soft tissue calcifications and increased risk of cardiovascular events.[28] Restriction of dietary phosphorus is the key to preventing these complications. Therefore, the *NKF/KDOQI Clinical Practice Guidelines for Bone Metabolism and Disease* recommends a phosphorus restriction of 800–1000 mg/day for individuals with CKD Stages 3 and 4 when serum phosphorus levels are greater than 4.6 mg/dL. This is feasible with a diet low in animal protein, dairy, and processed foods, which would be a vegetable-based protein diet, high in fresh foods.[29] Dietary sources of phosphorous containing foods are shown in Table 11-7.

Many patients with CKD Stages 4 and 5 will need a phosphate binder, which interferes with the absorption of phosphate in the small intestine, keeping the serum

Table 11-6 Foods with High And Low-To-Medium Potassium Content

High Potassium Vegetables	High Potassium Fruits and Juices
Artichokes	Apricots, apricot nectar
Beans (navy, lentil, kidney, pinto)	Avocados
Broccoli	Bananas
Brussels sprouts	Cantaloupe melons
Carrots, raw	Dates
French fries	Figs
Greens	Honeydew melons
Lima beans	Mangos
Parsnips	Nectarines
Potato, baked	Oranges, orange juice
Pumpkin	Papayas
Spinach	Prunes, prune juice
Sweet potato	Raisins
Tomato, tomato juice	Rhubarb
Winter squash (butternut, acorn)	Watermelon
Vegetable juices	

Other High Potassium Foods

Bran Cereal	Nuts
Chocolate	Potato Chips
Milk (more than 4–8 oz/day)	Salt substitutes (containing KCL)
Molasses	

Low-To-Medium Potassium Vegetables*	Low-To-Medium Potassium Fruits and Juices*
Asparagus	Apples, apple juice
Beets	Apple sauce
Cabbage	Blueberries
Carrots, cooked	Cherries
Cauliflower	Cranberries, cranberry juice
Celery	Fruit cocktail
Corn	Grapefruits, grapefruit juice (only 4oz/day)
Cucumber	Grapes, grape juice
Eggplant	Lemons
Green beans	Limes
Green peppers	Peaches, fresh (small)
Kale	Pears, fresh (small), pear nectar
Lettuce	Pineapples, pineapple juice (only 4 oz/day)
Okra	Plums
Onions	Raspberries (1 cup)
Peas	Strawberries (1 cup)
Potato (only when double-boiled)	Tangerines
Radishes	
Wax beans	
Zucchini	

*Low-to-medium potassium foods must be consumed in limited amounts. Generally, three servings of fruits and three servings of vegetables for a potassium restricted diet.
Source: Hark L, Morrison G (Eds), *Medical Nutrition and Disease: A Case-based Approach*, 4th edition. Wiley-Blackwell, Malden, MA, 2009.

Table 11-7 Phosphorus Content of Selected Foods

Foods	Portion Size	Phosphorus Content (mg)
Dairy		
Cheese, cheddar	1 oz	145
Cheese, cream	1 tbsp	15
Frozen yogurt	½ cup	95–100
Half-and-half	½ cup	110
Ice cream	½ cup	70–100
Milk (whole, low fat, skim)	8 oz	220–230
Pudding (vanilla/chocolate dry mix regular made with 2% milk)	½ cup	115–135
Pudding (chocolate dry mix instant made with 2% milk)	½ cup	350
Pudding, (vanilla/chocolate/tapioca/rice-ready-to-eat)	½ cup	45–75
Yogurt (all kinds)	8 oz	215–350
Protein foods		
Beef, cooked	3 oz	150–200
Eggs, whole	1 large	95
Liver, beef (panfried)	3 oz	410
Peanut butter	1 tbsp	55
Sardines, Atlantic, canned in oil	3 oz	415
Tuna	3 oz	140–265
Vegetables		
Baked beans and pork and beans	½ cup	95–150
Dried beans	½ cup	130
Chickpeas	½ cup	110–140
Lentils, boiled	½ cup	180
Soybeans, green boiled	½ cup	140
Soybeans, mature boiled	½ cup	210
Bread and cereals		
Barley, pearled cooked	1 cup	85
Bread, white	1 slice	25
Breads whole grain	1 slice	60
Cornbread (from mix)	1 piece	225
Raisin Bran	1 cup	225
Miscellaneous		
Chocolate	1 oz	70
Nuts, mixed, dry	1 oz	125
Peanuts, dry roasted	1 oz	100
Beverages*		
Beer	12 oz	50
Coffee, brewed	6 oz	5
Colas	12 oz	60

*Please note that inorganic phosphates contained in preservatives found in many beverages are absorbed 100%, even if total phosphorus content does not seem high. Check labels for any ingredient containing "phos-" and avoid these products if following a low phosphorus diet.
Source: USDA National Nutrient Database for Standard Reference, Release 20.

Table 11-8 Selected Phosphate-Binding Medications

Medication	Dose	Ca² (mg) (elemental)	Al (mg)	Manufacturer
Calcium carbonate*				
Calcium carbonate, 1250 mg	1 tab	500	0	Roxane Labs
Oscal 500	1 tab	500	0	GlaxoSmithKline
Tums (regular)	1 tab	200	0	GlaxoSmithKline
Tums (extra-strength)	1 tab	300	0	GlaxoSmithKline
Ultra	1 tab	400	0	GlaxoSmithKline
500	1 tab	500	0	GlaxoSmithKline
Calcium acetate				
PhosLo	1 tab	169	0	Fresenius Medical Care
Calphron	1 tab	169	0	Nephro-Tech
Calcium acetate	1 tab	169	0	Hillestad Pharmaceuticals
Calcium acetate	1 tab	169	0	Generic
Phoslyra	5 ml	0	0	Fresenius Medical Care
Sevelamer HCL				
Renagel 800 mg	1 tab	0	0	Genzyme
Renagel 400 mg	1 tab	0	0	Genzyme
Sevelamer carbonate				
Renvela 800 mg	1 tab	0	0	Genzyme
Renvela powder-0.8 g	1 pkt	0	0	Sanofi-Aventis
Renvela powder-2.4 g	1 pkt	0	0	Sanofi-Aventis
Lanthanum carbonate				
Fosrenol 1000 mg	1 tab	0	0	Shire
Fosrenol 750 mg	1 tab	0	0	Shire
Fosrenol 500 mg	1 tab	0	0	Shire

*Calcium carbonate is now rarely used for phosphate-binding due to its calcium content relative to current suggested guidelines for calcium intake in CKD.
Source: Hark L, Morrison G (Eds), *Nutrition and Disease: A Case-based Approach*, 4th edition. Wiley-Blackwell, Malden, MA, 2009.

phosphate levels within normal range. Available phosphorus binders include calcium acetate, sevelamer hydrochloride, sevelamer carbonate, and lanthanum carbonate as shown in Table 11-8.

Serum calcium levels vary depending on the stage of CKD. When GFR falls below 30 mL/min, hypocalcemia may occur due to impaired vitamin D metabolism and reduced calcium reabsorption in the GI tract.[21] The *KDOQI Clinical Practice Guidelines for Bone Metabolism and Disease* recommends 1.5–2.0 g of calcium (including dietary and supplemental calcium) for hypocalcemia in CKD Stages 3–4 and 1.5–1.8 g for Stages 4–5, not yet receiving dialysis. The goal is to keep serum calcium levels at the lower level of the normal range (8.4–9.5 mg/dL).[29]

If plasma intact PTH is above the target range for the stage of CKD, serum 25-hydroxyvitamin D should be measured at first encounter. If it is normal, repeat annually; if <30 ng/mL (75 nmol/L), supplementation with vitamin D$_2$ (ergocalciferol) should be initiated.[29] Because of the kidney's inadequate conversion of vitamin D from 25 hydroxycholecalciferol [25(OH)D] to its active form, 1,25-dihydroxycholecalciferol [1,25(OH)$_2$D], supplementation of vitamin D as an analog may also be required if PTH levels do not normalize.[29]

Water Balance and Fluid Restriction

Fluid intake for individuals with CKD should be in proportion to their daily urine output. If edema is present, prescribing loop diuretics will increase sodium and water excretion to assist in maintaining balance. Sodium restriction, in addition to pharmacologic therapy will aid in the control of volume maintenance.

Vitamins

Protein and mineral restrictions to manage CKD often result in a diet deficient in essential vitamins. Supplementation with a renal specific vitamin, or water-soluble vitamins that contain at least the recommended dietary allowance for B-complex vitamins and ascorbic acid may be necessary.[30]

Adjunctive Therapy

Most individuals with CKD develop anemia primarily because of the kidney's decreased production of the endogenous hormone erythropoietin. Many individuals will need to begin treatment with erythropoietin stimulating agents (ESAs) in the

---

Case 1 Part 1

Shawn, a 19-year-old African-American student, presented to the emergency room with headaches and shortness of breath. Over the past year, he has gained 10 lb (4.5 kg), although his diet has not changed. He reports a decreased appetite over the past 3 months, difficulty concentrating, and fatigue. He has no history of asthma, rheumatologic or hematologic disorders, or diabetes. He has no family history of renal disease. His father has high blood pressure.

PHYSICAL EXAMINATION: Height: 69″ (176 cm). Current weight: 170 lb (77.3 kg). Usual weight: 155 lb (70.5). Heart rate: 96 b.p.m. Blood pressure: 200/120 mmHg. Cardiac: regular rate and rhythm, S3 gallop. Lungs: faint crackles bilateral bases. Extremities: 2+ peripheral edema bilateral legs.

LABORATORY VALUES: Sodium: 135 mEq/L. Potassium: 4.4 mEq/L. Calcium: 7.5 mg/dL. Adjusted calcium: 8.1 mg/dL. Phosphorus: 5.9 mg/dL. Estimated GFR 25 mL/min/1.73 m^2, Hemoglobin: 9.3 g/dL.

DIAGNOSTIC STUDIES: Chest X-ray: congestive heart failure.

QUESTION: Based on these findings, Shawn is diagnosed with Stage 4 CKD. He requires nutrition therapy. Based on physical examination, should his current body weight be used to estimate his caloric and protein needs?

ANSWER: No. Due to the evidence of volume overload, his caloric and protein requirements should be calculated based on his usual/ideal body weight. Referral to a registered dietitian to educate Shawn on a protein restricted diet that will provide adequate calories is advised.

form of epoetin alfa or darbepoetin alfa prior to initiating dialysis. To promote quality red blood cell production, correcting iron deficiency with either intravenous, intramuscular, or oral supplementation is necessary as well.[31]

Nephrotic Syndrome

Nephrotic syndrome refers to renal disease associated with large quantities of protein spilling in the urine (greater than 3.5 g/day). In all cases, proteinuria is a consequence of glomerular basement membrane damage that results in increased permeability to protein. Patients diagnosed with nephrotic syndrome often exhibit poor appetite, muscle wasting, and malnutrition (primarily protein deficiency). Patients with nephrotic syndrome also exhibit edema or anasarca due to decreased serum albumin and decreased plasma oncotic pressure. Hyperlipidemia, with elevations either in serum cholesterol and/or triglycerides, also occurs in nephrotic syndrome and correlates with the degree of proteinuria. Screening for proteinuria is recommended for all patients with a family history of renal disease, hypertension, or diabetes, as early detection and treatment can slow glomerular damage and the progression to CKD.[32]

Nutrition Therapy for Nephrotic Syndrome
Protein

A moderate protein restriction is recommended for all patients in the early diagnosis of nephrotic syndrome to reduce the amino acid load to the glomerulus. Diminishing the quantity of albumin crossing the damaged glomerular membrane will allow time for glomerular reabsorption of protein and decreased wasting. A moderate protein restriction intake at 0.8–1.0 g/kg/day is recommended. This amount may need to be adjusted based on nutritional status and degree of proteinuria. Vegetarian diets utilizing soy protein, rather than meat-based protein, may also be beneficial for patients with nephrotic syndrome.[21,32]

Energy

Nephrotic syndrome is generally a condition associated with weight loss secondary to protein loss.[32] Adequate calories from non-protein sources are needed to utilize protein and promote weight maintenance. Small frequent meals may be better tolerated if ascites or early satiety is present. Caloric needs for weight maintenance are estimated at 35 kcal/kg/day. Because these patients are often edematous, dry weight should be used for calorie determination.

Lipids

Dyslipidemia due to altered lipoprotein structure and reduced clearance is common in patients with nephrotic syndrome. Elevated very-low-density lipoprotein (VLDL), intermediate-density lipoprotein, LDL-C, total cholesterol, and triglyceride levels warrant a dietary fat restriction to less than 30% of total calories. Dietary cholesterol should be limited to less than 200 mg/day. Pharmacologic therapy (statins) may be necessary if diet alone is ineffective at controlling lipid levels listed or if nephrotic syndrome persists.[32]

Sodium and Fluid

Controlling edema via sodium restriction and diuretics is essential in the management of nephrotic syndrome. Since hypoalbuminemia, high oncotic pressure, third spacing of fluid, and sodium retention are associated with nephrotic syndrome, restricting sodium intake to less than 2 g/day is recommended. The exact level of restriction must be individualized based on the degree of edema. Fluid restriction is not generally recommended unless the patient is hyponatremic.[32] Dietary sources of sodium are listed in Table 11-5.

Potassium

Abnormal potassium levels may occur in patients with nephrotic syndrome depending on the diuretic prescribed to control their volume status or if ACE inhibitors are used to control proteinuria. Monitoring serum potassium levels is essential to determine whether a low, moderate, or high potassium diet is recommended. Dietary sources of potassium listed in Table 11-6.

Calcium and Vitamin D

Hypocalcemia is often seen in the presence of hypoalbuminemia in patients with nephrotic syndrome. Serum calcium levels, both free and corrected, should be monitored periodically. Since serum albumin will cause a falsely decreased serum calcium value, a corrected calcium must be calculated. This will provide an accurate assessment of calcium status in a number of these patients. A concurrent vitamin D deficiency may lead to inadequate calcium absorption; therefore, vitamin D levels should be checked and vitamin D supplementation is recommended.[32] The following equation is used to correct the serum calcium level in relation to degree of hypoalbuminemia:[33]

Corrected Calcium = [(Normal albumin − serum albumin) × (correction factor)]
$\qquad\qquad\qquad$ + serum calcium
Correction factor = 0.8
Normal albumin   = 4.0 mg/dL

Renal Replacement Therapy

Once a patient reaches Stage 5 CKD, one of the following forms of RRT must be initiated: hemodialysis (HD), both in-center or at home; peritoneal dialysis (PD), both continuous ambulatory peritoneal dialysis (CAPD) or continuous cycling peritoneal dialysis (CCPD).

Nutrition Therapy for Dialysis
Protein

The loss of amino acids, the catabolic stress of dialysis, and the advisably low level of protein intake in the pre-dialysis period contribute to poor protein status in the chronic dialysis patient. For this reason, protein intake is not restricted in patients undergoing maintenance dialysis. A protein allowance of 1.2 g/kg/day for in-center HD patients and 1.2–1.3 g/kg/day for home hemodialysis (HHD) or PD patients should be adequate to maintain a positive nitrogen balance, and replace the amino acids lost during dialysis.[22]

During episodes of peritonitis, patients receiving peritoneal dialysis have increased dietary protein needs due to greater losses of protein across an inflamed peritoneum. If patients show clinical or diagnostic signs of protein deficiency, such as weight loss or hypoalbuminemia, supplemental nutrition drinks, bars, or powders are recommended to meet daily protein requirements.[22]

Energy
Caloric recommendations for dialysis patients are estimated in order to maintain a patient's ideal body weight. If the diet is lacking sufficient calories from carbohydrates and fat, endogenous protein is used for energy production. This results in accumulation of uremic toxins and loss of valuable muscle mass. In PD, calories are constantly absorbed from the high glucose dialysate. These "empty calories" must be factored in to the daily caloric intake when making recommendations to prevent weight gain and obesity (Table 11-3).[18] Patients on both HD and PD, however, may also require nutritional supplements to meet caloric as well as protein needs. Enteral nutrition may also be required if oral intake with liquid supplements is insufficient to prevent weight loss. Also, intradialytic parenteral nutrition (IDPN) for HD patients, in which a solution of amino acids, dextrose, and possibly lipids is infused through the venous line during dialysis, may be an acceptable means of nutrition support. For PD, intra-peritoneal nutrition (IPN), in which one bag of a solution containing amino acids is substituted for a dextrose-containing solution, is a possible form of protein nutrition support as well.[34] Patients undergoing either form of dialysis must be referred to a home infusion company and meet specific criteria to be approved for payment through their insurance. A referral to the registered dietitian should be made and this process will then be initiated.

Lipids
As mentioned previously, dyslipidemia is prevalent in patients with CKD and ESRD. Patients undergoing HD often present with normal or high total choles-terol, LDL-C, and triglyceride levels. Patients on PD frequently have high total cholesterol, LDL-C, and triglyceride levels as well as low HDL-C levels. Nutrition therapy is aimed at normalizing cholesterol and triglyceride levels without adversely affecting protein and overall caloric intake in dialysis patients. Pharmacologic therapy for dyslipidemia is often initiated in order to avoid further restrictions to an already complex diet regimen; however, they may not be effective in preventing cardiac events.[35]

Sodium and Fluid
Sodium balance continues to be one of the main challenges for patients undergoing dialysis therapy due to the high sodium content of today's typical diet. Since the body strives to maintain a certain osmolality, a large sodium load causes increased thirst, increased fluid consumption, and resulting fluid overload. For patients on HD, sodium intake is generally restricted to 2–3 g/day, with a fluid allowance of 1000 mL/day plus the amount of urine output, if any.[33] This will allow an acceptable fluid weight

gain of approximately 1 kg or 2.2 lb per day. Sodium and water may be removed more easily with PD because it is performed daily or continuously. This is also true for home HD because it is usually done five to six times per week. A more liberal sodium and water intake is therefore possible for PD and home HD patients. When considering fluid balance, each case must be managed individually. For instance, if a PD patient consistently requires a higher glucose dialysate to remove large volumes of fluid, he/she must be counseled to decrease sodium and fluid intake in order to avoid the negative effects of the additional glucose exposure, namely, peritoneal membrane insufficiency and solid weight gain.[36,37]

Potassium

Potassium intake for patients receiving dialysis must be individualized to maintain normal serum potassium levels. Patients on maintenance HD usually can maintain serum potassium levels between 3.5 and 5.5 mEq/L with diets containing 2–3 g/day (50–75 mEq/day). Persistent hyperkalemia, despite dietary counseling can be treated by lowering the dialysate potassium content. In the case of persistent hypokalemia, usually seen in patients with malnutrition, dietary potassium intake may be liberalized and/or dialysate potassium content increased. This is especially important for patients receiving digoxin therapy, as it may further lower potassium levels and lead to cardiac arrhythmias.[6] Patients on maintenance PD usually maintain a normal serum potassium level without restricting potassium intake. If serum potassium levels fall below normal, dietary potassium is increased, and if unsuccessful, potassium supplements may be required. For those on home HD, dietary potassium may be liberalized depending upon frequency and amount of dialysis performed. Being specific with dietary recommendations and following lab values after implementing an intervention is critical to avoid hyperkalemia.

Calcium, Phosphorus, PTH, and Vitamin D

Phosphorus is used as a preservative in many foods and is found naturally in meats, poultry, fish, and dairy products (Table 11-7). As renal function diminishes, phosphorus excretion decreases and a dietary phosphorus restriction is necessary. The goal of nutrition therapy for patients on dialysis is to allow adequate protein intake, which contains about 1000–1200 mg of phosphorus per day, while maintaining a serum phosphate level of approximately 3.5–5.5 mg/dL or even closer to the normal range.[38] It is also necessary to read labels on many beverages and pre-packaged foods to identify phosphorus-based additives, as such additives should be avoided.[39]

Controlling serum phosphorus by diet alone is difficult if the patient is consuming recommended protein levels (1.2–1.3 g/kg/day). Further, phosphorus is poorly removed by dialysis. Therefore, most dialysis patients are prescribed phosphate binders, such as calcium acetate, sevelamer hydrochloride, sevelamer carbonate, or lanthanum carbonate as shown in Table 11-8. These medications are taken with meals and snacks to promote phosphate-binding in the gut, aimed at decreasing phosphorus absorption. Non-calcium binders may be better choices for phosphate-binding than calcium-containing binders consistent with efforts to avoid excessive calcium intake and the potential increased risk of soft tissue and cardiovascular calcification. The *K/DOQI Clinical Practice Guidelines for Bone Metabolism in Disease* recommend keeping serum calcium levels between 8.4

and 9.5 mg/dL.[29] Calcium-based binders are acceptable in certain situations, for example, post-parathyroidectomy or in patients with hypocalcemia.

Dialysis patients often require active vitamin D (1,25 (OH)$_2$D) administered either orally or parenterally to suppress high levels of parathyroid hormone (PTH). Intermittent or daily doses of oral calcitriol, doxercalciferol, or paracalcitol are generally utilized for PD and home HD. Intravenous doses are generally used for HD patients and administered during the treatment. These may be used in conjunction with the calcimimetic medication cinacalcet to suppress elevated PTH levels. Cinacalcet also assists in lowering serum calcium and phosphorus levels.[6] Patients prescribed cinacalcet require careful monitoring of serum calcium levels at regular intervals to reduce the risk of hypocalcemia. Intravenous calcitriol is not generally used for the suppression of PTH for HD patients due to increased risk of hypercalcemia. However, it may be used for patients who have had parathyroidectomies in order to maintain normal serum calcium levels.

CASE 1 Part 2

Shawn eventually progressed to Stage 5 CKD, requiring dialysis. He elected to begin in-center hemodialysis. Current lab values: albumin: 3.2 g/dL; adjusted calcium: 9.4 mg/dL; phosphorus: 6.4 mg/dL. He has been taking calcium acetate 667 mg 1 tablet three times per day with meals to correct hypocalcemia and hyperphosphatemia.

QUESTION: What is the recommendation for daily protein allowance now that hemodialysis has been initiated?

ANSWER: Shawn no longer requires a protein restricted diet since dialysis will remove nitrogenous wastes. The catabolic state of dialysis will also contribute to increased protein losses requiring increased protein intake; at least 1.2 g/kg/day.

QUESTION: Would you recommend any changes in the phosphorus binding regimen?

ANSWER: Yes. Due to persistent hyperphosphotemia and a rising calcium level, you may elect to change to an increased dose of a non-calcium containing binder. Change to a non-calcium containing binder may also reduce the risk of soft tissue calcification.

Vitamins and Iron

Dialysis patients generally receive folic acid supplementation (1 mg/day), pyridoxine (10 mg/day), B-complex (at RDA levels), and ascorbic acid (60–100 mg/day) due to potential dietary deficiencies and losses during dialysis. There are many forms of renal specific vitamins available that contain these water-soluble vitamins. Recent research shows that reducing homocysteine levels with folic acid in patients with ESRD does not decrease cardiovascular events.[40]

Iron supplementation for patients receiving either PD or HD is usually necessary if they are receiving erythropoietin stimulating agents (ESAs) for anemia. Periodic (weekly or monthly) doses of intravenous preparations of iron gluconate or iron sucrose are given to maintain a serum iron saturation greater than 20% and ferritin level greater than 200 ng/mL.[31] Iron dextran is rarely used now due to potential adverse reactions and oral iron is not recommended due to poor absorption and GI side effects. Current *NKF/KDOQI Clinical Practice Guidelines for Anemia* state that there is insufficient evidence to supplement iron when the ferritin levels are above 500 ng/mL.[31] However, more recent research shows that repleting iron stores when ferritin levels range from 200 to 1200 ng/mL and the iron saturation is less than or equal to 25% will improve the body's response to ESAs and increase hemoglobin.[41] Further, "when ferritin levels are above 500 ng/mL, decisions regarding i.v. iron administration should consider ESA responsiveness, hemoglobin and transferrin saturation levels, and the patient's clinical status".[31] Due to a lack of evidence on when iron supplementation may cause deleterious effects, such as hemachromatosis, there are no current guidelines for when iron supplements should be initiated.

Renal Transplantation

Many kidney transplant programs now require a body mass index (BMI) of $< 35–40 \, kg/m^2$ for eligibility of active status on the transplant list in efforts to avoid surgical complications. However, recent research indicates that central obesity, measured as waist/hip ratio (WHR), is a stronger predictor of all-cause mortality and cardiovascular death than body mass index (BMI) alone in the general population and in renal transplantation patients.[42,43] The goal of nutrition therapy for patients who have undergone renal transplantation is to provide optimal nutrition without exacerbating the metabolic side effects of immunosuppressive drugs and other medical therapy. Nutritional goals will vary depending on the length of time post-transplant. In the early post-transplant phase, emphasis is placed on ensuring adequate protein intake, encouraging weight gain/maintenance depending on weight status prior to transplant, and avoidance of raw or fresh foods (due to risk of infection while on high doses of immunosuppressants). Blood glucose control while on steroid therapy is also essential. In the event of acute tubular necrosis (ATN) and/or organ rejection, nutrient modifications may be necessary to prevent hyperkalemia and control hypertension and circulating blood volume.

Nutrition Therapy for Renal Transplant
Protein
Protein catabolism occurs in the immediate post-operative period secondary to the stress of surgery and increased catabolic effects of high doses of steroids and other immunosuppressive medications such as cyclosporine and tacrolimus. Recommended protein intake for these patients is 1.3–2.0 g/kg/day.[44] Many of the short-term and long-term side-effects of corticosteroid use have been eliminated by minimizing their use.[45,46] Once the kidney is functioning well and immunosuppression is reduced, protein intake is based on the RDA at 0.8–1 g/kg/day.

Energy
In addition to protein, adequate calories are necessary in the post-operative period in order to promote wound healing and prevent opportunistic infection. Recommended caloric intake for these patients is 30–35 kcal/kg/day, based on usual body weight

(UBW).[44] Because increased appetite is a common side effect of steroid therapy, the long-range goal is weight maintenance. It has been shown that early intensive nutrition counseling and follow-up can successfully prevent unwanted weight gain in the first year post-transplant.[47]

Carbohydrate

Hyperglycemia frequently occurs post-transplant as a consequence of exposure often referred to high-dose steroids and other immunosuppressive drugs, often referred to as steroid-induced diabetes or steroid-induced hyperglycemia.[48] Insulin is commonly prescribed in the immediate post-transplant period and patients will require a carbohydrate controlled diet. Hyperglycemia often resolves as steroid doses decrease, but if a patient was pre-diabetic prior to transplantation, they may require long-term insulin therapy. Medical and nutritional management of diabetes and obesity are essential to post-transplant care. In addition, collaboration with an endocrinologist is valuable in order to optimize therapy.

Lipids

Dyslipidemia occurs after renal transplantation as a side effect of immunosuppressive therapy or secondary to obesity. Consequently, chronic care recommendations are to limit total dietary fat with emphasis on decreasing saturated fat and substituting monounsaturated and polyunsaturated fats. Fish oil supplements have shown some benefit as well.[49]

Sodium, Fluid, and Potassium

It is critical to closely monitor sodium, fluid, and potassium in the post-transplant period. Recommendations vary depending on length of time from transplant. The incidence of hyponatremia in the first 90 days post-transplant is very high in patients receiving tacrolimus and cyclosporine with infusions of normal saline solution. Hyponatremia resolves in nearly every case after the first 90 days and once the body adjusts to immunosuppression.[50] Volume restriction to correct hyponatremia may cause renal hypoperfusion and transplant allograft damage and is not recommended. Checking sodium levels is critical in the first months post-transplant. As patients progress, a sodium-restricted diet is often recommended in order to control hypertension and prevent end-organ damage secondary to hypertension.

Potassium levels should also be closely monitored in the first few months post-transplant. Immunosuppression can occasionally cause hyperkalemia, though it is uncommon.[50] Patients on ACE inhibitors or diuretics may still experience potassium disturbances, warranting serum potassium monitoring. Generally, potassium restriction post-transplant is not required once a patient's transplant is functioning well. Adequate intake of potassium should be encouraged in order for patients to avoid hypokalemia.

Fluid is generally not restricted post-operatively, as encouraging renal perfusion and filtering is of utmost importance. Even in the case of acute tubular necrosis, when a patient may be distinctly oliguric, fluid intake, either intravenously or by mouth, is encouraged to prompt the kidney to filter. Monitoring for symptoms of volume overload is important during the early post-transplant phase and if severe, fluid intake may be slightly reduced or diuretics may be prescribed. Generally patients with a transplanted kidney can drink fluid without restriction, as long as they are not experiencing allograft rejection.

Calcium and Phosphate

Generally, neither dietary phosphate restriction nor phosphate-binding medication is necessary post-transplant. In fact, hypophosphatemia due to increased phosphate excretion and bone uptake sometimes develops in the acute post-transplant period and may require a high-phosphorus diet and/or phosphate supplementation. Also, steroid therapy interferes with calcium absorption and osteoporosis is common for many kidney transplant recipients, especially for those on long-term steroid therapy.[51] Calcium and vitamin D supplementation may also be required longer term for post-transplant patients.

Herbal and Dietary Supplement Use in CKD

In recent years, complementary or alternative medicine (CAM) has become very popular in industrialized countries. Patients in all stages of CKD and post-transplant must be very cautious when considering the use of herbal remedies and dietary supplements.[52] These products are not FDA regulated and many are carcinogenic, hepatotoxic, or nephrotoxic. Therefore, products may not contain what the label advertises. Laboratory analyses have identified products lacking the stated ingredients or being contaminated with pesticides, poisonous plants, heavy metals, or conventional drugs.[52] Nurse Practitioners who care for these patients should be aware of CAM therapies and treatments and appropriately advise patients (Table 11-9).

Herbal supplements are also dangerous due to their unpredictable pharmacokinetics. For example, St John's Wort may interfere with the bioavailability of cyclosporine and tacrolimus, and cause transplant rejection. Echinacea should also be avoided by kidney transplant recipients due to its stimulation of the immune system which could counteract the effectiveness of immunosuppressants.[53–55]

Fish oils must be used with caution when prescribed with anticoagulants or antiplatelet medications, as they can increase the risk of bleeding. Some bulk-forming laxatives, such as flaxseed and fiber require a large fluid intake to be effective. Therefore, they should be used with caution for patients requiring fluid limitations. Noni juice, a beverage supplement used for various indications, should be avoided in

Table 11-9 When to Refer to a Registered Dietitian

- Assessment of nutrition status and calculation of nutrients is needed for a patient; all types of kidney disease (inpatient/outpatient).*
- Determination of oral vs enteral/parenteral nutrition is needed (inpatient/outpatient).*
- Recommendation for compostion of enteral/parenteral nutrition is needed (inpatient).
- Specific oral diet modification is needed; specific diet order, especially whether protein restriction is appropriate (inpatient/outpatient).*
- Education of the patient for modification of nutrient needs is required (inpatient/outpatient).*

---

*For referral to an RD for an outpatient with CKD Stages 1–4, utilize outpatient hospital nutrition services if available, or go to www.eatright.org to locate an RD. For patients receiving outpatient HD or PD, refer to RD in the facility providing these services.

CKD patients at risk for hyperkalemia due to its high potassium content.[52–55] It is therefore very important that Nurse Practitioners question renal patients about their use of herbs and dietary supplements, especially those with CKD.

Summary: Role of Nurse Practitioners

The primary focus of nutrition therapy for renal disease includes management of appropriate protein and calorie intake, fluid and electrolyte balance, as well as the need for specific vitamins and minerals, especially vitamin D and iron. Since recommendations for each of these elements varies according to the type and stage of renal disease, Nurse Practitioners should have a general knowledge of the guidelines within each disease state. Nurse Practitioners can manage renal patients and support the nutritional recommendation and treatment plan developed by the dietitian. Nurse

Table 11-10 Educational Resources For Patients and Professionals

Organization	Type of Information	URL
The National Kidney Foundation (NKF)	Information/education materials for various stages of CKD, types of dialysis, transplant, nutrition, and kidney stones.	www.kidney.org
Davita, Inc.	Information about kidney disease, treatment options, education articles, recipes, online kidney diet meal planner, dialysis center locator.	www.davita.com
American Kidney Fund (AKF)	Information about financial assistance grants for kidney patients (in English and Spanish).	www.kidneyfund.org
Kidney School	Information for patients about kidney function, treatment options, and nutrition (with meal plans).	kidneyschool.org
American Association of Kidney Patients	Information for patients about chronic kidney disease, dialysis, transplant, advocacy.	www.aakp.org
Kidney Options	Information about kidney disease, treatment options, nutrition, social services, recipe and question of the week, dialysis center locator.	www.kidneyoptions.com
Renal Support Network (RSN)	Education, advocacy, resources, social networking, and forums for patients.	http://www.rsnhope.org
National Center for Complementary and Alternative Medicines (NCCAM)	Government agency dedicated to exploring CAM practices, consumer information.	http://nccam.nih.gov/
National Institutes of Health (NIH) Office of Dietary Supplements-Relevant Links	Links to dietary supplement fact sheets, dietary supplement use and safety; nutrient recommendations.	http://ods.od.nih.gov/

Practitioners and registered dietitians should collaborate to optimize nutrition therapy for patients with renal disease. The dietitian should assist in formulating a patient specific treatment plan that will provide each individual with the appropriate amounts of the aforementioned nutrients. Educational resources for patients and professionals are shown in Table 11-10.

References

1. Cadieux PA, Burton JP, Devillard E, et al. *Lactobacillus* by-products inhibit the growth and virulence of uropathogenic *Escherichia coli. J Physio Pharm* 2009;Suppl 6:13–18.
2. National Guideline Clearinghouse (NGC). Guideline synthesis: diagnosis and management of lower urinary tract infection, January 2008 (revised April 2011).
3. Gupta K, Chou MY, Howell A, et al. Cranberry products inhibit adherence of p-fimbriated Escherichia coli to primary cultured bladder and vaginal epithelial cells. *J Urol* 2007;177: 2357–2360.
4. Pinzón-Arango PA, Liu Y, Camesano TA. Role of cranberry on bacterial adhesion forces and implications for escherichia coli-uroepithelial cell attachment. *J Med Food* 2009;12:259–270.
5. Terris MK, Issa MM, Tacker JR. Dietary supplementation with cranberry concentrate tablets may increase the risk of nephrolithiasis. *Urology* 2001;57:26–29.
6. Turkoski, BB, Lance, BR, Bonfiglio, MF. *Drug Information Handbook for Advanced Practice Nursing*, 8th edition. Lexi-comp Inc., Hudson, 2007.
7. Reid G. Probiotic agents to protect the urogenital tract against infection. *Am J Clin Nutr* 2001;73:437S–443S.
8. National Yogurt Association. Live & active culture yogurt. www.aboutyogurt.com/index.asp. Accessed 2012.
9. Beetz R. Mild dehydration: a risk factor of urinary tract infections? *Eur J Clin Nutr* 2003;Suppl 2: S52–S58.
10. Orfeas L, Jaber BL. Kidney stones. In: Byham-Gray LD, Burrowes JD, Cherow GM (Eds), *Nutrition in Kidney Disease*. Humana Press, Totowa. 2008:513–530.
11. Borghi L, Meschi T, Maggiore U, et al. Dietary therapy in idiopathic nephrolithiasis. *Nutr Rev* 2006;64:301–312.
12. Hark L, Deen D, Pruzansky A. Overview of nutrition assessment in clinical care. In: Hark L, Morrison G (Eds), *Medical Nutrition and Disease: A Case-based Approach*. Wiley-Blackwell, Malden, MA, 2009:39–57.
13. Himmelfarb J, Ikizler TA. Acute kidney injury: changing lexicography, definitions, and epidemiology. *Kidney Int* 2007;71:71–76.
14. Gervasio JM, Cotton AB. Nutrition support therapy in acute kidney injury: distinguishing dogma from good practice. *Curr Gastroenterol Rep* 2009;14:325–331.
15. Druml W. Acute renal failure. In: Byham-Gray LD, Burrowes JD, Chertow M. *Nutrition in Kidney Disease*. Humana Press: Totowa, 2008:87–502.
16. Hung C-C, Bonventre JV. Acute kidney injury. In: Singh AK (Ed.), *Educational Review Manual in Nephrology*. Castle Connolly Graduate Medical, New York, 2008:51–90.
17. *Mosby's Medical Dictionary*, 8th edition. Elsevier, Philadelphia, 2009.
18. Burkhart J. Metabolic consequences of peritoneal dialysis. *Semin Dial* 2004;17:498–504.
19. NKF K/DOQI Clinical Practice Guidelines for Chronic Kidney Disease: Evaluation, Classification, and Stratification. *Am J Kidney Dis* 2002;39:S37–S75, S112–S155, S170–S212.
20. Fouque D, Aparicio M. Eleven reasons to control the protein intake of patients with chronic kidney disease. *Nat Clin Pract Nephrol* 2007;3:383–392.
21. Schiro-Harvey K. Nutrition and pharmacologic approaches. In: Byham-Gray LD, Burrowes JD, Chertow M. *Nutrition in Kidney Disease*. Humana Press, Totowa, 2008:191–226.

22. NKF K/DOQI Clinical Practice Guidelines for Nutrition in Chronic Renal Failure. *Am J Kidney Dis* 2000;35:S58–S61.

23. National Kidney Foundation. K/DOQI clinical practice guidelines and clinical recommendations for diabetes and chronic kidney disease. *Am J Kidney Dis* 2007;49:S62–S73.

24. Harper CR, Jacobson TA. Managing dyslipidemia in chronic kidney disease. *J Am Coll Card* 2008:51:2375–2384.

25. NKF K/DOQI Clinical Practice Guidelines for hypertension and antihypertensive agents in chronic kidney disease. *Am J Kidney Dis* 2004;43:S16–S230.

26. Allon M. Disorders of potassium metabolism. In: Greenberg A (Ed.), *Primer on Kidney Diseases*, 4th edition. Elsevier, Philadelphia, 2005:110–119.

27. Moe S, Drueke T, Cunningham J. Definition, evaluation, and classification of renal osteodystrophy: a position statement from Kidney Disease: Improving Global Outcomes (KDIGO). *Kidney Int* 2006;69:1945–1953.

28. McCullough, PA, Sandberg, KR, Dumler, F, et al. Determinants of coronary vascular calcification in patients with chronic kidney disease and end-stage renal disease: a systematic review. *J Nephrol* 2004;17:205.

29. NKF K/DOQI Clinical practice guidelines for bone metabolism and disease in chronic kidney disease. *Am J Kidney Dis* 2003;42:S29–S91.

30. Wiggins KL. Guideline 2, nutrition care of adult dialysis patients. In: *Guidelines for Nutrition Care of Renal Patients*, 3rd edition. American Dietetic Association, Chicago, 2002:5–18.

31. NKF-DOQI *Clinical Practice Guidelines for the Treatment of Anemia of Chronic Renal Failure.* National Kidney Foundation, New York, 2006.

32. Yeun JY, Kaysen GA. The nephrotic syndrome. In: Byham-Gray LD, Burrowes JD, Chertow GM (Eds), *Nutrition in Kidney Disease*. Humana Press, Totowa, 2008: 503–512.

33. The Clinician's Ultimate Reference. Corrected calcium calculator. www.globalrph.com/calcium.cgi. Accessed 2012.

34. Wiesen K, Mindel G. Dialysis. In: Byham-Gray L, Burrowes J, Chertow G (Ed.), *Nutrition in Kidney Disease*. Humana Press, Totowa, 2008:231–257.

35. Marrs JC, Saseen JJ. Effects of lipid-lowering therapy on reduction of cardiovascular events in patients with end-stage renal disease requiring hemodialysis. *Pharmacotherapy* 2010:30:823–829.

36. Heimberger O, Stenvinkel P, Lindholm B. Nutritional effects and nutritional management of chronic peritoneal dialysis. In: Kopple JD, Massry SG. *Nutritional Management of Renal Disease*, 2nd edition. Lippincott Williams & Wilkins, Philadelphia, 2004:477–512.

37. Ikizler TA. Nutritional and peritoneal dialysis. In: Mitch WE, Klahr S. *Handbook of Nutrition and the Kidney*. Lippincott Williams & Wilkins, Philadelphia 2005:228–244.

38. Moe SM, Drueke TB, Block GA, et al. KDIGO clinical practice guideline for the diagnosis, evaluation, prevention, and treatment of chronic kidney disease-mineral and bone disorder (CKD-MBD). *Kidney Int* 2009;76(Suppl 113):Sv–Svi.

39. Kalantar-Zadeh K, Gutekunst L, Mehrotra R, et al. Understanding sources of dietary phosphorus in the treatment of patients with chronic kidney disease. *Clin J Am Soc Nephol* 2010;5:519–530.

40. Heinz J, Kropf S, Luley C, et al. Homocysteine as a risk factor for cardiovascular disease in patients treated by dialysis: a meta-analysis. *Am J Kidney Dis* 2009;54:478–489.

41. Coyne DW, Kapoian T, Suki W, et al. and the DRIVE Study Group. Ferric gluconate is highly efficacious in anemic hemodialysis patients with high serum ferritin and low transferring saturation: results of the dialysis patients' response to IV iron with elevated ferritin (DRIVE) study. *J Am Soc Nephrol* 2007;18:975–984.

42. Postorino M, Marino C, Tripepi G. Abdominal obesity and all-cause and cardiovascular mortality in end-stage renal disease. *J Am Coll Cardiol* 2009;53:1265–1272.

43. Orazuo L, Armstrong K, Banks M, et al. Central obesity is common in renal transplant recipients and is associated with increased prevalence of cardiovascular risk factors. *J Nutr Diet* 2007;64:200–206.

44. Blue LS. Adult kidney transplantation. In: Hasse JM, Blue LS (Eds), *Comprehensive Guide to Transplant Nutrition*. American Dietetic Association, Chicago, 2002:49.

45. Woodle ES, First MR, Pirsch J, et al. A prospective, randomized double-blind, placebo-controlled multicenter trial comparing early (7 day) corticosteroid cessation versus long-term, low-dose corticosteroid therapy. *Ann Surg* 2008;4:564–577.

46. Jaber JJ, Feustel PJ, Elbahloul O, et al. Early steroid withdrawal therapy in renal transplant recipients: a steroid-free sirolimus and CellCept-based calcineurin inhibitor-minimization protocol. *Clin Transplant* 2007;21:101–109.

47. Lopes IM, Martin M, Errasti P, et al. Benefits of a dietary intervention on weight loss, body composition and lipid profile after renal transplantation. *Nutrition* 1999;15:7–10.

48. Danovitch G. Immunosuppressive medications and protocols for kidney transplantation. In: Danovitch G (Ed.), *Handbook of Kidney Transplantation*, 4th edition. Lippincott Williams & Wilkins, Philadelphia, 2005:72–110.

49. Lim AKH, Manley KJ, Roberts MA, et al. Fish oil for kidney transplant recipients. *Cochrane Database of Systematic Reviews* 2007, Issue 2. Art. No.: CD005282. DOI: 10.1002/14651858.CD005282.pub2.

50. Higgins R, Ramalyan TD, Kanji H, et al. Hyponatremia and hyperkalemia are more frequent in renal transplant recipients treated with tacrolimus than with cyclosporine. Further evidence for differences between cyclosporine and tacrolimus nephrotoxicities. *Nephrol Dial Transplant* 2003;19:444–450.

51. Massari PU. Disorders of bone and mineral metabolism after renal transplantation. *Kidney Int* 1997;52:1412–1421.

52. Colson CE, DeBroe ME. Kidney injury from alterative medicines. *Adv Chronic Kidney Dis* 2005;12:261–275.

53. Burrowes JD, Van Houten G. Use of alternative medicine by patients with stage 5 chronic kidney disease. *Adv Chronic Kidney Dis* 2005;12:312–325.

54. Radler DR. Dietary supplements. In: Byham-Gray L, Burrowes J, Chertow G (Ed.), *Nutrition in Kidney Disease*. Humana Press, Totowa, 2008:531–542.

55. Nowack R, Balle C, Birnkammer F, et al. Complementary and alternative medications consumed by renal patients in Southern Germany. *J Ren Nutr* 2009;19:211–219.

12 Cancer Prevention and Oncology Care

Tamara B. Kaplan, MD
Maureen Huhmann, DCN, RD, CSO
Theresa P. Yeo, PhD, MPH, MSN, AOCNP

OBJECTIVES

- Discuss the role of dietary and lifestyle factors in the prevention of cancer.
- Evaluate the impact of cancer on nutritional status of individuals with cancer.
- Examine the nutrition-related side-effects of cancer therapy.
- Discuss the role of nutrition therapy in the treatment of cancer and during survivorship.

Introduction

Cancer is a major chronic disease that contributes significantly to both morbidity and mortality, accounting for 12% of all deaths worldwide.[1] Cancer will affect one in every three people before the age of 75.[1] While genetics certainly play a role in predisposing one to cancer, lifestyle factors have a significant influence on cancer risk.[2] It is estimated that 50% of cancer incidence and 30–35% of cancer mortality in Americans is related to poor diet, obesity, and excessive alcohol intake.[3] Therefore, the purpose of this chapter is twofold: (1) to discuss the important role that Nurse Practitioners play in assisting patients to assess and reduce their risk of cancer and (2) to address the nutritional issues in patients diagnosed with cancer and those undergoing treatment and living with cancer.

Obesity and Cancer

Obesity is strongly associated with an increased risk of colon, kidney, pancreatic, esophageal, endometrial, and post-menopausal breast cancer.[4-6] The idea that excess weight may be linked to cancer risk is supported by evidence that calorie restriction protects against various types of tumors. The American Institute for Cancer Research (AICR) published the report *Food, Nutrition, Physical Activity and the Prevention of Cancer: A Global Perspective* which reviewed over 7000 research studies and conclusively established the link between obesity and cancer.[3] Several mechanisms have been proposed to explain how obesity affects cancer. One important factor is

The Nurse Practitioner's Guide to Nutrition, Second Edition. Edited by Lisa Hark, Kathleen Ashton and Darwin Deen.
© 2012 John Wiley & Sons, Inc. Published 2012 by John Wiley & Sons, Inc.

that excess adipose tissue causes alterations in hormone metabolism. One hypothesis is that high levels of insulin and insulin-related growth factors in obese people may promote tumor development. Insulin stimulates multiple cellular mechanisms that may potentially lead to uncontrolled cell growth and ultimately cancer.

Breast Cancer

Scientists first suggested a link between excess body weight and breast cancer in the 1970s. Since that time, studies have demonstrated that there is a strong relationship between obesity and increased breast cancer risk in post-menopausal women,[7] although this link was not found in pre-menopausal women.[8] Post-menopausal women who gain a considerable amount of excess weight also dramatically increase their risk of breast cancer.[9] Cohort studies have shown that post-menopausal women whose BMI is in the top quartile increase their breast cancer risk by about 40%. In the Women's Health Study (1999–2004), women with a BMI greater than 40 kg/m^2 had a 60% higher risk of dying from cancers of all causes compared with women with a normal BMI. This increased risk is independent of other factors such as lifestyle and physical activity.[10] According to the National Cancer Institute (NCI), weight gain during adulthood is the strongest predictor of breast cancer risk.[11]

Endometrial Cancer

Unlike breast cancer there seems to be a positive and linear relationship between endometrial cancer and obesity. This positive correlation is true for both pre-menopausal and post-menopausal women. Studies show overweight and obese women are two to four times more likely to develop uterine cancer.[12]

Colon Cancer

Colon cancer, is a largely a preventable disease with a high cure rate associated with early detection. Colon cancer risk is associated with certain genetic alterations, a family history of colon cancer and the development of adenomatous polyps, and certain environmental factors, such as cigarette smoking, moderate to heavy alcohol consumption, obesity, and a sedentary lifestyle.[13] Approximately 90% of the disease occurrence is in persons over the age of 50. Familial colon cancers account for 5% of all colon cancers. Familial colon cancers can demonstrate a Mendelian pattern of inheritance and include the familial adenomatous polyposis (FAP) and hereditary non-polyposis colorectal cancer (HNPCC) types. In addition, 15–30% of sporadic colon cancers occur in persons at increased risk due to a personal history of adenomatous polyps or having a first-degree relative diagnosed with colon cancer before the age of 60. Men with high BMI levels (>35 kg/m^2) consistently show an increase risk of colon cancer; however, the evidence for women is not quite as strong.[14,15] The National Cancer Institute estimates that the calculated risk of colon cancer increases 11% with a BMI>30 kg/m^2.[11]

The location of excess body weight may influence this risk.[16] Abdominal fat seems to play a significant role in the risk of developing colon cancer. Overweight men tend to collect fat in their abdomen, while in women fat is more likely to be distributed in the hips, thighs, and buttocks. Thus, it will be important for researchers to define the relationship between colon cancer and waist-to-hip ratio or waist circumference.

According to the American Cancer Society, a diet high in fat increases the production of bile salts which are converted into potential carcinogens by the intestinal flora.[1] Red meats (beef, lamb, or liver) and processed meats (hot dogs and luncheon meats) can increase colorectal cancer risk. Cooking meats at very high temperatures (frying, broiling, or grilling) creates carcinogens that increase cancer risk. Factors found to be slightly protective against colon cancer include: vigorous physical activity, daily multivitamin use, use of calcium supplements, and low intake of fat from red meat.

Recent research shows an inverse relationship between vitamin D levels and the risk of colon and rectal cancers. Researchers found up to a 33% decrease in risk for these cancers among the patients with the highest levels of vitamin D intake. The lower risk was attributed to increased levels of vitamin D from both dietary sources and supplements.[17]

Pancreatic Cancer

A meta-analysis of 21 prospective studies in persons with pancreatic cancer found that for every 5-unit increase in BMI, the relative risk of developing pancreatic cancer increased 10% in women and 16% in men.[6] The population-attributable risk percentage of obesity-associated pancreatic cancer is estimated at 26.9% in the US, compared with the population-attributable risk for cigarette smoking of 25%.[18] A recent case-control study of 841 pancreatic cancer patients and 754 healthy controls found that persons who were overweight and between the ages of 14 and 39 years and those who were obese and between 20 and 49 years had an increased risk of developing pancreatic cancer. This increased risk was independent of having diabetes.[19] Furthermore, obese patients had higher mortality rates among both resected and unresected cases.

Nutrition and Cancer Prevention
Meat and Protein

According to the AICR, there is strong evidence that red meat intake from beef, pork, lamb, and processed meats, such as bacon, sausage, hot dogs, salami, bologna, ham, and pepperoni significantly increases the risk of colorectal cancer.[3] It is recommended that patients eat a maximum of **18 oz of cooked red meat** per week and avoid processed meat if possible. Each additional ounce of processed meat consumed per day increases the risk of developing colorectal cancer. Processed meats have also been linked to a higher incidence of stomach cancer. This increased risk may be due to the nitrates and nitrosamines. Nitrites and nitrates react with amino acids to form cancer-causing nitrosamines. These compounds are used to provide a pink hue to cured meat without which the meat would turn brown during storage.

There are also concerns about cooking methods that use high temperatures such as frying, broiling, or barbecuing. When meats such as beef, pork, poultry, and fish are cooked at high temperatures, the amino acids and creatine may form carcinogenic compounds called heterocyclic amines (HCAs). Case-control studies from the NCI found that people who consumed medium-well or well-done beef increased their risk of stomach cancer threefold in comparison to those who consumed rare or medium-rare beef.[11] Other NCI studies have also shown that a high intake of well-done, fried, or barbecued meats is associated with an increased risk of developing colorectal, pancreatic, and breast cancer.

Carbohydrates, Fiber, and Whole Grains

The protective effects of eating whole grains to prevent cancer has not been clearly established. However, many case-controlled studies have shown an association between high intake of whole grains and a low incidence of several types of cancer.[20] A meta-analysis of 40 case-control studies that looked at 20 different types of cancer found that those with high whole grain intake had a 34% lower overall cancer risk compared with those with low whole grain intake. While a decreased risk of gastrointestinal (GI) cancers is most commonly associated with whole grain intake, the lignans in whole grains (phytoestrogens) may also affect hormone-dependent cancers as well.[21]

Fiber is known to provide many health benefits such as reducing the risk of heart disease and diabetes and preventing constipation. Because fiber increases stool bulk and speeds the transit time of food through the colon, scientists hypothesize that this decreased transit time may help reduce the exposure of colon mucosa to carcinogens. However, recent studies have failed to support this hypothesis.[22] The Nurse's Health Study followed 80,000 female nurses for 16 years and found no strong association between dietary fiber and a reduced risk for colon cancer.[23] In contrast, many case-control studies conducted prior to 1990 did find a lower incidence of colon cancer in people with high fiber intake. These discrepancies indicate that more research is needed before conclusions may be drawn about the relationship between fiber intake and cancer risk. It is important to note that the type and amount of fiber consumed varied among the different studies.[24]

Fats

While total fat intake does not seem to alter cancer risk, diets high in animal fats are associated with the development of colorectal and prostate cancer. In contrast, some oils such as those that contain omega-3 fatty acids (DHA and EPA) can have a beneficial effect. Omega-3 fatty acids are converted to anti-inflammatory prostaglandins, which may reduce tumor growth.[25] While omega-3 fatty acids from fish oils may be beneficial, omega-6 fatty acids (from vegetable oils) may actually be harmful and promote prostate cancer.[26]

Omega-6 fatty acids cause the production of a family of eicosanoids including prostaglandins, which affect immunity and promote inflammation. The health impact of these various fatty acids is determined by the ratio of omega-6 to omega-3 fatty acids consumed. Interestingly in the US, 60 years ago, people consumed a dietary ratio of omega-6 to omega-3 that was about 2:1. Today, the ratio is roughly 25:1, due to the high intake of vegetable oils and low intake of fish.

Phytochemicals

Phytochemicals are compounds found in plants that have the ability to protect plants against diseases caused by bacterial or fungal infections. These compounds may also play an important role in preventing tumor growth in humans.[27] Over 4000 different types of plant phytochemicals have been identified as shown in Table 12-1. The two

Table 12-1 Common Phytonutrients

- Carotenoids.
- Flavonoids (Polyphenols), including Isoflavones (Phytoestrogens).
- Inositol Phosphates (Phytates).
- Lignans (Phytoestrogens).
- Isothiocyanates and Indoles.
- Phenols and Cyclic Compounds.
- Saponins.
- Sulfides and Thiols.
- Terpenes.

Source: Darwin Deen, MD, MS, and Lisa Hark, PhD, RD, 2012. Used with permission.

Table 12-2 Food Sources of Common Phytochemicals

Family	Examples	Foods
Carotenoids	Beta-carotene	Leafy green and yellow vegetables (broccoli, sweet potato, pumpkin, carrots)
	Lycopene	Tomatoes and tomato products, guava, pink grapefruit, watermelon
	Lutein	Spinach, kale, cabbage, Swiss chard, broccoli, Brussels sprouts, turnips, and collard greens
	Zeaxanthin	Carrots, peaches, green oranges, mango, corn, eggs, citrus fruits
	Beta-cryptoxanthin	Citrus, peaches, apricots
Flavonoids	Resveratrol	Red grapes, red wine
	Anthocyanidins	Blueberries, raspberries, Acai, eggplant, red grapes, blackcurrant
	Quercetins	Kale, apples
	Isoflavones	Soybeans, tofu, soymilk, soy products
	Catechin	Tea, wine
Sulfur compounds	Sulphoraphane	Broccoli
	Indoles	Cruciferous vegetables
	Ellagic acid	Strawberries, blueberries, raspberries
	Alliins (sulfur compounds)	Onions, garlic, scallions, leeks, chives
	Glucosinolates	Cruciferous vegetables

Source: Darwin Deen, MD, MS, and Lisa Hark, PhD, RD, 2012. Used with permission.

main classes of phytochemicals include the carotenoids and the flavonoids. The other families of phytochemicals include various other polyphenols, sulfur compounds, and saponins.

Food sources of common phytochemicals are listed in Table 12-2. Flavonoids are found in grapes, apples, berries, green tea, and red wine, and many other foods which have been described as "cancer fighting foods". The chemical structure of these polyphenols makes them ideal for absorbing free radicals and serving as effective antioxidants. Free radicals are unstable molecules produced by the cell that ultimately lead to cell damage which can contribute to the development of cancer. Antioxidants interact with and stabilize free radicals and thus prevent them from causing harm to cells.

Soy and Breast Cancer

Soybeans are legumes that are used to make tofu, soy milk, miso, tempeh, soy burgers, soy sauce, and soy nut butter. Soy contains a class of phytochemicals called isoflavones. The main isoflavones in soybeans are genistein and daidzein. These compounds are similar in structure to human estrogen. Thus, isoflavones are often referred to as phytoestrogens. Researchers originally associated soy with reduced breast cancer risk after observations of diet differences in Eastern and Western cultural diets.[28]

It has been suggested that the lower rates of endometrial and breast cancer found in Asian women may be due to their high consumption of soy. Based on these initial observations, several studies have examined the influence of soy on breast cancer risk.[29] The prevailing hypothesis is that phytoestrogens compete with estradiol for the binding sites on estrogen receptors.[30] These phytoestrogens are acting as selective estrogen receptor modulators (SERMs). For example, when genistein binds to estrogen receptors, it produces a weaker cellular response compared with estrogen. When genistein binds to the receptor it blocks estrogen from reaching the receptors – therefore, potentially protecting women from developing breast cancer.

Several studies have shown that consumption of soy (55 g per day or more) reduces women's risk of developing breast cancer. Studies have found that pre-menopausal women may benefit from eating soy foods since their natural estrogen levels are high. However, other studies have shown conflicting results. These contrasting effects may be due to the amount of isoflavone consumed in the studies or the timing of soy consumption (e.g. ingestion during adolescence). There may also be a certain threshold needed for soy consumption before the protective effects are realized. A key factor that may influence the effect of soy on breast cancer risk is the age at which soy is introduced into the diet. Most studies have shown strong evidence for a decrease in breast cancer occurrence in women who consumed soy before puberty and during adolescence.

Researchers are still actively investigating the protective effects of soy against the development of breast cancer. AICR and the American Cancer Society (ACS) suggest that data on soy and breast cancer are inconclusive.[1,3] More information is needed before any dietary recommendations can be made. The exception is for women who have estrogen-receptor positive breast cancer or those taking anti-estrogen medications such as tamoxifen or aromatase inhibitors. According to AICR, patients taking such medication should limit or avoid soy intake until further studies are conducted.[3]

Soy and Prostate Cancer

The role of soy phytoestrogens in prostate cancer is also controversial.[31,32] While estrogen is used to treat established cases of prostate cancer because it inhibits cancer growth, estrogens have also been associated with the development of benign prostatic hyperplasia and prostate cancer.[33] Over the last 30 years, studies have shown conflicting results regarding the impact of soy on prostate cancer. Men who consumed a soy-enriched diet have lower prostate-specific antigen (PSA) levels compared with controls. One study demonstrated that adding 2 oz of soy grits per day to the diets of men diagnosed with prostate cancer resulted in reductions in PSA levels.[34] The increased incidence of prostate cancers in the West compared with the East may be attributable, in part, to the differences in diet and lifestyle.[33]

Fruits and Vegetables
Berries
Blackberries, raspberries, strawberries, blueberries, cranberries, gogiberries, pomegranates, and lingon berries have high flavonoid content. Berries also contain a unique phytochemical compound known as ellagic acid that may have the capacity to interfere with tumorigenesis.[35] Ellagic acid is a polyphenol antioxidant found in high concentrations in raspberries, pomegranates, and strawberries. Ellagic acid may work by preventing the activation of carcinogenic substances in the body. It may also be a powerful inhibitor of angiogenesis which allows for the increased blood supply necessary for tumor growth.

Raspberries and blueberries contain another class of polyphenol compounds called anthocyanidins, which are responsible for the blue and red colors of berries. Anthocyanidins are among the most potent antioxidants ever discovered. In the laboratory, anthocyanidins have been shown to stop cells from synthesizing DNA which resulted in apoptosis.[36] Anthocyanidins may also inhibit angiogenesis.[37] Other laboratory studies have shown that these phytochemicals can selectively inhibit the growth of lung, colon, and leukemia cancer cells without affecting the growth of healthy cells. This evidence supports promoting the consumption of berries as strategy in fighting cancer.

Vegetables
Both the ACS and AICR recommend consuming a diet rich in fruits and vegetables to reduce the risk of cancer. In particular, several cohort studies suggest that fruits and vegetables may protect against cancers of the oropharynx, esophagus, stomach, colon, rectum, and lungs.[38] However, the results of studies linking cancer prevention to fruit and vegetable consumption have been inconclusive and inconsistent.[39] There is significant evidence that consuming large amounts of cruciferous vegetables may reduce cancer risk.[40,41] Cruciferous vegetables contain high concentrations of a group of sulfur compounds called glucosinolates. The breakdown of these beneficial compounds may be accomplished when these vegetables are chopped or chewed.

Indoles and isothiocynates, which are also found in cruciferous vegetables, may help prevent cancer by eliminating carcinogens and by changing the metabolism and activity of certain hormones.[42] For example, one study showed that consumption of 250 g/day broccoli and 250 g/day of Brussels sprouts caused an increase in the urinary excretion of a substance thought to be a possible carcinogen found in well-done meat.[43] This suggests that high dietary intake of cruciferous vegetable may decrease cancer risk by helping to eliminate carcinogens found in food. A list of the most common cruciferous vegetables are shown in Table 12-3.

Two other molecules have received attention for their potential cancer-fighting properties: sulforaphane and indole-3-carbinol (I3C). Studies show that sulforaphane, an isothiocynate found in high concentrations in broccoli, has the ability to both cause excretion of toxic, cancer-causing substances from the body as well as promote

Table 12-3 Key Dietary Sources of Cruciferous Vegetables

• Cabbage	• Arugula
• Broccoli	• Bok choy
• Brussels sprouts	• Chinese cabbage
• Cauliflower	• Rutabaga
• Collard greens	• Radishes
• Kale	• Turnips
• Mustard	

Source: Darwin Deen, MD, MS, and Lisa Hark, PhD, RD, 2012. Used with permission.

the death of tumor cells.[44] Indole-3-carbinol is produced by the hydrolysis of glucosinolates but contains no sulfur atoms. Research has focused on I3Cs ability to influence estrogen metabolism. I3C may play an important role in cancers that are dependent on estrogen such as breast, cervical, and uterine cancers.

Several factors must be considered in order to maximize the indole and isothiocyanate nutrient content in cruciferous vegetables. Glucosinolates are extremely water-soluble and boiling cruciferous vegetables in water for more than 10 minutes may reduce the amount of glucosinolates by half. Steaming or stir-frying is a more effective way to maximize the amount of cancer-fighting compounds present in these vegetables. While NCI recommends consuming 5–9 servings of fruits and vegetables, there is currently no specific recommendation on cruciferous vegetable consumption.

Tomatoes

Tomatoes have a high concentration of the carotenoid lycopene. Carotenoids are the molecules in fruits and vegetables that are responsible for their vibrant red, orange and yellow colors.[45] Some carotenoids, such as beta-carotene, are precursors to vitamin A. Lycopene, although not a precursor to vitamin A, may be the carotenoid with the greatest cancer fighting potential.[46] The association between lycopene and prostate cancer comes from observations that in countries where there is high tomato consumption such as Italy, Spain, and Mexico, have lower rates of prostate cancer have been observed compared with the US or England.[47] Several studies have shown that individuals who consume large amounts of tomato products have a reduced risk of developing prostate cancer.[48] However, different tomato products contain variable concentrations of lycopene. For example, while tomato paste may contain 29.3 mg/100 g, canned tomatoes may contain only 9.7 mg/100 g. This variability makes it difficult to come to any definitive conclusions linking tomato products and prostate cancer prevention.[49]

Not all carotenoids demonstrate promising anticancer effects. Beta-carotene is a carotenoid found in many foods that are orange in color, including sweet potatoes, carrots, cantaloupe, squash, apricots, pumpkin, and mangos. In 1994, a cancer prevention study known as the Alpha-Tocopherol (Vitamin E)/Beta-Carotene Cancer Prevention Study (ATBC) found that lung cancer rates of male smokers increased in those who received beta-carotene supplements.[50] Thus smokers should be warned not to take beta-carotene supplements.

Garlic

Garlic is part of a larger group of vegetables known as the Allium family, which includes onions, scallions, leeks, and chives. Allium vegetables possess a sulfur-containing compound called alliin that is converted to allicin when raw garlic is crushed, chewed, or chopped by an enzyme known as allinase. Allicin then quickly converts to a number of other compounds including diallyl sulfide (DAS), diallyl disulfide (DADS), and ajoene. Garlic seems especially protective against cancers caused by nitrosamines, which are chemical compounds commonly found in preserved meat products such as salami, bacon, and sausage. In addition to garlic's action on carcinogenic substances, researchers believe that garlic may have the ability to directly attack and destroy tumor cells. Cancer is characterized by unregulated cell division, and organosulfur compounds such as DADS and ajoene have the ability to induce cell cycle arrest when added to cancer cells in cell culture. Additionally, DAS may induce apoptosis in cancer cells grown in culture.[51] While more studies are needed before dietary recommendations can be made, garlic continues to be listed as a cancer-fighting food.

Case 1

Keisha is a 33-year-old African-American woman who presents to your clinic for a complete physical examination after learning that her 35-year-old brother has been diagnosed with colon cancer. Her brother's physician advised the family that all the siblings should have a screening physical examination and a colonoscopy.

LIFESTYLE: Keisha does not have any symptoms suggestive of colon cancer, such as progressive fatigue, change in bowel habits or stool patterns, cramping or abdominal pain, black tarry stools or bright red blood in her stools, abdominal distention and bloating, jaundice, feeling of incomplete bowel evacuation or a previous history of cancer. She drinks hard liquor on the weekend (usually three to four gin and tonic beverages or whiskey on Friday and Saturday nights). She quit smoking 3 years ago; she smoked one pack per day for 15 years. She has poor dietary patterns — frequently eats fast food, fatty and fried foods, salty snacks, and drinks two to three Coca-Colas per day in addition to two cups of coffee every morning. Her weight has been steadily increasing since the birth of her last child 10 years ago. She walks on occasion but is limited in activity by her weight. She is 5'2" and weighs 230 lb (BMI: 42.1 kg/m²). She is employed as a file clerk in a law office and considers her job to be stressful. She is married and has two children; a boy age 10 and a daughter age 14. She monitors her blood pressure at home and reports that it is usually about 140/92 mmHg.

ADVICE: The occurrence of colon cancer in Keisha's 35-year-old brother increases her risk two- to threefold the usual incidence rate. It will be important to determine if her brother had a hereditary syndrome or a sporadic type of colon cancer. The American Cancer Society's screening guidelines vary based on the risk category of the individual. At a minimum for having sporadic cancer in a first-degree member, Keisha is considered at *Increased Risk* and may be counseled to have a screening colonoscopy every 5 years beginning at age 40, or 10 years before the youngest case in the immediate family, whichever is earlier.

Therefore, the approach to addressing Keisha's concerns is multi-dimensional and involves obtaining a thorough family history to determine if she should begin colon cancer screening at an earlier age. As part of this process it is essential to evaluate her family medical history not just for colon cancer and polyps, but for any other type of cancer. A history of cancer in aunts, uncles, grandparents, nieces, nephews, and cousins is important. Depending on the pathologic characterization of her brother's tumor as a hereditary condition or a sporadically occurring cancer, she may benefit from genetic counseling. Lifestyle modifications are critical to Keisha's future health. She can reduce her risk of obesity-related cancers, diabetes, metabolic syndrome, and cardiovascular disease by beginning a program of gradual weight loss and increased physical activity. The American Cancer Society recommends these lifestyle changes in order to lower one's risk of developing colon cancer:

- Get to and stay at a healthy weight. Be physically active.
- Eat a diet with plenty of fruits and vegetables, whole grains, and less red or processed meats.
- Limit the amount of alcohol you drink. Colon cancer has been linked to moderate to heavy alcohol use. Alcohol should be limited to no more than 1 drink a day for women.
- Don't use tobacco in any form.
- Referral to a smoking cessation program if Keisha resumes her smoking habit.

In Keisha's situation, she will need to gradually reduce her weight. Daunting as this may seem, with the addition of fruits and vegetables and a reduction in alcohol and red meat consumption plus a progressive walking program it can be achieved over a few years. It is important for Keisha to understand and accept that this is a long-term plan and that it may take 1 to 2 years to achieve her goals.

Vitamins and Cancer Prevention

Research on the anti-cancer effects of vitamin supplements has been mixed. Some studies have shown either no benefit from vitamins or an increased incidence of cancer in those taking certain supplements. The ATBC Cancer Prevention Study found that 50 mg a day of alpha-tocopherol, a form of vitamin E, had no effect on lung cancer incidence. They also found that 20 mg of beta-carotene, a precursor of vitamin A, increased lung cancer incidence in smokers by 18%.[50]

On the other hand, there is some research to suggest that vitamin D may possess cancer fighting properties.[52] Vitamin D is produced by the body but also found in a variety of foods. "Vitamin D" refers to both vitamin D_3 (also known as cholecalciferol), created by skin cells after exposure to UVB light, and vitamin D_2 (ergocalciferol). Vitamin D_2 comes from a plant sterol and is slightly structurally different from vitamin D_3. Neither compound is biologically active in the body. First, these compounds must be modified by hydroxylase enzymes and converted to 25-hydroxyvitamin D (25(OH) D) and then to 1,25-dihydroxyvitamin D (1,25(OH)$_2$D).

People who live in the northern regions of the US and Europe do not receive as much sunlight and are more prone to vitamin D deficiencies. In the northern parts of the United States, the population rates of cancers of the bladder, breast, colon, ovary, and rectum are twice what they are in southern regions. Race also plays a role because the higher levels of melanin in dark skin prevent UV penetration and thus vitamin D synthesis. In fact, individuals with white skin synthesize vitamin D six times faster than those with dark skin. A review of 63 observational studies examining the protective effects of vitamin D on breast, ovarian, prostate, and colon cancers, showed that vitamin D protects against cancer.[17,52] This review suggests that taking 1000 international units (IU) (or 25 µg) of vitamin D_3 per day lowers the risk of developing colon cancer by 50%. It may also decrease the risk of developing breast and ovarian cancer by 30%.

In laboratory studies, mice were induced with cancer and then treated with a synthetic compound that mimicked $1,25(OH)_2D$. The compound reduced tumor growth in mice by about 80%. $1,25(OH)_2D$ may inhibit the uncontrolled growth of tumor cells and thus stop cancer. Clinical interventions will ultimately provide the best evidence to determine vitamin D's role in cancer prevention, but until those studies have been completed, an adequate dose of vitamin D is indicated.

Minerals

Selenium is an essential micronutrient for all people and is found in Brazil nuts, red meat, poultry, and fish. Selenium is thought to help control cell damage that may lead to cancer because it boosts the body's antioxidant capacity. Most people do not obtain the recommended dose of 200 µg a day from their typical diet. Selenium has been shown in multiple studies to be an effective tool in warding off various types of cancer, including breast, esophageal, stomach, prostate, liver, and bladder cancers. Several studies have also shown that when selenium is used in conjunction with vitamin C, vitamin E, and beta-carotene, it blocks free radical formation.[53] Several promising studies have shown potential benefit of selenium in the prevention of prostate cancer. One epidemiological study suggested that men with high blood levels of selenium were about half as likely to develop advanced prostate cancer as the men with lower blood selenium. While selenium may be an important mineral for preventing cancer, it may also be helpful for those suffering from cancer. Some believe that the use of selenium during chemotherapy in combination with vitamin A and vitamin E can reduce the toxicity of chemotherapy drugs.[53]

Alcohol and Wine

Excessive alcohol consumption is linked to an increased risk of cancer of the mouth, throat, larynx, esophagus, breast, and liver. According to ACS, alcohol users experience oral cancers six times more often than non-alcohol users. Alcohol is also the primary cause of liver cancer. Findings from the Women's Health Study (1999–2004) suggest that moderate alcohol consumption also increases the risk of breast cancer and the higher the alcohol consumption, the greater the risk of breast cancer.[54] Additionally, studies have shown a strong correlation between high-alcohol and low-folate intake with an increased cancer risk.[55]

While excessive alcohol intake has been shown to have detrimental consequences for human health, moderate alcohol intake may have beneficial effects. There are specific compounds in certain wines that may protect against cancer.[56] For example, resveratrol, a cancer-fighting polyphenol found in nature, is produced by some plants when under attack from bacteria and fungi. Resveratrol is able to inhibit the initiation, promotion, and progression of cancer by triggering cell death and slowing the growth of cancer cells.[56] Resveratrol is also a potent antioxidant and may possess anti-angiogenic properties. Studies associating red wine consumption and cancer in humans are in their preliminary stages.

This antibacterial chemical is found in the skin of grapes and is a small component of red wine. There are distinctive properties of red wine that are due to the long process of grape fermentation, which allows certain polyphenols to be extracted from the grape's skin and allows the wine to absorb resveratrol. In addition, Nurse Practitioners should continue to advise patients that consumption of large amounts of alcoholic beverages may actually increase the risk of some cancers. Therefore, patients who drink alcohol should do so in moderation — one drink or less per day for women and two drinks per day for men.

Cancer Prevention Guidelines
Maintain a healthy weight throughout life
- Balance calorie intake with physical activity.
- Avoid excessive weight gain throughout life.
- Achieve and maintain a healthy weight if currently overweight or obese.

Adopt a physically active lifestyle
- *Adults*: engage in at least 30 minutes of moderate to vigorous physical activity, on 5 or more days of the week; 45–60 minutes of physical activity are preferable.
- *Children and adolescents*: engage in at least 60 minutes per day of moderate to vigorous physical activity at least 5 days per week.

Eat a healthy diet, with an emphasis on plant sources
- Choose foods and drinks in amounts that help achieve and maintain a healthy weight.
- Eat five or more servings of a variety of vegetables and fruits each day.
- Choose whole grains over processed (refined) grains.
- Limit intake of processed and red meats.

If you drink alcoholic beverages, limit your intake
- Drink no more than one drink per day for women or two per day for men.

Source: American Cancer Society. (www.cancer.org)

Physical Activity Recommendations

Being physically active is a key component of a healthy lifestyle and recommended for the prevention of many chronic diseases, including cancer.[41] A sedentary lifestyle is associated with weight gain. Being overweight or obese increases the risk of developing certain cancers.[4,5,41] Regular physical activity is an important component of cancer prevention. AICR and the American Cancer Society recommend that all individuals incorporate moderate levels of physical activity, equivalent to brisk walking, for at least 30 minutes every day.[1,3] As fitness levels improve, individuals should aim for 60 minutes or more of moderate, or 30 minutes or more of vigorous physical activity every day.

Oncology Care
Introduction
Nutrition issues for patients with cancer include: malnutrition, malabsorption, weight loss, weight gain, nutrition and mineral deficiencies, changes in appetite, and changes in protein metabolism due to chemotherapy and radiation therapy. Nurse Practitioners working with oncology patients who are knowledgeable about these issues should consider employing the recommended nutrition therapies to improve patient outcomes. It is also critical for oncology Nurse Practitioners to work closely with registered dietitians who support these patients.

Malnutrition in Cancer Patients
Malnutrition is prevalent among patients with certain types of cancer, including GI, pancreatic, head/neck, and lung cancers. Thirty to 90% of patients with cancer face some degree of clinical malnutrition. At the time of diagnosis, approximately 75% of cancer patients are malnourished.[57–59] Malnutrition and loss of fat-free body mass have been correlated with a decreased response to cancer therapy, poor survival, and a diminished quality of life.[59–63] Malnutrition can also affect surgical outcomes and complication rates. In fact, 20–40% of cancer patients die each year from the effects of malnutrition and its complications rather than malignancy.[58] Maintaining good nutritional status during cancer treatment is critical to increasing the likelihood of successful completion of prescribed therapies and to improve patients' quality of life.[57–59]

The impact of cancer on basal energy expenditure is variable. Cancer patients may have reduced, normal, or increased energy expenditure.[64,65] This variability is caused by individual responses to the tumor, body composition, and type and stage of the tumor.[62] In addition, byproducts of the tumor can also affect metabolism.[66] Because of this variability, it is hard to predict energy requirements for cancer patients. Patients with Stage III/IV disease may have significant reductions in their energy and protein intake, which may be a consequence of cancer-related symptoms such as anorexia, taste changes, dysphagia, nausea, vomiting, and diarrhea. Poor intake may also be due to other disease and treatment-related factors, such as recovery from major surgery.[67] A reduction in nutrient intake can result in impairments in the physical structure, function, and well-being of the cancer patient and may contribute to the underlying malnutrition that is commonly observed in these patients. The factors that may affect the nutritional status of cancer patients are shown in Table 12-4. Managing these factors is crucial in order to manage the disease and improve the quality of life of the cancer patient.

Weight Loss
Weight loss is a key outcome parameter that can be utilized in assessing the nutritional status of patients with cancer. The prevalence of weight loss in oncology patients ranges from 31 to 100%, depending upon tumor site, stage, and treatment.[57,59,68–70] Even minimal weight loss, in the range of 5%, is associated with increased mortality.[59] A study conducted with ambulatory patients with cancer showed that 59% had decreased appetite, 67% had decreased food intake, and 54% were underweight.[71]

Table 12-4 Common Side-Effects of Anti-cancer Treatment

• Pain	• Stomatitis
• Fatigue	• Dysphagia/Esophagitis
• Weakness	• Nausea/vomiting
• Anorexia	• Gustatory changes
• Weight loss	• Myalgias/arthralgias
• Lack of energy	• Dermatitis
• Xerostomia	• Hyperpigmentation
• Constipation	• Anxiety
• Dyspnea	• Depression
• Diarrhea/Constipation	• Insomnia and sleep disturbances
• Neutropenia	• Anemia
• Infection	• Bone marrow suppression

Organ Dysfunction
- Cardiac and pulmonary toxicities
- Neurotoxicity, particularly peripheral neuropathies and chemobrain
- Nephrotoxicity
- Hepatotoxicity

Source: Maureen Huhmann, DCN, RD, CSO and Theresa P. Yeo, PhD, MPH, ACNP, 2012. Used with permission.

The frequency of weight loss ranges from 31% in patients with non-Hodgkin's lymphoma to 87% in patients with gastric cancer.[59] Other selected reports of weight loss include those for tumors of the esophagus (57%), stomach (50%), and larynx (47%).[72] Pancreatic cancer patients frequently will have lost 10–20% of their body weight at the time of diagnosis. Additionally, patients with malignant solid tumors of the colon, prostate, lung, pancreas, or GI tract experience weight loss, starting in the pre-diagnosis phase and which is often exacerbated by surgery, chemotherapy, and radiation therapy.

Weight loss is greater in patients with Stage III/IV disease than in those with Stage I/II disease. The weight loss observed in cancer patients may be progressive if appropriate interventions are not implemented to prevent and/or slow the rate. Multiple factors contribute to the weight loss experienced by cancer patients.[62,63] Some additional factors not discussed previously include physiological changes associated with the development of the tumor itself, the host response to the tumor, and the side-effects of cancer treatments. These are outlined in Table 12-5.

Cancer Cachexia
Cancer Cachexia Syndrome (CCS) refers to the characteristic wasting seen in 50–80% of cancer patients with advanced disease and is most prevalent among patients with GI and lung cancers.[73,74] With the exception of breast cancer, patients with solid tumors are at greater risk of developing CCS.[75] Features of cancer cachexia include weight loss, anorexia, fatigue, early satiety, depression, reduced quality of life, and asthenia.[64,76] CCS is a complex metabolic state which leads to depletion of energy and muscle stores.

Table 12-5 Causes of Weight Loss in Cancer Patients

Metabolic Change	Side-Effect
Physiologic abnormalities associated with the tumor	• Malabsorption • Obstruction • Diarrhea • Vomiting
Host response to the tumor	• Anorexia • Altered metabolism
Side-effects of anti-cancer treatment	• Mucositis • Radiation enteritis • Xerostomia • Nausea, vomiting and diarrhea • Alteration in sense of taste

Source: Maureen Huhmann, DCN, RD, CSO and Theresa P. Yeo, PhD, MPH, ACNP, 2012. Used with permission.

CCS has features of malnutrition that are distinct from those found in starvation states. Unlike patients who experience starvation, patients experiencing CCS lose both adipose and skeletal muscle mass, while preserving visceral muscle mass and increasing hepatic mass.[74] Also unlike starvation, the weight loss associated with CCS cannot be reversed with increases in nutrients.[78]. In the presence of CCS, weight loss will continue despite increased administration of nutrients.[77] Muscle wasting in the presence of significant weight loss is a hallmark of cachexia. CCS should be suspected when an involuntary weight loss of greater than 5% of pre-morbid weight is observed within 1 month.

The loss of lean tissue leads to reduced organ functional capacity and weakness, which ultimately results in immobility and death due to loss of respiratory muscle function. A weight loss of greater than 15% in cancer patients typically causes impaired physiological function, with death occurring in up to 30% of patients. Many of the changes in body composition associated with severe weight loss in cancer cachexia are thought be the result of tumor-induced pathophysiological changes in normal metabolism. In particular, the effects may result from changes in cytokine and hormone levels. Pro-inflammatory cytokines, such as tumor necrosis factor, interferon-γ, and interleukins 1 and 6 are considered important mediators of CCS. In addition, tumor byproducts such as proteolysis inducing factor, lipid mobilizing factor, and mitochondria uncoupling proteins 1, 2, and 3 exhibit specific effects on nutrient metabolism.[66] This leads to increased energy requirements which impair the normal adaptive response to starvation. These include an altered insulin sensitivity, increased protein use, and increased cytokine synthesis. These cytokines and tumor byproducts can cause hypermetabolism and anorexia. The increased metabolic rate and reduced food intake contribute to an overall negative energy balance and accelerated weight loss in cancer patients.

Weight Gain
Although the development of advanced cancers is often associated with weight loss and CCS, weight gain has been associated with certain types of cancer treatments.

Weight gain has been reported in 50–96% of breast cancer patients receiving adjuvant cancer treatment.[79] A significant number of these patients gain more than 20 lb.[79,80] Weight gain has also been observed in prostate cancer patients who receive androgen deprivation therapy.[81] The weight is gained in the form of sarcopenic obesity, or weight gain in the absence of lean tissue gain.[80] Weight gain may be related to increased food intake to manage symptoms. It may also be related to decreased physical activity, or a modification of metabolic rate.[79] Weight gain and being overweight have been associated with increased risk of cancer recurrence and mortality in breast cancer survivors.[82] Current interventions for weight gain in patients include calorie restriction and exercise training.[81]

Substrate Metabolism

Cancer patients experience an increased rate of body protein breakdown (50–70%) as protein synthesis fails to keep up with protein breakdown. Muscle wasting contributes to the fatigue, weakness, asthenia, and respiratory complications observed in patients with advanced cancer.[83] These individuals are unable to conserve body protein stores. They break down muscle protein to provide energy for use in glucose synthesis by the liver.[84] In healthy patients, the body attempts to spare proteins by using carbohydrates and fats as preferred sources of energy. However, the breakdown of protein in cancer patients occurs in an excessive manner. The tumor byproduct, proteolysis inducing factor (PTF), has been implicated in the increased turnover of body protein stores and appears to induce protein degradation and inhibit protein synthesis.[85] A loss of 30% body weight has been correlated with a decrease of 75% of skeletal muscle mass due to protein degradation.[64]

Cancer patients may also experience an increased rate of lipolysis, or the breakdown of fat, and turnover of glycerol and fatty acids. Adipose tissue is broken down to provide energy as the disease progresses; the loss of adipose tissue accounts for the greatest reduction in body mass. The increased breakdown of body fat can result in elevated blood lipid levels in cachectic patients. Lipid mobilizing factor, a tumor byproduct, may be responsible for this increased rate of lipolysis and seems to act directly on adipocytes, causing a release of free fatty acids and glycerol.[84]

Cancer patients may also suffer from abnormal glucose metabolism. Glucose intolerance and abnormal insulin response have been frequently observed in patients with cancer-induced weight loss.[65] In addition, insulin resistance has also been observed in patients with GI cancers, possibly due to insulin resistance or decreased pancreatic function.[86] Tumors use glucose to produce large amounts of lactate which is converted back into glucose through gluconeogenesis in the liver (Cori cycle).[84] This process requires adenosine triphosphate (ATP) in order to function. This contributes to hypermetabolism and further weight loss.

Diagnosing Malnutrition in Cancer Patients

Markers of nutrition status (serum albumin, total lymphocyte count, immune competence, anthropometric changes, body composition) may be affected by the cancer and may serve to give an indication of the severity of the nutritional impact of the disease. Unfortunately, an acute phase response associated with the inflammatory effects of cancer may alter the levels of certain markers and this may limit their reliability. Current weight and weight history are the parameters most commonly used. However, this can also be unreliable in cancer patients due to fluid shifts and resultant edema.

Nutrition screening, should be employed to identify those patients who should undergo a more formal nutrition assessment, in order to identify early malnutrition. The American Society for Parenteral and Enteral Nutrition (ASPEN) and the American Dietetic Association (ADA) recommend that all cancer patients undergo nutrition screening as a component of their initial evaluation in order quickly to identify individuals at nutritional risk[87,88] A clear picture of the patient's nutritional status and objective and subjective data should be incorporated into the nutrition screening.[88] The use of a single laboratory parameter or the use of current weight alone are not specific and should be combined with subjective measures to diagnose nutritional issues.[88,89]

Several evidence-based nutrition screening tools have been used in cancer patients to identify those who are at greatest risk for developing nutritional problems. The Patient Generated Subjective Global Assessment (PG-SGA) tool is a modification of the Subjective Global Assessment tool.[90,91] It is divided into two sections; the first is completed by the patient and includes weight history, symptoms, dietary intake, and activity level, and the second is completed by the Nurse Practitioner and evaluates metabolic demand, disease in relation to nutritional requirements, and a physical assessment. A numeric score is calculated by adding the points obtained in sections one and two. The numeric scores can be used as a triage system to initiate a formal nutrition assessment, intervention, and follow-up.[92] The PG-SGA numeric score, when repeated at subsequent time points, is useful to demonstrate small improvements or deteriorations in nutritional status.[93]

Nutrition-Related Side-Effects of Cancer Treatment

Maintenance of nutritional status during cancer treatment is essential to increase the likelihood of successful completion of prescribed cancer therapies and to improve the patient's quality of life during and after treatments. Adequate and appropriate nutrition therapy can help slow or minimize reduction in body weight, reduce cancer treatment-associated side-effects, improve quality of life, diminish the risk of other co-morbid diseases, and increase the likelihood of survival[94,95] (Table 12-6).

Each anti-cancer treatment modality (surgery, chemotherapy, and radiation therapy) presents risks to patients' nutritional integrity. Eating problems experienced during chemotherapy are perceived by patients as being highly stressful.[96] Surgery causes metabolic stress which can lead to hypermetabolism. This hypermetabolism contributes to muscle and fat breakdown leading to weight loss post-operatively.[97] Decreased dietary intake secondary to diet restriction and poor appetite add to this weight loss.[63] Surgical resection that results in a change in anatomy of the GI tract may present mechanical barriers to food ingestion. Colon resections can lead to diarrhea, malabsorption, and dehydration. Pancreatic surgery can affect pancreatic enzyme and insulin secretion, leading to metabolic consequences.[63]

Chemotherapy is highly toxic to rapidly dividing cells such as those that line the GI tract.[63] Side-effects related to chemotherapy administration vary greatly. These drugs may impair food intake directly via "stomatoxic" reactions such as mucositis, diarrhea,

Table 12-6 Key Nutrition Therapy Goals for Patients with Cancer

- Reverse prior episodes of poor nutrition.
- Prevent further nutritional decline.
- Improve stamina and strength.
- Maintain weight.
- Support adequate calorie and nutrient intake.
- Prevent weight loss and promote weight gain.
- Prevent malnutrition, anorexia, and cachexia.
- Reverse malnutrition and weight loss that have already occurred.
- Improve body composition.
- Enhance immune function.
- Maximize tolerance to cancer therapies.
- Improve functional or performance status.
- Reduce fatigue.
- Improve physical functioning and quality of life.

Source: Maureen Huhmann, DCN, RD, CSO and Theresa P. Yeo, PhD, MPH, ACNP, 2012. Used with permission.

and vomiting. Chemotherapy may also indirectly affect food intake due to issues of fatigue, pain, food aversions, and taste changes. Nausea and vomiting are among the most distressing side-effects associated with chemotherapy.[63] Symptoms can occur prior to treatment, during treatment, or 1–2 weeks later and can last from several hours to days.[63]

Similar to chemotherapy, radiation therapy is most toxic to cells with a high turnover rate.[63] Radiation to any portion of the GI tract can cause extreme susceptibility to malnutrition. Greater that 70% of patients who receive radiation to the pelvic area experience acute inflammatory intestinal changes, including diarrhea, abdominal pain, and nausea.[98] In some patients, this can progress to chronic radiation enteritis requiring lifelong medicating and dietary changes. Treatment-related side-effects of radiation to the head and neck, such as mucositis, xerostomia, taste change, and dysphagia peak two-thirds of the way through treatment and, in some cases, can become permanent.[99] Radiation therapy in the area of the thyroid can cause permanent thyroid damage leading to changes in metabolism.[100] Table 12-7 presents nutrition-related interventions for common treatment side-effects experienced by cancer patients.[101] These approaches are most effective when combined with multidisciplinary intervention which includes pharmaceuticals.

Nausea and vomiting are the two of the most distressing side-effects of cancer treatment, occurring in 21–68% of advanced cancer patients. Nausea and vomiting are also the most likely side-effects of radiation treatment to affect nutrition status by decreasing the amounts and types of food patients can eat during treatment. Uncontrolled nausea and vomiting can also interfere with the patient's ability to receive cancer treatment. Medical management of nausea has greatly improved in the last decade.

Nausea is best treated prophylactically. Once vomiting has commenced it is more difficult to control.[102] Prescribing a combination of several classes of anti-emetics is currently recommended as prophylaxis in the setting of highly emetogenic chemo-therapy (American Society of Clinical Oncology and the Antiemetic Subcommittee

Table 12-7 Key Nutrition Interventions for Cancer Treatment Side-Effects

Symptom	Intervention
Taste Changes	• Rinse mouth with baking soda prior to eating • Use plastic cutlery and dishes • Eat cool or room temperature foods • Tart foods, flavorful seasonings, and marinated foods
Xerostomia	• Fluids with meals, moisten and/or puree foods • Oral moistening mouthwash/gel • Papaya juice • *Avoid*: caffeine, alcohol, commercial mouthwashes
Stomatitis/Mucositis	• Bland, soft foods, easy to swallow foods • Cook food (especially vegetables) until they are soft and tender • Cut food into small pieces, or puree food in blender • Mix food with broth, gravies, or sauces to make them easier to swallow • Capsaicin candy • *Avoid*: Acidic, spicy, rough, and salty foods
Diarrhea	• BRAT Diet (Bananas, Rice, Apple sauce, Toast) • Initially low fiber → slowly increase soluble fiber • Temporary avoidance of milk products (with the exception of yogurt) • Increase fluid intake (including juice and broth) • Prophylactic use of probiotics to prevent radiation-induced diarrhea • *Avoid*: High fat foods, caffeine, alcohol, tobacco, strong spices
Dumping Syndrome	• Small, frequent meals (every 2 hours) • Increase protein and fat content of meals • Fluids between meals • Limit simple carbohydrates
Constipation	• Gradually increase fiber rich foods (whole grains, bread, bran cereals, fruits and vegetables) • 8–10 glasses of fluid daily • 4–8 oz of prune juice once or twice a day • Increase physical activity • Fiber supplement → Stool softener → Laxative
Nausea	• Fluids between meals • Cold foods may be better tolerated • *Avoid*: Foods with strong odors, high fat foods, strong spices
Vomiting	• NPO → Clear Liquid → Full Liquid → Soft • Maintain fluid intake (including juice and broth)
Early Satiety	• Limit excessive intake of fat and fiber • Small, frequent meals (every 2 hours) • Increase protein and carbohydrate content of meals • Fluids between meals
Bloating and gas	• Avoid gas forming foods: cabbage, onions, gum, beans, corn • Eat low fat and reduced fat foods

Source: Maureen Huhmann, DCN, RD, CSO and Theresa P. Yeo, PhD, MPH, ACNP, 2012. Used with permission.

of the Multinational Association of Supportive Care in Cancer).[103] There are also a variety of treatment regimens for anticipatory nausea and refractory or breakthrough nausea and vomiting. As nausea may be induced by smell, opening of food trays outside of the patient's room may reduce the impact of the smell prior to eating.

Other GI complications of cancer treatments (constipation, diarrhea, and bowel obstruction) are common problems in cancer patients. The causes of these symptoms can sometimes be hard to decipher. For example, diarrhea in a patient post-Whipple with pancreatic cancer receiving concurrent chemotherapy and radiation may be a result of malabsorption secondary to pancreatic enzyme deficiency. It may also be due to dumping syndrome as a result of gastric and upper GI surgery. Finally, it may occur as a side-effect of chemotherapy and radiation. Multidisciplinary intervention with a combination of dietary and pharmaceutical interventions can assist with the management of these symptoms. It is important to be realistic in the treatment plans of these patients as to what symptoms can be managed with dietary interventions alone and which require a multi-modal approach.

Cancer patients may also develop treatment-induced oral or intestinal mucositis, which is an inflammation of the lining of the mouth and GI tract and is a common side-effect of cancer chemotherapy and/or radiation therapy. Severe inflammation that leads to the development of lesions, ulceration, and bleeding can occur in the mouth, esophagus, and intestine. Patients can experience intense pain, cramping, nausea, and gastroenteritis. The severity and nature of the mucositis varies based on the patient's treatment regimen. Among patients with mucositis, food and fluid intake may be drastically limited and nutrient absorption may be reduced. Clinically significant oral mucositis negatively impacts virtually all head and neck cancer patients receiving radiation therapy. It also affects approximately 50% of hematologic stem cell transplant (SCT) patients and up to 25% of patients with epithelial malignancies treated with cycled chemotherapy.[104–106] A patient who develops mucositis in a previous cycle of chemotherapy is estimated to be four times more likely to develop mucositis in subsequent cycles. Oral mucositis related pain affects the patient's ability to eat, drink, speak, and sleep.[106] Table 12-7 summarizes key nutrition interventions for many of these common treatment-induced side-effects.

Maintaining Energy and Protein Intake

Nutritional status has an important effect on the patient's quality of life and their tolerance of anti-cancer treatments. Early and sustained nutritional intervention is one of the most valuable adjuncts for the optimal management of cancer. Nurse Practitioners should work with patients to prevent weight loss, reduce muscle wasting, and avoid nutrient deficiencies. Weight management and prevention of weight loss should be considered primary goals for cancer patients. Preventing weight loss is simpler, safer, and less expensive than trying to regain weight. Sufficient calories and protein should be provided to meet the nutritional and energy needs of each patient and to minimize protein catabolism and use of stored energy reserves.

In order to support protein synthesis, prevent the loss of lean body mass, and minimize the magnitude of the nitrogen deficit, sufficient protein should be provided. Requirements for protein in most patients range from 1.0 to 1.5 g/kg/day. Carbohydrates should provide the primary source of energy and fat should represent

25–30% of calories, including sources of the essential fatty acids. The diet should also include adequate amounts of protein, vitamins, minerals, and trace elements. In addition adequate dietary fiber and fluid intake should be ensured in order to manage constipation and diarrhea. For patients with inadequate *ad libitum* food intake, high-protein and energy-dense oral nutritional supplements may serve to increase energy and protein intake, improve nutritional status, and increase body weight and quality of life. They may serve to reduce the incidence and severity of anorexia, diarrhea, and radiation toxicity and treatment.[107]

Germ-Free (Neutropenic) Diet

Many chemotherapeutic agents cause myelotoxicity, which subsequently results in neutropenia. Historically, a very restrictive, germ-free or neutropenic diet has been employed in neutropenic patients. These diets eliminated foods such as fresh fruits, vegetables, and yogurt.[108,109] Recent data indicate no benefit to adherence to these diets.[110-113] The use of the Food and Drug Administration (FDA)-approved food safety guidelines have been found to be more effective in preventing infection in neutropenic patients. Adherence to these guidelines is also higher than with very restrictive diets. These guidelines recommend proper food handling, especially frequent hand washing. Food Safety tips to reduce risk of infection are listed in Table 12-8.

Table 12-8 Food Safety Tips for Cancer Patients to Reduce Risk of Infection

- Fastidious cleaning of food preparation areas and surfaces.
- Frequent hand washing and vigilant personal hygiene.
- Wash hands before handling food, between handling raw and cooked food, and between dirty and clean dishes.
- Wash hands after using the restroom, handling garbage, touching the garbage pail, coughing, sneezing, touching the hair or face, and after eating.
- Cook all meats thoroughly.
- Avoid serving meat on platters that held raw meat.
- Avoid foods containing eggs if proper refrigeration was not maintained.
- Avoid eating meats stored in a refrigerator for more than 48–72 hours.
- Work surfaces and kitchen utensils should be disinfected frequently by washing with hot, soapy water.
- Do not keep perishable foods such as milk, yogurt, and sandwiches at room temperature for more than 2 hours.
- Hot food should be kept hot (above 165 °F), and cold food cold (under 40 °F).
- Use chilled ingredients to prepare salads.

Source: Maureen Huhmann, DCN, RD, CSO and Theresa P. Yeo, PhD, MPH, ACNP, 2012. Used with permission.

Summary: Role of Nurse Practitioners

Nurse Practitioners, in collaboration with dietitians, play an important role in the nutritional management of cancer patients. Inadequate nutrition intake and subsequent malnutrition are associated with increased mortality, poor treatment tolerance, and poor response to treatment. The identification and management of cancer and treatment-related symptoms are vital to provide the best environment for adequate nutrient intake during and after treatment.

Case 2

James is a 61-year-old Causcasian man who has recently undergone a pancreaticoduo-denectomy, also known as the "mini-Whipple", for pancreatic adenocarcinoma. He returns to the clinic with his wife, Nancy, to see the Nurse Practitioner. He is 8 weeks post-surgery and has not yet begun adjuvant chemo-radiation therapy. Nancy is concerned because he continues to experience poor appetite (though his weight has stabilized at 142 lb), and he has frequent malodorous stools that seem to float in the toilet. They both thought that he would be "better" by now. What advice can you offer James and Nancy?

ADVICE: The most comforting information that you can offer this couple is to explain that what he is experiencing is "usual" at this stage of recovery from pancreatic cancer surgery. Patients often expect a quick recovery period. Let him know that it may take up to one year for him to feel "normal" in terms of his appetite and bowel pattern and that his appetite and bowel problems may temporarily worsen during adjuvant therapy. It is important to check the amount of pancreatic enzyme supplements he is using daily. One or more capsules should be taken immediately before eating all meals and snacks. This will improve the breakdown of fat, protein, carbohydrate, and thus improve absorption, while reducing the volume and density of his stools. He can titrate the number of capsules per meal (some patients require three per meal and one with a snack) until he achieves the desired effect. It is also important to inform James that over time his need for enzyme supplements will decrease and pancreatic enzyme replacement may not be necessary.

With regard to his diet, James may begin to eat the foods he seems to enjoy or that he is craving. The goal is to avoid weight loss and to begin to build muscle strength and endurance which will be needed during adjuvant treatment. He should be encouraged to eat small, frequent meals of calorie-rich/nutrient-dense foods, such as yogurt, milkshakes, and pudding. Cool to room temperature foods are better tolerated. Probiotic granules and products will also improve his digestion. Liquid nutritional supplements may be prescribed, if these appeal to him. He should monitor his weight daily and watch for leg edema, which may indicate too much sodium intake. Advise James and Nancy to gradually add back his favorite foods by observing how his digestive system handles the food.

References: Pancreatic Cancer Action Network,[114] The Lusgarten Foundation[115]

References

1. American Cancer Society Statistics 2011. www.cancer.org/Research/CancerFactsFigures. Accessed 2012.
2. Beliveau R, Gingras D. *Foods to Fight Cancer*. Dorling Kindersley: New York, 2007.
3. American Institute for Cancer Research (AICR). Food, Nutrition, Physical Activity and the Prevention of Cancer: a Global Perspective. Second Expert Report. www.aicr.org. Accessed 2012.
4. Bianchini D, Kaaks R, Vainio H. Overweight, obesity, and cancer risk. *Lancet Oncology* 2002;3:565–574.

5. Calle EE, Rodriquex C, Walker-Thurmond K, et al. Overweight, obesity, and mortality from cancer in a prospectively studied cohort of U.S. adults. *N Engl J Med* 2003;348:1625–1638.

6. Larsson SC, Orsini N, Wolk A. Body mass index and pancreatic cancer risk: a meta-analysis of prospective studies. *Int J Cancer* 2007;120:1993–1998.

7. Linos E, Willett WC. Diet and breast cancer risk reduction. *J Natl Compr Canc Network* 2007;5:711–718.

8. Michels KB, Mohllajee AP, Roset-Bahmanyar E, et al. Diet and breast cancer. A review of the prospective observational studies. *Cancer* 2007;109(12 Suppl):2712–2749.

9. Huang ZSE, Hankinson GA, Colditz, et al. Dual effects of weight and weight gain on breast cancer risk. *JAMA* 1997;278:1407–1411.

10. Ogden CL, Carroll MD, Curtin LR, et al. Prevalence of overweight and obesity in the United States,1999–2004. *JAMA* 2006;295:1549–1555.

11. National Cancer Institute. Nutrition in Cancer Care (PDQ®). www. cancer.gov. Accessed 2012.

12. Tanabe K, Utsunomiya H, Tamura M, et al. Expression of retinoic acid receptors in human endometrial carcinoma. *Cancer Sci* 2008;99:267–271.

13. Ryan-Harshman M, Aldoori W. Diet and colorectal cancer: review of the evidence. *Can Fam Physician* 2007;53:1913–1920.

14. Beresford SAA, Johnson KC, Ritenbaugh C, et al. Low-fat dietary pattern and risk of colorectal cancer. The Women's Health Initiative Randomized Controlled Dietary Modification Trial. *JAMA* 2006;295:643–654.

15. Rennert G. Prevention and early detection of colorectal cancer – new horizons. *Recent Results Cancer Res* 2007;174:179–187.

16. Doyle VC. Nutrition and colorectal cancer risk: a literature review. *Gastroenterol Nurs* 2007;30:178–182.

17. Ma Y, Zhang P, Wang F, et al. Association between vitamin D and risk of colorectal cancer: a systematic review of prospective studies. *J Clin Oncol* 2011;29:3775–3782.

18. Calle EE, Kaaks R. Overweight, obesity and cancer: epidemiological evidence and proposed mechanisms. *Nat Rev Cancer* 2004;4:579–591.

19. Li D, Morris JS, Liu J, et al. Body mass index and risk, age of onset, and survival in patients with pancreatic cancer. *JAMA* 2009;301:2553–2562.

20. Schatzkin A, Mouw T, Park Y, et al. Dietary fiber and whole-grain consumption in relation to colorectal cancer in the NIH-AARP Diet and Health Study. *Am J Clin Nutr* 2007;85: 1353–1360.

21. Slavin JL. Mechanisms for the impact of whole grain foods on cancer risk. *Am Coll Nutr* 2000;19(3 Suppl):300S–307S.

22. Lin J, Zhang SM, Cook NR, et al. Dietary intakes of fruit, vegetables, and fiber, and risk of colorectal cancer in a prospective cohort of women (United States). *Cancer Causes Control* 2005;16:225–233.

23. Park Y, Hunter DJ, Spiegelan D, et al. Dietary fiber intake and risk of colorectal cancer. A pooled analysis of propsective cohort studies. *JAMA* 2005;294:2849–2857.

24. Fuchs C, Giovannucci E, Colditz G, et al. Dietary fiber and the risk of colorectal cancer and adenoma in women. *N Engl J Med* 1999;340:169–176.

25. MacLean CH, Newberry S, Mojica WA, et al. Effects of omega-3 fatty acids on cancer risk. A systematic review. *JAMA* 2006;295:403–415.

26. Pandalai PK, Pilat MJ, Yamazaki K, et al. The effects of omega-3 and omega-6 fatty acids on in vitro prostate cancer growth. *Anticancer Res* 1996;16:815–820.

27. Lanza E, Jartman TJ, Albert PS, et al. High dry bean intake and reduced risk of advanced colorectal adenoma recurrence among participants in the Polyp Prevention Trial. *J Nutr* 2006;136:1896–1903.

28. Linseisen J, Piller R, Hermann S, et al. Dietary phytoestrogen intake and premeno-pausal breast cancer risk in a German case-control study. *Intern J Cancer* 2004;110: 284–290.

29. Wu AH, Yu MC, Tseng CC, et al. Epidemiology of soy exposures and breast cancer risk. *Br J Cancer* 2008;98:9–14.

30. Duffy C, Perez K, Partridge A. Implications of phytoestrogen intake for breast cancer. *CA Cancer J Clin* 2007;57:260–277.

31. Parsons JK, Newman V, Mohler JL, et al. The Men's Eating and Living (MEAL) Study: a cancer and leukemia group B pilot trial of dietary intervention for the treatment of prostate cancer. *J Urol* 2008;72:633–637.

32. Holzbeierlein JM, McIntosh J, Thrasher JB. The role of soy phytoestrogens in prostate cancer. Preventive and alternative medicine. *Curr Opin Urol* 2005;15:17–22.

33. Berkiw SE, Barnard ND, Saxe GA. Diet and survival after prostate cancer diagnosis. *Nutr Rev* 2007;65:391–403.

34. Perabo FG, Von Low EC, Ellinger J, et al. Soy isoflavone genistein in prevention and treat-ment of prostate cancer. *Prostate Cancer Prostatic Dis* 2008;11:6–12.

35. Singletary KW, Jung KJ, Giusti M. Anthocyanin-rich grape extract blocks breast cell DNA damage. *J Med Food* 2007;10:244–251.

36. Tulio AZ Jr, Reese RN, Wyzgoski FJ, et al. Cyanidin 3-rutinoside and cyanidin 3-xylosylrutinoside as primary phenolic antioxidants in black raspberry. *J Agric Food Chem* 2008;56:1880–1888.

37. Zafra-Stone S, Yasmin T, Bagchi M, et al. Berry anthocyanins as novel antioxidants in human health and disease prevention. *Mol Nutr Food Res* 2007;51:675–683.

38. Miller MF, Bellizzi KM, Sufian M, et al. Dietary supplement use in individuals living with cancer and other chronic conditions: a population-based study. *J Am Diet Assoc* 2008;108: 483–494.

39. Pierce JP, Natarajan L, Caan BJ, et al. Influence of a diet very high in vegetables, fruit, and fiber and low in fat on prognosis following treatment for breast cancer. The Women's Healthy Eating and Living (WHEL) Randomized Trial. *JAMA* 2007;298:289–298.

40. Kirsh VA, Peters U, Mayne ST, et al., on behalf of the Prostate, Lung, Colorectal and Ovarian Cancer Screening Trial. Prospective study of fruit and vegetable intake and risk of prostate cancer. *J Natl Cancer Inst* 2007;99:1200–1209.

41. Kushi LH, Byers T, Doyle C, et al., and The American Cancer Society 2006 Nutrition and Physical Activity Guidelines Advisory Committee. American Cancer Society guidelines on nutrition and physical activity for cancer prevention: reducing the risk of cancer with healthy food choices and physical activity. *CA Cancer J Clin* 2006;56:254–281.

42. Fimognari C, Lenzi M, Hrelia P. Chemoprevention of cancer by isothiocyanates and anthocyanins: mechanisms of action and structure-activity relationship. *Curr Med Chem* 2008;15:440–447.

43. Walters DG, Young PJ, Agus C, et al. Cruciferous vegetable consumption alters the metabo-lism of the dietary carcinogen 2-amino-1-methyl-6-phenylimidazo[4,5-b]pyridine (PhIP) in humans. *Carcinogenesis* 2004;25:1659–1669.

44. Zhang Y, Tang L. Discovery and development of sulforaphane as a cancer chemopreventive phytochemical. *Acta Pharmacol Sin* 2007;28:1343–1354.

45. Farwell WR, Gaziano MJ, Norkus EP, et al. The relationship between total plasma carotenoids and risk factors for chronic disease among middle-aged and older men. *Br J Nutr* 2008;100:883–889.

46. Schnabele K, Briviba K, Bub A, et al. Effects of carrot and tomato juice consumption on fecal markers relevant to colon carcinogenesis in humans. *Br J Nutr* 2008;99:606–613.

47. Givannucci E, Rimm EB, Liu Y, et al. A prospective study of tomato products, lycopene, and prostate cancer risk. *J Natl Cancer Inst* 2002;94:391–398.

48. Grainger EM, Schwartz SJ, Wang S, et al. A combination of tomato and soy products for men with recurring prostate cancer and rising prostate specific antigen. *Nutr Cancer* 2008;60:145–154.

49. Huang CS, Liao JW, Hu ML. Lycopene inhibits experimental metastasis of human hepatoma SK-Hep-1 cells in athymic nude mice. *J Nutr* 2008;138:538–543.

50. Omenn GS, Goodman GE, Thornquist MD, et al. Effects of a combination of beta carotene and vitamin A on lung cancer and cardiovascular disease. *N Eng J Med* 1996;334:1150–1155.

51. Ngo SN, Williams DB, Cobiac L, et al. Does garlic reduce risk of colorectal cancer? A systematic review. *J Nutr* 2007;137:2264–2269.

52. Thorne J, Campbell MJ. The vitamin D receptor in cancer. *Proc Nutr Soc* 2008;67: 115–127.

53. Lippman SM, Klein EA, Goodman PJ, et al. Effect of selenium and vitamin E on risk of prostate cancer and other cancers: the Selenium and Vitamin E Cancer Prevention Trial. *JAMA* 2009;301:39–51.

54. Zhang S, Lee I, Manson J, et al. Alcohol consumption and breast cancer risk in the women's health study. *Am J Epid* 2007;165:667–676.

55. Mason JB, Cole BF, Baron JA, et al. Folic acid fortification and cancer risk. *Lancet* 2008;371:1335.

56. Athar M, Back JH, Tang X, et al. Resveratrol: a review of preclinical studies for human cancer prevention. *Tox Applied Pharm* 2007;224:274–283.

57. Bozzetti F. Rationale and indications for preoperative feeding of malnourished surgical cancer patients. *Nutrition* 2002;18:953–959

58. Bozzetti F. Screening the nutritional status in oncology: a preliminary report on 1000 outpatients. *Support Care Cancer* 2009;17:279–284.

59. Dewys WD, Begg C, Lavin PT, et al. Prognostic effect of weight loss prior to chemotherapy in cancer patients. Eastern Cooperative Oncology Group. *Am J Med* 1980;69: 491–497.

60. Murry DJ, Riva L, Poplack DG. Impact of nutrition on pharmacokinetics of anti-neoplastic agents. *Int J Cancer Suppl* 1998;11:48–51.

61. Hammerlid E, Wirblad B, Sandin C, et al. Malnutrition and food intake in relation to quality of life in head and neck cancer patients. *Head Neck* 1998;20:540–548.

62. Martin C. Calorie, protein, fluid and micronutrient requirements. In: McCallum P, Polisena C (Eds), *The Clinical Guide to Oncology Nutrition*. American Dietetic Association, Chicago, 2000:45–52.

63. Capra S, Ferguson M, Ried K. Cancer: impact of nutrition intervention outcome–nutrition issues for patients. *Nutrition* 2001;17:769–772.

64. Tisdale MJ. Pathogenesis of cancer cachexia. *J Support Oncol* 2003;1:159–168.

65. Barber M. The pathophysiology and treatment of cancer cachexia. *Nutr Clin Pract* 2002;17:203–209.

66. Tisdale MJ. Tumor-host interactions. *J Cell Biochem* 2004;93:871–877.

67. Hutton JL, Martin L, Field CJ, et al. Dietary patterns in patients with advanced cancer: implications for anorexia-cachexia therapy. *Am J Clin Nutr* 2006;84:1163–1170.

68. Linn BS, Robinson DS, Klimas NG. Effects of age and nutritional status on surgical outcomes in head and neck cancer. *Ann Surg* 1988;207:267–273.

69. Nguyen TV, Yueh B. Weight loss predicts mortality after recurrent oral cavity and oropharyngeal carcinomas. *Cancer* 2002;95:553–562.

70. Haugstvedt TK, Viste A, Eide GE, et al. Factors related to and consequences of weight loss in patients with stomach cancer. The Norwegian Multicenter experience. Norwegian Stomach Cancer Trial. *Cancer* 1991;67:722–729.

71. Tchekmedyian NS. Costs and benefits of nutrition support in cancer. *Oncology* (Williston Park) 1995;9:79–84.

72. Segura A, Pardo J, Jara C, et al. An epidemiological evaluation of the prevalence of malnutrition in Spanish patients with locally advanced or metastatic cancer. *Clin Nutr* 2005;24:801–814.

73. Tisdale MJ. Mechanisms of cancer cachexia. *Physiol Rev* 2009;89:381–410.

74. Tisdale MJ. Cancer cachexia. *Curr Opin Gastroenterol* 2010;26:146–151.

75. von Haehling S, Anker SD. Cachexia as a major underestimated and unmet medical need: facts and numbers. *J Cachex Sarcopenia Muscle* 2010;1:1–5.

76. Barber MD. The pathophysiology and treatment of cancer cachexia. *Nutr Clin Pract* 2002;17:203–209.

77. Tisdale MJ. Cachexia in cancer patients. *Nat Rev Cancer* 2002;2:862–871.

78. MacDonald N, Easson AM, Mazurak VC, et al. Understanding and managing cancer cachexia. *J Am Coll Surg* 2003;197:143–161.

79. Costa LJ, Varella PC, del Giglio A. Weight changes during chemotherapy for breast cancer. *Sao Paulo Med J* 2002;120:113–117.

80. Demark-Wahnefried W, Peterson BL, Winer EP, et al. Changes in weight, body composition, and factors influencing energy balance among premenopausal breast cancer patients receiving adjuvant chemotherapy. *J Clin Oncol* 2001;19:2381–2389.

81. Holzbeierlein JM, Castle E, Thrasher JB. Complications of androgen deprivation therapy: prevention and treatment. *Oncology* (Huntingt) 2004;18:303–309; discussion 10, 15, 19–21.

82. Ingram CDR, Brown JKPFR. Patterns of weight and body composition change in premenopausal women with early stage breast cancer: has weight gain been overestimated? *Cancer Nurs* 2004;27:483–490.

83. Ravasco P, Monteiro-Grillo I, Vidal PM, et al. Nutritional deterioration in cancer: the role of disease and diet. *Clin Oncol* (R Coll Radiol) 2003;15:443–450.

84. Inui A. Cancer anorexia-cachexia syndrome: current issues in research and management. *CA Cancer J Clin* 2002;52:72–91.

85. Tisdale MJ. Metabolic abnormalities in cachexia and anorexia. *Nutrition* 2000;16: 1013–1014.

86. Nebeling L. Changes in carbohydrate, protein, and fat metabolism in cancer. In: McCallum P, Polisena C (Eds), *The Clinical Guide to Oncology Nutrition*. American Dietetic Association, Chicago, 2000:53–60.

87. Committee CoPCQM. Identifying patients at risk: ADA's definitions for nutrition screening and nutrition assessment. *J Am Diet Assoc* 1994;94:838–839.

88. August DA, Huhmann MB. ASPEN clinical guidelines: nutrition support therapy during adult anticancer treatment and in hematopoietic cell transplantation. *J Parenter Enteral Nutr* 2009;33:472–500.

89. Sarhill N, Mahmoud F, Walsh D, et al. Evaluation of nutritional status in advanced metastatic cancer. *Support Care Cancer* 2003;11:652–659.

90. Ottery FD. Definition of standardized nutritional assessment and interventional pathways in oncology. *Nutrition* 1996;12:S15–S19.

91. Detsky AS, McLaughlin JR, Baker JP, et al. What is subjective global assessment of nutritional status? *J Parenter Enteral Nutr* 1987;11:8–13.

92. Luthringer S, Kulakowski K. Medical nutrition therapy protocols. In: McCallum P, Polisena C (Eds), *The Clinical Guide to Oncology Nutrition.*American Dietetic Association, Chicago, 2000:24–44.

93. Ferguson M. Patient-generated subjective global assessment. *Oncology* 2003;17: 13–14.

94. Lacey K, Pritchett E. Nutrition care process and model: ADA adopts road map to quality care and outcomes management. *J Am Diet Assoc* 2003;103:1061–1072.

95. Ravasco P, Monteiro-Grillo I, Camilo ME. Does nutrition influence quality of life in cancer patients undergoing radiotherapy? *Radiother Oncol* 2003;67:213–220.

96. McGrath P. Reflections on nutritional issues associated with cancer therapy. *Cancer Pract* 2002;10:94–101.

97. Bosaeus I, Daneryd P, Svanberg E, et al. Dietary intake and resting energy expenditure in relation to weight loss in unselected cancer patients. *Int J Cancer* 2001;93:380–383.

98. McGough C, Baldwin C, Frost G, et al. Role of nutritional intervention in patients treated with radiotherapy for pelvic malignancy. *Br J Cancer* 2004;90:2278–2287.

99. Isenring EA, Capra S, Bauer JD. Nutrition intervention is beneficial in oncology outpatients receiving radiotherapy to the gastrointestinal or head and neck area. *Br J Cancer* 2004;91:447–452.

100. Jereczek-Fossa BA, Alterio D, Jassem J, et al. Radiotherapy-induced thyroid disorders. *Cancer Treat Rev* 2004;30:369–384.

101. Huhmann MB, Cunningham RS. Identification and nutritional treatment of cancer related weight loss. *Lancet Oncology* 2005;6:334–343.

102. Einhorn LH, Grunberg SM, Rapoport B, et al. Antiemetic therapy for multiple-day chemotherapy and additional topics consisting of rescue antiemetics and high-dose chemotherapy with stem cell transplant: review and consensus statement. *Support Care Cancer* 2011;19(Suppl. 1):S1–S4.

103. Naeim A, Dy SM, Lorenz KA, et al. Evidence-based recommendations for cancer nausea and vomiting. *J Clin Oncol* 2008;26:3903–3910.

104. Vera-Llonch M, Oster G, Hagiwara M, et al. Oral mucositis in patients undergoing radiation treatment for head and neck carcinoma. *Cancer* 2006;106:329–336.

105. Woo SB, Sonis ST, Monopoli MM, et al. A longitudinal study of oral ulcerative mucositis in bone marrow transplant recipients. *Cancer* 1993;72:1612–1617.

106. Sonis ST, Elting LS, Keefe D, et al. Perspectives on cancer therapy-induced mucosal injury: pathogenesis, measurement, epidemiology, and consequences for patients. *Cancer* 2004;100:1995–2025.

107. Odelli C, Burgess D, Bateman L, et al. Nutrition support improves patient outcomes, treatment tolerance and admission characteristics in oesophageal cancer. *Clin Oncol.* 2005;17:639–645.

108. Carter LW. Bacterial translocation: nursing implications in the care of patients with neutropenia. *Oncol Nurs Foru.* 1994;21:857–867.

109. Smith LH, Besser SG. Dietary restrictions for patients with neutropenia: a survey of institutional practices. *Oncol Nurs Forum* 2000;27:515–520.

110. Jubelirer SJ. The benefit of the neutropenic diet: fact or fiction? *Oncologist* 2011;16:704–707.

111. Moody K, Finlay J, Mancuso C, et al. Feasibility and safety of a pilot randomized trial of infection rate: neutropenic diet versus standard food safety guidelines. *J Pediatr Hematol Oncol* 2006;28:126–133.

112. Tabori U, Jones H, Malkin D. Low prevalence of complications in severe neutropenic children with cancer in the unprotected environment of an overnight camp. *Pediatr Blood Cancer* 2007;48:148–151.

113. Larson E, Nirenberg A. Evidence-based nursing practice to prevent infection in hospitalized neutropenic patients with cancer. *Oncol Nurs Forum* 2004;31:717–725.

114. Pancreatic Cancer Action Network. Diet and Nutrition: Nutritional concerns with pancreatic cancer. http://www.pancan.org. Accessed 2012.

115. The Lusgarten Foundation. Understanding Pancreatic Cancer. A Guide for Patients and Caregivers. The Lustgarten Foundation for Pancreatic Cancer Research, New York, 2007.

13 Enteral and Parenteral Nutrition Support

Jennifer M. Dolan, MS, RD, CNSC
Nancy Sceery, LD, RD, CNSC
Nancy Stoner, RN, MSN, CNSC

OBJECTIVES

- Describe the indications and contraindications for enteral nutrition (EN) and parenteral nutrition (PN).
- Identify the appropriate enteral formula to meet a patient's requirements.
- Identify the most appropriate route for tube feeding administration based on a patient's clinical condition.
- Select appropriate monitoring tools and methods to identify, prevent, and treat complications of tube feeding.
- Determine the composition of parenteral nutrition formulas and how the macronutrient, micronutrient, and fluid requirements are calculated.
- Describe appropriate methods for monitoring and management of the complications associated with PN support including home PN.

Introduction

Nurse Practitioners working in acute, chronic, and home-care settings are in key positions to identify patients that require specialized nutrition support and to work with the nutrition support team to optimize nutritional outcomes. Nurse Practitioners typically assess nutritional status, recommend appropriate routes for nutrition support, outline nutritional goals, and translate these recommendations into enteral nutrition (EN) and parenteral nutrition (PN) orders. This chapter provides Nurse Practitioners with a comprehensive overview of both EN and PN, including indications, contraindications, types of formulas, administration methods, and appropriate monitoring tools and methods to identify, prevent, and treat complications of EN. The chapter also describes the composition of PN formulas, macronutrient, micronutrient, and fluid requirements, methods for monitoring and managing complications associated with PN, and metabolic needs of patients receiving PN.

The Nurse Practitioner's Guide to Nutrition, Second Edition. Edited by Lisa Hark, Kathleen Ashton and Darwin Deen.
© 2012 John Wiley & Sons, Inc. Published 2012 by John Wiley & Sons, Inc.

Enteral Nutrition Support

Enteral nutrition (EN) is a method of providing nutrition support to patients who have a functioning gastrointestinal (GI) tract. Short-term tube feeding is often used in acute-care settings for patients who are unable to maintain adequate oral intake due to impaired mental status, poor appetite, or other therapies that prevent eating such as mechanical ventilation. Guidelines established by the American Society of Parenteral and Enteral Nutrition (ASPEN) recommend initiating nutrition support when patients are expected to (or have) not received adequate oral intake for at least 7 days.[1] However, patients who are malnourished or stressed may require earlier initiation of nutrition support. All patients should have EN initiated within 24–48 hours of intensive care unit (ICU) admission.[2] Most institutions provide nutrition screening for patients so that nutrition support can be initiated when appropriate.

Indications and Advantages of Tube Feeding

Patients with inadequate oral intake or for whom oral intake is contraindicated can be fed with a feeding tube. Careful assessment of GI functionality is crucial and should be documented before starting EN. Both the length (at least 100 cm) and the functional capacity of the small bowel contribute to the success of EN.[1] Advances in tube feeding have made EN possible in conditions previously thought to be contraindications, such as acute pancreatitis and high-output proximal enterocutaneous fistulae.[1,3] GI impairment can be subtle; a cautious trial of tube feeding may be appropriate before initiating PN[2] (see Table 13-1 for indications and contraindications for EN).

Enteral nutrition offers many potential advantages over PN including lower rates of infections, fewer metabolic complications, decreased hospital length of stay, and reduced cost.[2,4] It has been proposed that the benefits of EN are, in part, due to a preservation of gut integrity.[5] Studies in critically ill patients have demonstrated decreased morbidity in those receiving EN compared with those given PN, and

Table 13-1 Indications and Contraindications for Enteral Nutrition

Indications for EN	Contraindications for EN
Impaired swallow function (e.g., neurological disease or oropharyngeal dysphagea)	Diffuse peritonitis

Inadequate oral intake
  Poor appetite
  Increased metabolic needs (e.g., trauma, burns, wounds)
	Intestinal obstruction

Acute pancreatitis	Intractable vomiting or diarrhea
High output proximal fistula	Paralytic ileus Gastrointestinal ischemia Short bowel syndrome Severe malabsorption Distal high output fistula Severe gastrointestinal bleed Refusal of nutrition support by the patient

Source: Jennifer M. Dolan, MS, RD, CNSC, 2012. Used with permission.

several meta-analyses studies demonstrate the superiority in outcomes of feeding with EN compared with PN across most disease states.[6] EN should therefore be the nutrition support therapy of choice when feasible and safe.[2]

Nutritional Content of Tube Feeding Formulas

Enteral formulas are available in powder or liquid form and can be delivered in an open or closed system. Sterile liquid enteral formulas should be used in preference to powdered reconstituted formulas whenever possible.[7]

Caloric densities range from 1–2 kcal/mL. Most patients' nutrient needs will be met using a 1–1.2 kcal/mL formula. More concentrated formulas are indicated for patients with volume constraints (e.g., heart or liver failure) or with very high calorie requirements (e.g., cystic fibrosis). Most products contain 70–85% water. Additional water to meet fluid requirements can be administered as water flushes through the tube during the day[1] (see Case 13-1 for how to calculate the water flush requirement). Use of purified water or sterile water for formula reconstitution, medication dilution, and flushes should be considered in at-risk patients.[7]

EN formulas generally have osmolalities that are easily tolerated when administered correctly and therefore there is no reason to dilute a formula.[7] Formulas with osmolalities over 1000 mOsm may contribute to diarrhea but EN formulas of ≤ 700 mOsm (majority of tube feeding formulas) should not contribute to increased stool output.[8]

Carbohydrate

Carbohydrate and fat are the primary source of calories in EN formulas. Most patients will tolerate a standard formula that is 40–50% carbohydrate and 25–35% fat. EN formulas are lactose and gluten-free. Specialty formulas designed to improve glucose control in diabetic patients contain a lower concentration of carbohydrate and are supplemented with fiber. These formulas are useful in those patients with diabetes who cannot be controlled with insulin and a standard formula since they tend to be higher in fat and are more expensive. Speciality diabetic formulas are not required for all individuals with diabetes.[1]

Protein

Protein in EN formulas can be supplied as whole protein (polymeric), partially hydrolyzed protein (peptide-based), or fully hydrolyzed protein (crystalline amino acids) and range in content from 11 to 25% of total calories. Most patients tolerate polymeric formulas. Partially hydrolyzed formulas should be reserved for patients with malabsorption (e.g., pancreatitis, Crohn's disease, or cystic fibrosis). Fully hydrolyzed formulas should be reserved for those with malabsorption who have failed a trial of partially hydrolyzed formulas. Substituting a hydrolyzed formula for a polymeric formula has not been shown to be effective in reducing diarrhea in patients without documented malabsoprtion.[6]

Formulas with a specific amino acid composition or a low protein to calorie ratio formulas are available for patients with organ failure (e.g., high branched chain amino acid formulas for patients with liver failure or low protein formulas for patients with renal failure on dialysis.[2] Recently, glutamine and arginine have been added to some EN formulas to meet the needs of "conditionally essential" amino acids. Glutamine is

Table 13-2 Enteral Nutrition Properties

Formula Type	Calories per Liter (average)	Protein per Liter (average)	Water Content of Formula (average)	Characteristics	Sample Patient Population
Polymeric standard	1000–1500	40–65	85%	Whole protein, polysaccharide, and mixture of fat sources. Some have added fiber	Well- nourished individuals on chronic tube feeding.
Nutrient dense High calorie Fluid restricted	2000	80	70	Polymeric with reduced water	Heart failure or anyone with very high calorie requirements or very limited water requirement.
Low calorie	1000	60	85	Low calorie to nitrogen ratio	Obesity.
High protein	1500	70	75	Over 15% of calories as protein	Most hospitalized patients; those with high protein requirements to support wound healing.
Partially or fully hydrolyzed	1000–1300	50	85	Oligo-peptides and free amino acids (elemental) in place of whole proteins, low fat, and/or high concentrations of medium chain triglycerides	Malabsorption; pancreatitis.
Specialty formulas	1300–1500	40–70	70–85	Added glutamine, arginine, marine oils, antioxidants, branched chain amino acids, low electrolytes, low carbohydrate	Critically-ill surgical patients, liver failure, renal failure not on dialysis, diabetes uncontrolled with insulin.

Source: Jennifer M. Dolan, MS, RD, CNSC and Nancy Evens-Stoner, MSN, RN, 2012. Used with permission.

essential for proliferation of mucosal cells and it can act as a respiratory fuel. Arginine is a nitric oxide precursor and may enhance wound healing and immune function. Patients with trauma, burns, and GI cancer requiring surgery seem to benefit most from glutamine-containing formulas.[2,9] Surgical patients and those with wounds benefit most from arginine. Arginine supplemented formulas should be used very cautiously in patients with severe sepsis.[2] Again, these special products are more expensive so it is best to use them only when needed.

Fat

The fat content of EN formulas varies. Formulas designed for patients with malabsorption are low in long-chain fats or are supplemented with medium chain triglycerides (MCT) since these are more easily absorbed.[10,11] High-fat formulas have been designed to limit carbohydrate intake for patients with diabetes and respiratory insufficiency; they contain 55% of total calories as fat. Historically, it was thought that low carbohydrate/high fat formulas resulted in less carbon dioxide production, but the data show that it is the total calorie load that affects carbon dioxide production more than individual macronutrient content.[12]

The fat component of EN formulas has recently been the focus of much research. Most tube feeding formulas now contain a mixture of omega-6- and omega-3-fatty acids in order to reduce inflammation.[10,11,13] Single center studies have shown a benefit of formulas supplemented with marine oils, but multi-center trials have shown no benefit of fish oil in the treatment of acute respiratory distress syndrome (ARDS) or sepsis.[13-16]

Fiber

Some formulas contain added fiber (up to 15 g/L). Many contain a mixture of fibers, both soluble and insoluble. Soluble fiber may reduce diarrhea by increasing stool bulk and providing a source of energy for colonocytes. Fiber has also been promoted for blood sugar control in patients with diabetes. Fiber increases the viscosity of formulas and can contribute to the clogging of feeding tubes, so fiber-containing formulas should be administered through a tube that is at least 10 French in diameter.[1] Insoluble fiber should be avoided in critically ill patients, and both soluble and insoluble fiber should be avoided in patients at-risk for bowel ischemia or severe dysmotility.[2]

Vitamins, Minerals, and Trace Elements

Vitamins, minerals, and trace elements are all included in standard EN formulas. Most formulas meet the RDA for these nutrients in 1–1.5 liters. A vitamin and mineral supplement is appropriate for patients receiving less than the necessary volume to meet the requirements. Additional antioxidants (vitamin C and E) have been added to some formulas to treat specific diseases associated with oxidative stress.

Selecting Tube Feeding Formulas

Most institutions create a formulary that offers a few select formulas to meet most patients' needs while limiting inventory. Modular components are available to supplement EN formulas thereby modifying calorie and protein content better to meet many patients' needs.

The type and quantity of macronutrients (carbohydrate, protein, fat, and fiber) and micronutrients (vitamin, minerals, and trace elements) can vary among EN formulas. Formulas should be selected after defining a patient's nutrient and fluid requirements (taking into consideration gut function and disease state).

Selecting Tube Feeding Route

It is important for Nurse Practitioners to consider the potential duration of tube feeding prior to selecting the EN access device. Patients requiring only 4–6 weeks of therapy should be managed with an oro/nasogastric or oro/nasoenteric tube, which can be placed with little risk to the patient.[7,17] Patients who require long-term tube feeding should have a gastrostomy, jejunostomy, or gastrostomy with jejunal extension. This can be done percutaneously (PEG, PEJ, PEG-J) without general anesthesia by a gastroenterologist or an interventional radiologist. Surgically placed tubes require anesthesia, so they are often inserted in conjunction with other surgeries such as tracheostomy. All of these methods of tube placement carry some risks which are minimized when an experienced physician is performing the procedure and the patient's clinical and nutritional status is not severely compromised. PEG tubes may be utilized for feeding within 3 hours of placement in adults but there may be a delay in using surgically placed tubes.[18] Contraindications for placement of gastrostomy and jejunostomy tubes include significant ascites, peritoneal dialysis, and recent ventriculoperitoneal shunt.[17,19] Obesity may preclude endoscopic placement of feeding tubes.

Feeding into the stomach is most consistent with GI physiology and allows feeding to be administered without a pump.[19] Gastric tubes are common in patients who receive home EN. Small bowel tubes, which are ideally placed past the ligament of Treitz, are used for patients with gastroparesis, gastric outlet obstruction, recurrent aspirations, severe pancreatitis, proximal enteric fistulas, and post-operative anastamotic gastroenteric stenosis.[19] Either gastric or small bowel feeding is acceptable in the ICU setting. Small bowel feeding is preferred in patients with intolerance to gastric feeding (e.g., gastric residual > 500 mL). Feeding tubes can be manually advanced into the small bowel at the bedside by trained staff. Radiologic and endoscopic techniques are also used for small bowel tube placement. Finally, if a patient is undergoing abdominal surgery, naso-enteric feeding tubes should be directly placed in the operating room post-operatively to facilitate early enteral feeding. Radiographic confirmation of tube position should be made using a plain film of the abdomen prior to initiating EN. This is also the case when a tube is repositioned.[7,17,19] The tube type, tip location, and external markings should be documented in the medical record and re-checked prior to each feeding.[7] The exit site of naso-enteric feeding tubes should be marked at the time of the initial radiograph. If there is uncertainty regarding placement, a radiograph should be considered to determine tube location.[7]

Ordering and Administering Tube Feeding

Standardized order forms should be developed for EN regimens to aid prescribers in meeting each patient's nutritional needs and to improve order clarity. EN orders should include five elements: two patient identifiers, the formula, the enteral access device, the administration method, and rate. Order protocols may incorporate feeding advancement, transitional orders, and implementation of ancillary orders. The use of generic terms to describe EN formulas is encouraged. Patient transfer between and within healthcare environments requires clinician-to-clinician communication to promote the accurate transfer of the EN prescription.[7]

Tube feeding schedules should be designed around the patient's clinical condition, physical activity, and the access device. Gastric feeding allows a large volume (200–500 mL) of formula to be administered via a syringe or gravity drip.[20] Patients may prefer to administer their tube feeding over a short period of time, three to five times daily, in a manner similar to eating meals. This method, referred to as intermittent gravity feeding, requires minimal equipment and encourages independence for patients receiving home EN. The small bowel cannot tolerate large volumes, so small bowel tube feedings must be administered with a pump over a prolonged time period (8–24 hours).[19] Critically ill patients generally receive tube feeding continuously over 24 hours. Patients who are more mobile are good candidates for tube feeding that is cycled nocturnally. This also allows patients who are transitioning to oral intake to avoid appetite suppression during the day.

Intermittent feedings are usually initiated at 100–200 mL over 20–40 minutes. The feeding is then advanced by 50–100 mL with every feeding until the eventual goal volume is tolerated. Continuous tube feeding is generally initiated at 20–30 mL/hour. The feeding volume is increased in a stepwise fashion by 10 mL/hour, every 6–8 hours, to a goal rate by the second or third day, depending on patient tolerance. Mild bloating and loose bowel movements are common when tube feeding is initiated. If the patient shows any signs of severe feeding intolerance, such as diarrhea (>500 mL per shift), elevated gastric residuals (>500 mL), or vomiting, the administration should not be further advanced and may be discontinued temporarily during an appropriate clinical evaluation.[1,3]

Administering Medications

It is imperative that Nurse Practitioners understand safe practice guidelines and proper medication administration principles to ensure optimal medication and tube feeding absorption.[19-21] Medication Administration guidelines are shown in Table 13-3.

Table 13-3 Medication Administration Guidelines

- Consult the pharmacy regarding availability of liquid medication and safety of crushing tablets.
- If crushing a medication, crush finely and disperse in warm water if clinically appropriate.
- Do not crush enteric coated, sustained released, or timed-released tablets or capsules.
- Use the liquid form of medication whenever possible.
- Do not mix medications together.
- Each medication should be administered separately.
- Medications should not be mixed with enteral formulas.
- Flush the feeding tube before and after each medication is administered and one final time prior to resuming enteral nutrition.
- Consult the pharmacy on the timing of medications in relationship to the feeding to avoid drug-nutrient reactions.
- Consult the pharmacy before administering drugs through a small bowel feeding tube.
- Identify medications that require an acidic stomach pH for proper absorption.

Source: Jennifer M. Dolan, MS, RD, CNSC, 2012. Used with permission.

Table 13-4 Monitoring Guidelines and Prevention/Treatment of Complications

Metabolic	Gastrointestinal	Mechanical
Reassess calorie requirements weekly based on weight changes; indirect calorimetry best reflects metabolic rate, though this technology is often limited to academic health centers.	Abdominal evaluation for distention, tenderness, nausea, vomiting, diarrhea, or constipation every shift in hospitalized patients and daily in home patients.	Aspiration precautions: maintain head of bed elevation at least 30 degrees and preferably 45 degrees when EN is being administered.
Electrolytes daily until stable in ICU patients, monthly in home patients.	Check gastric residual every shift; hold EN for gastric residual >500 ml. Consider promotility agent or advancement of tube to the post-pyloric position if residual persistently >500 ml.	Clogged tubes: for prevention, flush tube every 4–6 hours, at any time EN is held, and before/after administration of each medication. Use warm water or pancreatic enzymes if tube clogged. Avoid colas, cranberry juice
Glucose at least daily and up to every 4h.	Diarrhea: likely cause is sorbitol-containing, antibiotic, or other hyperosmolar liquid medications, *C. difficile* colitis, or underlying GI disorders and rarely the EN formula. Consider soluble-fiber containing formula or the use of a probiotic. Do not start an antidiarrheal until infectious etiology has been ruled out.	Dislodged tubes: Nasoenteric: secure nasoenteric tubes to skin with tape; radiographically confirm placement if dislodged Percutaneous: place temporary tube in ostomy site to avoid closure. If tract is new/immature, replacement should be done in radiology; avoid placement of catheters or tubes not intended for use as EN devices such as urinary or GI drainage tubes can lead to enteral misconnection and tube migration with potential for GI obstruction.
	Constipation (common in immobile patients and those receiving high dose pain medication): ensure adequate water is provided. Consider soluble fiber-containing formula.	Leaking tubes: ensure adequate fixation and proper skin care. Avoid replacement with a larger diameter tube.
Nitrogen balance, as requested by a dietitian, in patients with suspected hypercatabolism (e.g., trauma).	Dehydration (common in patients receiving diuretic therapy or those with high fluid losses from drains, diarrhea, or emesis). For hospitalized patients, evaluate daily intake/output, weight, blood pressure, heart rate, electrolytes, and skin turgor.	

Source: Jennifer M. Dolan, MS, RD, CNSC, 2012. Used with permission.

Monitoring and Complications

Nurse Practitioners are typically responsible for the ordering and monitoring of nutrition support in acute, chronic, and home-care settings, which may also include annual follow-up visits in the primary care setting. Morbidity, mortality, length of hospital stay, and costs are important outcome measures to monitor the efficacy of EN support. Feedings received should be compared with prescribed calorie and protein goals. Adjustments in prescriptions should be based on changes in clinical status and activity. In critically-ill patients, there is no difference in outcome between those who receive trophic (i.e., < 20 mL/hour) vs. full energy nutrition for the first week.[22] Efforts to provide greater than 50–65% of caloric goals by the second week results in maximal clinical benefit of EN.[2] Clinical monitoring of patients receiving tube feeding should include metabolic, GI, and mechanical assessment as described in Table 13-4.[2,7,19,20,23]

Enteral Nutrition Summary

Tube feeding offers a method of nutrition support to patients who are unable to consume adequate nutrition but have a functional GI tract. There are many advantages to EN over PN, and therefore EN should be used whenever feasible and clinically safe. There are a wide variety of formulas, tubes, and administration methods. Detailed assessment of the patient's clinical condition, nutrient requirements, and activity level will direct Nurse Practitioners in selecting the feeding route, formula, and administration method. Monitoring metabolic, mechanical, and GI tolerance to tube feeding will guide Nurse Practitioners in making adjustments in tube feeding therapy. Following these principles, tube feeding can support patients successfully for as long as the therapy is indicated.

Parenteral Nutrition Support

Parenteral nutrition (PN) is an intravenous form of nutrition indicated in patients requiring long-term therapy or who have extreme metabolic stress and high demand for nutrients who cannot sustain themselves with oral/EN. Macronutrient components include amino acids, dextrose (glucose), and lipids (long chain triglycerides). Micronutrients include vitamins, minerals, and trace elements. PN is formulated to provide complete nutrition with adjustments to support additional needs such as wound healing.

Nurse Practitioners working in hospital settings, especially GI surgery and surgical oncology services, are very involved in the management of patients receiving PN. These Nurse Practitioners typically order PN and determine the administration route, monitor all medical and nutritional indices, and provide discharge instructions. Nurse Practitioners working in out-patient settings also provide patient education and may admit patients with catheter-related bloodstream infections who are receiving home PN. This section aims to help Nurse Practitioners determine indications and contraindications for PN, the appropriate composition of PN formulas, and how the macronutrient, micronutrient, and fluid requirements are calculated. Nurse Practitioners will understand monitoring methods for and management of the complications associated with PN support, including home PN support.

Case 1: Enteral Nutrition Step-by-Step Approach

ST is a 76-year-old female who suffered a massive stroke. She had a G-tube placed. Plan is to discharge ST to a nursing home. She is 62" (157 cm) and 120 lb (54.5 kg). Her skin is intact.

Step	Formula	Patient Example
1. Calculate daily calorie requirement	Harris–Benedict: $[655 + 9.6 \text{ (Wt)} + 1.8 \text{ (Ht)} - 4.7 \text{ (age)}] \times 1.3$ or 25–30 kcal/kg	$[655 + 9.6 \ (54.5) + 1.8 \ (157) - 4.7 \ (76)] \times 1.3 = \sim 1400$ kcal 25 kcal/kg = ~1400 kcal/day
2. Calculate protein requirement	1 g/kg/day	~55 g protein per day
3. Calculate water requirement	100 mL/kg 1st 10 kg + 50 mL/kg 2nd 10 kg + 15 mL/kg remainder of weight	~2000 mL/day
4. Select enteral formula	See Table 13-2 for review of EN formulas	Standard polymeric formula with or without fiber
5. Calculate goal volume of formula needed to meet calorie goal	Kcal requirement ÷ kcal/L of formula = total L formula needed	1000 kcal/L ÷ 1400 kcal/day = ~1.4 L/day
6. Calculate amount of protein that will be provided from formula that was determined to meet calorie requirement	L standard polymeric formula × g protein/L	1.4 L standard polymeric formula × 40 g protein/l = 56 g protein
7. Determine if additional protein is required to meet protein goal	Protein requirement minus amount of protein in goal volume of formula needed to meet kcal requirement	55–56 g = negative 1 g
8. Calculate water content of goal EN	Total volume (mL) of formula × % water in formula	1400 × 0.85 = ~1200
9. Calculate additional water requirement	Water requirement minus water provided from formula	2000 – 1200 = 800 mL
10. Determine EN regimen	Intermittent: total volume ÷ 4 to 6 Continuous: total volume ÷ 12 to 24 h	1400 ÷ 4 = ~350 mL 4×/day 1400 ÷ 6 = ~235 mL 6×/day 1400 ÷ 12 = ~120 mL/h over 12 h 1400 ÷ 24 = ~60 mL/h over 24 h
11. Determine water bolus requirement	Additional water requirement divided every 4–6 h	800 ÷ 4 = 200 mL every 6 h or 800 ÷ 6 = 150 mL every 4 h

Source: Jennifer M. Dolan, MS, RD, CNSC, 2012. Used with permission.

Table 13-5 Indications and Contraindications for Parenteral Nutrition Support

Indications for PN	Contraindications for PN
Paralytic ileus	Expected therapy <7 days
Mesenteric ischemia	High-risk of line sepsis
Distal small bowel obstruction	Terminal prognosis where PN poses more risk than benefit or where goals of care are comfort only
High output distal intestinal fistula	Functioning gut
Malabsorption refractory to elemental gut feeding	Pancreatitis responsive to enteral feeds
Unable to obtain safe enteral access (e.g., uncorrectable coagulopathy, severe thrombocytopenia, severe neutropenia, anatomic defect)	Adaptive short gut where PO is adequate
Radiation enteritis	If a patient declines
Chronic intestinal pseudo-obstruction	
Short gut syndrome	
Refractory nausea and vomiting	
Stool output >1 liter	

Source: Nancy Lee Sceery, RD, LD, CNSD, 2012. Used with permission.

Indications and Contraindications

Oral/EN nutrition is always the preferred route to sustain nutrition and support immune function. However, adequate and consistent nutrition is paramount to healing, and when the gut cannot be used for full nutrition support, PN nutrition should be used to compensate. There are clear indications for chronic home PN, but controversy exists as to when to start PN for patients in the ICU.[2,24,25] PN is contraindicated when the GI tract is functional and safe for use, where prognosis is inconsistent with aggressive nutrition support, or in any condition where the risks outweigh the benefits.[1,26,27] Indications and contraindications for PN are shown in Table 13-5.

Determining Energy Requirements

Estimation of energy needs is difficult even in the healthy non-stressed individual, and becomes even more complex during illness and injury. Yet an accurate estimate of energy needs is critical in order to avoid the complications associated with over- and underfeeding. Starvation, a compensatory survival mechanism, is marked by reduced metabolic rate and protein preservation.[28] Stress and acute illness differ from starvation in the metabolic use of substrates associated with catabolism. The stress response is characterized by increased energy expenditure, protein catabolism to support gluconeogenesis (production of glucose from protein), and hyperglycemia related to catecholamine and glucocorticoid increase that outweighs an increase in hyperinsulinemia. A number of different methods and formulas have been derived to aid in determining energy expenditure and calorie needs for healing.[2,29,30] One of the most universally accepted formulas is 20–30 kcal/kg/day, which meets the majority of

Table 13-6 Daily Protein, Energy, and Fluid Requirements for the Adult

Protein	
Maintenance	0.8–1 g/kg
Catabolic patients	1.2–2 g/kg
Chronic renal failure (renal replacement therapy)	1.2–1.5 g/kg
Acute renal failure + catabolic	1.5–1.8 g/kg
Energy	
Total calories	20–30 kcal/kg
Fluid	30–40 ml/kg

Source: Mirtallo.[21] Used with permission.

patient's needs. Higher levels may be warranted with hypermetabolism. However, organ function must be monitored closely to assure tolerance to the increased metabolic load.[2,20,28,31,32] It is important to reassess energy requirements based on changes in clinical status on a regular basis, especially if there is an acute change in patient status. Daily protein, energy, and fluid requirements are shown in Table 13-6.

Macronutrients

PN solutions contain either all three macronutrients (dextrose, amino acids, and lipids — 3-in-1 — referred to as a total nutrient admixture [TNA]) or amino acids and dextrose (2-in-1) with intravenous fat emulsion (IVFE) administered separately. A mixed fuel system (carbohydrate, protein, and fat) best supports the overall nutritional needs of the human body.[1,33,34]

Carbohydrate

Carbohydrate, the body's primary fuel substrate, is supplied as dextrose monohydrate in PN solutions. The stock solution is 70%, but safe, final concentrations range from 5 to 25%.[33–36] Dextrose monohydrate yields 3.4 kcal/g. A 10% solution yields 100 g of carbohydrate per liter. The minimal need for central nervous system function, prevention of ketosis, and protein sparing is approximately 2 mg/kg/minute or 100 g dextrose per day. Higher dextrose concentrations can be used when fluid volumes need to be restricted.[26–28,37]

Dextrose infusion should be limited to 7 mg/kg/minute in stable patients and <4 mg/kg/minute in the critically ill patients to ensure substrate oxidation.[1,26,28,31] This includes dextrose from PN, IVF, and medication solvents. When the glucose oxidation rate is exceeded, undesirable fat synthesis occurs, resulting in hepatic steatosis which if left untreated, may progress to liver failure. Complications of overfeeding dextrose include hyperglycemia, excess carbon dioxide production, hepatic steatosis, and electrolyte aberrations. In general, overall carbohydrate should not exceed 60% of total kcal needs, 7 mg/kg/minute, or 350–400 g/24 hour bag.

Lipids

Intravenous fat emulsions (IVFE) are composed of aqueous suspensions of soybean or safflower oil, egg yolk phospholipid as the emulsifier, and glycerol in addition to phosphorus and vitamin K.[38] They supply the essential fatty acids (EFAs) (linoleic and α-linolenic acid), required for immune function, calories to spare protein for repletion or tissue synthesis, and are indicated where a reduction in carbohydrate load is desirable (e.g., persistent hyperglycemia).[26,37,39,40,41] Because of the egg yolk phospholipid, IVFE are contraindicated in patients with documented egg allergies. IVFE are also contraindicated in those with hypertriglyceridemia-induced pancreatitis or serum triglyceride values >400 mg/dL.

IVFE are available in 10, 20, and 30% concentrations. Ten and 20% concentrations are used for infusion with 2-in-1 solutions and 30% concentrations are used for compounding 3-in-1 solutions.[34,36,41] A 10% emulsion provides 1.1 kcal/mL, a 20% emulsion provides 2 kcal/mL, and a 30% emulsion provides 3 kcal/mL. Use of 20% IVFE may be beneficial in reducing the risk of hypertriglyceridemia.[41]

About 10% of calories per day (or 500 mL of 20% lipid weekly) from IVFE provides enough linoleic acid to prevent EFA deficiency (EFAD).[1,26,27] To reduce adverse events, limit IVFE to <1.5 g/kg/day, <0.11 g/kg/hour or <15–30% of total calories infused over 12–24 hours.[41] This includes lipid from propofol (10% IVFE). For patients receiving long-term PN, administering lipids every other day or two to three times a week may mitigate the potential for parenteral nutrition-associated liver disease (PNALD).

Protein (Amino Acids)

Protein is an essential substrate for tissue synthesis, wound repair, immune support, and lean body mass preservation. When calories are inadequate, protein will be broken down and used as an energy source. This can result in delayed wound healing. Enough protein should be provided to ensure nitrogen sparing, while dextrose and lipids are provided to meet energy expended.[1,28,39] Parenteral protein contains a mixture of essential and nonessential amino acids ranging in concentration from 3 to 20%. A 10% solution of amino acids supplies 100 g of protein per liter. Each gram of protein supplies 4 calories. In general, 15–20% of the total energy prescription should be supplied as protein, though protein is often prescribed based on body weight and stress level.[33,35,37,42] The average adult requires 0.8–1 g/kg/day for health maintenance. Critically ill patients with trauma, burns, sepsis, or those with wounds are hypercatabolic, so higher amounts of protein are indicated.[1,2,20,43,44] Calculations to determine nitrogen balance are shown in Table 13-7.

Providing more than 1.5 g/kg of protein has not been shown to significantly improve nitrogen retention, and excess protein can prompt azotemia, acid–base aberrations, and dehydration.[28,43,44] A rising BUN with normal creatinine may reflect impending or existing dehydration or protein overload. Nitrogen balance studies can be a useful tool in assessing protein needs and should be conducted on all patients where there is a concern for hypercatabolism. A negative nitrogen balance may indicate the need for

Table 13-7 Calculating Nitrogen Balance

Calculate nitrogen intake = Protein intake (g/day) ÷ 6.25

Calculate nitrogen output = 24 h urine urea nitrogen (g/day) + 4 g (insensible losses)
                                        + 2 g/L (diarrhea or wound vacuum drainage)

Calculate nitrogen balance = Nitrogen intake (g) – nitrogen output (g)

Source: Nancy Lee Sceery, RD, LD, CNSD, 2012. Used with permission.

more protein and/or more overall calories to spare protein. The goal is 2–4 g of positive nitrogen per day for anabolism, though this may not be achievable in severely hypercatabolic states. In this case, the goal shifts to minimizing negative nitrogen balance.

Fluid and Electrolyte Requirements

Once the macronutrient portion of the PN prescription has been established, the day-to-day management focuses on the fluid and electrolyte needs of the patient. Electrolytes are added to PN solutions in amounts sufficient to account for substrate metabolism. Electrolyte requirements will vary depending on the patient's fluid status, disease state, and organ function. Noting the electrolyte composition of hydration fluids and serum chemistry trends prior to PN implementation may be a useful guide in formulating the initial PN formula.[1,33] Exceeding thresholds for the electrolytes or minerals may alter the stability of the solution.

Some institutions use maximally concentrated PN formulations with additional IVF for hydration as needed since in-patients often receive other IVF for medication infusions. Otherwise, total volume should include maintenance fluid plus fluid to accommodate drainage (e.g., output from fistulas, ostomies, wounds, or fecal managers) and insensible losses from the skin and respiratory tract. Young adults require approximately 30–40 mL/kg/day, while older adults require approximately 20–30 mL/kg/day.[1,26,35] Daily weights are essential to assess fluid status. Weekly gain or loss greater than 3–4 lb (1.8 kg) generally represents fluid retention or loss and not tissue synthesis. Vital signs and physical examination changes (e.g., edema, ascites, and skin turgor) also offer evidence of fluid status. Daily mineral and electrolyte requirements in PN are shown in Table 13-8.

Table 13-8 Daily Mineral and Electrolyte Additions to Adult Parenteral Nutrition Formulations

Electrolyte	Standard requirement (per day)*	Sample starting dose (per day)	Max dose (per liter)	Max dose (per day)¶
Calcium	10–15 mEq	10 mEq	15 mEq	15 mEq
Magnesium†	8–20 mEq	16 mEq	16 mEq	40 mEq
Phosphorus‡	20–40 mmol	28 mmol (as either NaPhos or Kphos)‡	20 mmol	48 mmol
Sodium	1–2 mEq/kg+replacement	100 mEq/day§	150 mEq	150 mEq
Potassium	1–2 mEq/kg+replacement	70 mEq/day§	100 mEq	100 mEq
Acetate	As needed to maintain acid–base balance	Adjusted per patient need		
Chloride	As needed to maintain acid–base balance	Adjusted per patient need		

* Standard intake ranges based on healthy people with normal losses.
† Magnesium sulfate provides 8.12 mEq/g of magnesium.
‡ NaPhos contains 4 mEq sodium/ml and 3 mmol Phos/ml; Kphos contains 4.4 mEq potassium/ml and 3 mmol Phos/ml.
¶ Additional requirements should be reviewed with your nutrition support pharmacist to avoid unstable solutions.
§ Include the cation used for phosphate salt.
Source: Adapted from Mirtallo[21] and Mueller.[33]

Calcium, Phosphorus, and Magnesium

Calcium, phosphorus, and magnesium are cofactors for enzymes in the metabolism of macronutrients. When PN (or any dextrose containing IVF) is initiated, these three minerals may shift intra-cellularly especially in malnourished patients. Phosphorus and magnesium requirements are increased in patients with losses from fistulas or diarrhea. All three must be closely monitored and repleted prior to PN initiation and advancement.

Calcium is essential for normal muscle contraction, nerve function, blood coagulation, and bone mineralization. Typical calcium doses can range from 4.5 to 15 mEq/day. Sixty percent of serum calcium is bound to albumin. In the presence of low serum albumin levels, total serum calcium needs to be adjusted. A better method is to use serum ionized calcium as it is the most accurate way to assess calcium status. Calcium supplementation in the PN should be based on the ionized calcium level.

$$\text{Adjusted calcium} = [(4.0 - \text{serum albumin}) \times 0.8] + \text{serum calcium}$$

Phosphorus is an integral component of adenosine triphosphate (ATP). Severe hypophosphatemia can result in muscle, respiratory, or cardiac compromise, and ultimately to death if not monitored and repleted correctly.[42–46] Typical dosing ranges from 10 to 40 mmol/day. All electrolyte additions to a PN bag have limits due to stability; however, calcium and phosphorus are unique due to the potential for fatal calcium/phosphorus precipitates. It is imperative to follow safe guidelines for electrolyte additives and to consult with a pharmacist if any questions exist.[21,34,36]

Magnesium functions in all reactions involving ATP. Magnesium, also bound to albumin, can appear falsely low with hypoalbuminemia. Baseline dosing for magnesium sulfate is 8–20 mEq/day.

Sodium, Potassium, Chloride, and Acetate

Baseline sodium dosing is 1–2 mEq/kg. Requirements may be higher with excess nasogastric, urinary, ostomy, or fistula output, whereas restrictions may be warranted with renal, cardiac, or hepatic dysfunction.

Baseline potassium dosing is 1–2 mEq/kg. Hypokalemia may result from diuretics, amphotericin B, nasogastric suction, vomiting, excess stool output, and/or rapid refeeding of dextrose. Organ dysfunction and medications such as cyclosporine, bactrim, tacrolimus, and potassium-sparing diuretics may cause hyperkalemia. Potassium is given for the metabolism of substrates within the PN bag plus any ongoing losses. Acute deficits of potassium should be corrected by giving separate i.v. infusions of potassium.

Sodium and potassium may be added to PN in the form of chloride or acetate salts to maintain acid–base balance. In patients with upper GI losses, chloride needs are elevated, whereas acetate needs are elevated in those with lower GI losses. Acetate is converted to bicarbonate in the liver; bicarbonate should never be added to PN solutions since it is not compatible with other additives. A reasonable way to begin a PN formula is to split the acetate and chloride evenly (i.e., if the total PN sodium is 100 mEq, give 60 mEq NaCl and 40 mEq Na acetate, assuming normal acid-base balance) and then adjust daily as needed.

Vitamins, Minerals, and Trace Elements

Vitamins, minerals, and trace elements are essential cofactors for metabolism. Their routine addition to the PN solution is necessary to sustain endogenous levels and prevent deficiencies. Iron is not routinely recommended in patients receiving PN due to risk of infection, anaphylaxis and a potential for destabilization. However, in patients receiving long-term PN, or those with iron deficiency anemia, iron supplementation may be indicated at 25–50 mg/month (or 10 mg/week).[47] Iron dextran MUST be used as a test dose prior to administration. It is not recommended that i.v. iron be added to 3-in-1 solutions[21] (Tables 13-9 and 13-10). In the event that vitamin, mineral, or trace element deficiencies develop, or a patient presents for PN with pre-existing deficiencies, individual nutrients can be supplemented in the PN solution without exceeding the maximum dose.

Table 13-9 Adult Parenteral Multivitamins: Guidelines and Products

Vitamin	FDA requirements	MVI adult	Infuvite adult (10 ml)
A (retinol)	3300 USP units	3300 USP units	3300 USP units
D	200 USP units	200 UPS units*	200 USP units†
E	10 USP units	10 USP units	10 USP units
B$_1$ (thiamin)	6 mg	6 mg	6 mg
B$_2$ (riboflavin)	3.6 mg	3.6 mg	3.6 mg
B$_3$ (niacinamide)	40 mg	40 mg	40 mg
B$_5$ (dexpanthenol)	15 mg	15 mg	15 mg
B$_6$ (pyridoxine)	6 mg	6 mg	6 mg
B$_{12}$ (cyanocobalamin)	5 µg	5 µg	5 µg
C	200 mg	200 mg	200 mg
Biotin	60 µg	60 µg	60 µg
Folic acid	600 µg	600 µg	600 µg
K	0 units	150 µg	150 µg

*Vitamin D$_2$ (ergocalciferol) and
†Vitamin D$_3$ (cholecalciferol).
Source: Jennifer M. Dolan, MS, RD, CNSC and Nancy Lee Sceery, RD, LD, CNSD, 2012. Used with permission.

Table 13-10 Daily Trace Element Requirements

Trace Element	ASPEN Recommendations (per day)	GI Losses
Chromium	10–15 µg	20 µg/day
Copper	0.3–0.5 mg	0.5 mg/d
Manganese	60–100 µg	n/a
Selenium	20–60 µg	n/a
Zinc	2.5–5 mg*	12 mg/L of small bowel losses

*Additional 2 mg/day in hypermetabolic states.
Source: Mirtallo.[21] Used with permission.

Medications

PN solutions are designed to deliver nutrients, not medications. Therefore, PN is considered a medication in and of itself with stringent stability, sterility, and safety guidelines.[21,34,36,37] With a few exceptions, medications should not be added to the PN solution due to potential instability and incompatibility.[21,37] Heparin, insulin, H2 receptor antagonists, and octreotide are safe to add when necessary. Regular insulin is the only insulin that can be added and warrants frequent glucose monitoring.[1] All components of the PN solution should be added in the pharmacy rather than at the bedside to minimize the risk of infection and/or instability, though patients receiving home PN may add insulin and a multivitamin just prior to administering PN.[21]

Access

PN may be administered centrally or peripherally. The route of administration will depend on the length and goals of therapy, nutritional requirements, availability of i.v. access, severity of illness, and fluid status. Central access for administering PN can be obtained via the subclavian or jugular veins using a temporary central venous access device (CVAD) or via the basilic or cephalic vein using a peripherally inserted central catheter (PICC).[1] A tunneled catheter or implanted port may also be used for long-term access. The most common complications associated with the percutaneous placement of a CVAD are pneumothorax and arterial rupture. A chest X-ray should be obtained before using a newly placed CVAD to ensure that the line was correctly placed and no internal injuries occurred during insertion. The tip of a CVAD must be located in the distal superior vena cava adjacent to the right atrium to reduce the risk of catheter-related deep venous thrombosis.[26,48] With central line administration, the osmolarity is rapidly diluted by the high rate of blood flow returning to the heart, so there is no need to restrict substrate content.[1,48–50]

Substrate and electrolyte content is limited in peripheral PN (PPN) osmolarity due to constraints and the risk of phlebitis. Final dextrose concentration must be ≤10% and amino concentration between 3 and 4% to mitigate risk of phlebitis and maintain <900 mOsm/l.[1,49,50] PPN is reserved for short-term support (7–14 days) as a bridge back to oral/EN. PPN may not provide adequate calories and protein for hypermetabolic, fluid-restricted patients. However, it can prevent catabolism until GI function returns or central access is obtained.[20,21,26,37] The osmolarity of a PN solution can be estimated as follows:[50]

$$\text{Osmolarity (mOsmol/L)} = [(\text{grams dextrose/L} \times 5) + (\text{grams amino acid/L} \times 10) \\ + (\text{mEq cations/L} \times 2)]$$

The PN Prescription

The base solution can be specified by the actual grams of dextrose, fat, amino acids, and calories, or it can be prescribed as final concentrations. Individual electrolytes and minerals can be specified, or a selection can be made from several standard solutions. A reasonably safe starting formula (per liter) for most patients is 1 g amino acid per kg, 100 g dextrose, and 25–50 g lipid. In most institutions, the PN prescription is ordered for a 24-hour period. In most patients, the goal concentration can be achieved within the second to third day, depending on the patient's nutritional status and metabolic tolerance. Serum blood glucose levels should be controlled and all electrolytes within a reasonable limit of normal before advancing the PN concentration.[40,44,51]

All patients should first receive PN infused over 24 hours. Patients who are clinically and metabolically stable may then progress to cycled PN to allow for more physiologic feeding, freedom from the pump, increased ease of mobility, facilitation back to oral intake as GI status permits, and improved quality of life. A typical cycle runs over 10–16 hours. Cyclic PN facilitates the hepatic mobilization of synthesized fat by allowing insulin concentrations to decrease.[1,26,52,53]

Parenteral Nutrition Sample Taper Schedule

- Day 1: 24 hours.
- Day 2: 18 hours with a 1 hour taper up and 1 hour taper down.
- Day 3 (and thereafter): 12 hours with a 1 hour taper up and a 1 hour taper down.

As GI function returns, patients can be transitioned to EN or an oral diet. When EN/oral intake approaches 50% of estimated needs, calorie and protein levels in the PN can be decreased in a proportionate manner. Continue to wean down PN as oral/enteral intake increases, and discontinue PN once the patient is tolerating at least 75% of nutrient needs on a consistent basis.[1]

Monitoring and Management of Complications
Infectious Complications

Infection is a significant complication associated with the use of PN. A sudden change in the patient's temperature, especially in combination with new onset rigors, leukocytosis, or unexplained hyperglycemia, may be an indication of catheter-related blood stream infection (CRBSI). The catheter may be the primary source of infection or may be seeded by a remote source.[48,54] Ideally the access device should be removed and re-sited. For those patients with difficult access and/or on permanent PN, a long-term CVAD may be treated *in situ* providing the patient's symptoms improve after treatment is initiated. The main risk of leaving the catheter in place for patients who do initially respond to antibiotics is the risk of recurrent bacteremia. The prevalence of CRBSI can be reduced with proper catheter insertion technique and strict adherence to catheter care protocols.[54,55]

Metabolic Complications

Refeeding Syndrome Refeeding syndrome is a series of dangerous electrolyte aberrations and fluid shifts that can occur with rapid or high dose initiation of PN, primarily carbohydrate.[1,28,42,43,45,46] In any situation of prolonged, inadequate oral intake, refeeding nutrients promotes intracellular uptake of electrolytes and minerals for substrate metabolism that can result in decreased serum levels. This dramatic shift may cause generalized fatigue, lethargy, muscle weakness, cardiac dysfunction, and ultimately death if not prevented or if left untreated. The risk can be minimized with judicious monitoring and conservative initiation of PN. Fluid status, weights and serum potassium, phosphorus, and magnesium levels must be closely monitored and repleted aggressively as needed. This syndrome can also occur in severely malnourished patients when EN is initiated and patients are overfed.[2,32,35,43,45,46]

Glycemic Control Untreated, refractory hyperglycemia correlates with increased morbidity and mortality. Close monitoring and intervention have been shown to decrease the risk of infection and improve patient outcomes. Initially, blood glucose levels should be checked every four to six hours. A prudent goal is to maintain plasma glucose levels ≤150 mg/dL for critically ill patients and ≤180 mg/dL for non-critically ill patients. However, close collaboration with the medical team and/or endocrinology service is recommended.[40,52]

PN-associated hyperglycemia may be treated with a combination of basal, prandial, and correction insulin. Basal insulin is exogenous insulin required for patients with insulin deficiency to maintain blood sugar levels while NPO; it is typically provided as a long-acting insulin and administered subcutaneously once or twice daily. Prandial insulin is the insulin required to cover the dextrose in the PN (e.g., 0.1 units/g of dextrose); it is usually given in the form of regular insulin added directly to the PN solution. Insulin should be added to PN in a dose to cover only the dextrose; PN should not be used as a substitute for an insulin drip. Insulin should be added in incremental doses, and blood glucose should be monitored frequently until the appropriate dose is determined. Correction insulin is insulin given to treat unexpected hyperglycemia; it is usually given in the form of short-acting insulin administered subcutaneously based on a sliding scale. In some instances, it may be necessary to reduce dextrose calories and replace them with lipid calories to achieve glycemic control.[1]

Hypoglycemia may occur in patients if an excessive amount of insulin is added to the PN solution or after abrupt discontinuation of high-dextrose PN infusion ("rebound" hypoglycemia). Decreasing the PN rate of infusion by 50% over the 1 hour prior to discontinuation may prevent hypoglycemia, though some patients tolerate abrupt discontinuation if needed. Blood glucose level should be checked two hours after the PN solution is discontinued to rule out rebound hypoglycemia until glucose is stable.

Fluid and Electrolytes PN solutions can be maximally concentrated as needed for those with volume constraints or diluted to meet fluid requirement depending on institution-specific protocols. Any electrolyte abnormalities should be corrected prior to PN initiation. Close monitoring of electrolytes, especially potassium, magnesium, and phosphorus during the first few days of PN is essential. Correction of severe electrolyte imbalances must be made promptly with i.v. replacement to avoid serious complications as described previously. Table 13-11 lists recommended guidelines for monitoring patients receiving PN.[1,35,56]

Case 2: Parenteral Step-by-Step Approach

A 52-year-old female with a history of ulcerative colitis who had a total colectomy with ileostomy 15 years ago now admitted for repair of a para-stomal hernia complicated by recurrent small bowel obstruction. She is 64" (163 cm) and 160 lb (63 kg).

Step	Formula	Patient Example
1. Calculate non- protein calorie requirement	25–30 kcal/kg/day	25 kcal/kg × 63 kg = 1575 kcal/day 30 kcal/kg × 63 kg = 1890 kcal/day Goal: 1600–1900 kcal/kg/day
2. Calculate protein requirements*	1.5 g/kg	1.5 g/kg × 63 kg = 95 g protein/day
3. Calculate fluid requirement	25–30 mL/kg	25 mL × 63 kg = 1575 mL 30 mL/kg × 63 kg = 1890 mL
4. Calculate oxidative limits	Carbohydrate: 5 g/kg/day Lipid: 1 g/kg /day	5 g/kg/day × 63 kg = 315 g dextrose × 3.4 kcal/g = 1071 kcal dextrose 1 g/kg/day × 63 kg = 63 g lipid × 9 kcal/g = 567 fat kcal/day
5. Calculate carbohydrate requirement†	Non-protein kcal requirement X 60% carbohydrate	1600 non-protein kcal × 0.6 = 960 non-protein kcal. Round up to 1000 dextrose kcal/day
6. Calculate fat requirement‡	Non-protein kcal X 40% fat	1600 non-protein kcal × 0.4 = 640 lipid kcal. Round down to 600 lipid kcal
7. Select electrolytes¶	See Table 13-6	50 mEq NaCl 50 mEq Na acetate 30 mEq KCl
8. Select vitamins	Add multivitamin plus additional vitamin C if needed for wound healing	10 mL multivitamin, 250 mg vitamin C
9. Select minerals	See Table 13-6. Additional minerals if concerned for refeeding syndrome or losses from diarrhea/drains	10 mEq Ca gluconate 16 mEq magnesium sulfate 28 mmol Kphos 5 mg zinc for small bowel losses
10. Select trace elements	Add multi-trace element	1 mL multi-trace elements
11. Determine if additives are needed	Example: insulin (starting dose is usually 10 units/100 g CHO or 0.1 units/gram of dextrose)	Serum glucose normal, so additional insulin not indicated at this time
12. Select infusion time	For starter bag, always infuse over 24 h. Cycle prior to discharge	Infuse over 24 h until stable glycemic control on goal. Then change to 18 h × 1 day and advance to 12 h goal based on glycemic control

*Maintenance protein requirement ranges from 0.8 to 1.2 g/kg/day and repletion protein requirements range from 1.5 to 2 g/kg. Additional protein if tolerance demonstrated and nitrogen balance studies demonstrate need for higher protein load. Limited evidence to show therapeutic benefit >2 g/kg/day and can pose harm. †For acutely ill patients, minimum dextrose requirement is 3 g/kg/day and the maximum dextrose load is 5 g/kg. ‡Minimum fat requirement to prevent EFAD is 500 mL of 20% lipid weekly. Do not exceed 1 g/kg/day to avoid immunosuppression. ¶Acetate need in patients with small bowel losses. Source: Jennifer M. Dolan, MS, RD, CNSC, Nancy Lee Sceery, RD, LD, CNSD, and Nancy Evans-Stoner, MSN, RN, 2012. Used with permission.

Table 13-11 Recommended Guidelines for Monitoring Parenteral Nutrition

Chemistry	Start of Therapy	Acutely Ill Patients	Stable Patients	Home Patients (contingent upon status)
Electrolytes	Yes	Daily	1–2 times/week	Weekly or monthly
Ca^{++}, PO4$^-$, Mg^{++}	Yes	Daily	1– 2 times/week	Weekly or monthly
Triglycerides	Yes	Weekly	Every 2–4 weeks	Monthly
Prealbumin	Yes	Weekly	Every 2–4 weeks	Monthly
Liver function tests*	Yes	3 times per week	Every 1–4 weeks	Commensurate with electrolytes
Glucose	Yes	Every 4–6 h	At least daily	Commensurate with electrolytes
PT/PTT	Yes	Per MD request	Per MD request	Per MD request
Weight	Yes	Daily	1–2 times/week	Weekly
Intake and output	Yes	Daily	As needed	As needed
Nitrogen balance	No	Weekly until normal	Weekly until normal	No

*Contingent upon organ status.
Source: Jennifer M. Dolan, MS, RD, CNSC and Nancy Lee Sceery, RD, LD, CNSD, 2012. Used with permission.

Table 13-12 Key Steps to Prepare for Nutrition Support at Home

Step	Evaluate
1. Patient must be medically stable.	Assess for fever, white count elevation, pain assessment, fluid/electrolyte imbalance.
2. Identify reimbursement source for PN/EN.	Medicare requires clear documentation and need for therapy for >3 months.
3. Identify home PN/EN prescriber.	Patient must have a Nurse Practitioner or physician who will order PN/EN, monitor labs and response to therapy.
4. Select home infusion provider.	Discharge planner should identify home infusion provider.
5. Assess patient/caregiver ability and desire to administer home PN/EN.	Someone must learn to administer home PN/EN. Home nursing will not provide daily visits to administer PN/EN.
6. Adjust PN/EN infusion for home 48–72 hours before discharge.	PN — cycle PN from 24 hours to 18 hours to 12 hours. Assess blood glucose, daily electrolytes and I/O data EN — cycle small bowel feeds from 24 hours to 12 hours. Adjust gastric intermittent/bolus daytime feeds to mealtime schedule.
7. Monitor daily nutrition labs until discharge for PN patients.	Helps to define nutrient prescription prior to discharge including electrolytes and fluid requirements.
8. For patients with history of diabetes or glucose intolerance.	Consider endocrine consult to optimize regimen for blood sugar control.

Source: Nancy Evans-Stoner, MSN, RN, 2012. Used with permission.

Parenteral Nutrition Summary

Parenteral nutrition is a life-saving therapy that should be used to support, prevent, and/or treat under-nutrition in any condition where nutrient goals cannot be achieved by oral/enteral means. Nurse Practitioners should be very involved in all aspects of PN support and are integral members of the nutrition support team.

Home Nutrition Support

Patients who may require home EN or PN should be identified as early as possible to prepare and plan for this therapy.[56] Utilizing a multidisciplinary team involving the Nurse Practitioner, discharge planner, social worker, and nutrition support clinician will likely ensure a smooth transition. The discharge planner will evaluate the patient's insurance and determine if EN or PN is a covered service. The patient's and/or the caregiver's ability to participate in the care required to administer home nutrition support must be evaluated. Table 13-12 outlines the steps necessary to transition patients to home with EN or PN.

Summary: Role of Nurse Practitioners

Nurse Practitioners are in key positions to identify patients that require specialized nutrition support. The Nurse Practitioner's roles include: assessing nutritional status, selecting the appropriate route for nutrition, outlining nutritional goals and translating them into EN and PN orders. A good understanding of the metabolic needs of all patients is imperative to optimize nutritional outcomes in patients receiving EN and PN support in the hospital, nursing home, and home-settings.

References

1. Gottschlich MM, DeLegge MH, Mattox T, et al. *The ASPEN Nutrition Support Core Curriculum: A Case-Based Approach – The Adult Patient.* American Society Parenteral and Enteral Nutrition, Chicago, IL, 2007.
2. McClave SA, Martindale RG, Vanek VW, et al., the ASPEN Board of Directors and the American College of Critical Care Medicine. Guidelines for the provision and assessment of nutrition support therapy in the adult critically ill patient: Society of Critical Care Medicine (SCCM) and American Society for Parentral and Enteral Nutrition. *J Parenter Enteral Nutr* 2009;33:277–316.
3. McClave SA, Lukan JK, Stefater JA, et al. Poor validity of residual volumes as a marker for risk of aspiration in critically ill patients. *Crit Care Med* 2005;33:324–330.
4. O'Keefe SJD. A guide to enteral access procedures and enteral nutrition. *Nat Rev Gastroenterol Hepatol* 2009;6:207–215.
5. Schmidt H, Martindale R. The gastrointestinal tract in critical illness. *Curr Op Clin Nutr Metab Care* 2001;4:547–551.
6. Heyland DK, Dhaliwal R, Drover JW, Gramlich L, Dodek P, and the Canadian Critical Care Practice Guidelines Committee. Canadian clinical practice guidelines for nutrition support in mechanically ventilated, critically ill adult patients. *J Parenter Enteral Nutr* 2003;27:355–373.
7. Bankhead R, Boullata J, Bantley S, et al., the ASPEN Board of Directors. ASPEN Enteral Nutrition Practice Recommendations. *J Parenter Enteral Nutr* 2009;33:122–167.

8. Edes TE, Walk BE, Austin JL. Diarrhea in tube-fed patients: feeding formula not nessarily the cause. *Am J Med* 1990;88:91–93.

9. Houdijk APJ, Rijnsburger ER, Jansen J, et al. Randomised trial of glutamine-enriched enteral nutrition on infectious morbidity in patients with multiple trauma. *Lancet* 1998;352:772–776.

10. Abbott Nutrition for Health Professionals. http://abbottnutrition.com. Accessed 2012.

11. Nestle Health Science. http://www.nestle-nutrition.com. Accessed 2012.

12. Talpers SS, Pomberger DJ, Bunce SB, et al. Nutritionally associated increased carbon dioxide production: excess total calories vs. high proportion of carbohydrate calories. *Chest* 1992;203:551–555.

13. Pontes-Arruda A, Aragao AM, Albuquerque JD. Effects of enteral feeding with eicosapentaenoic acid, gamma-linolenic acid, and antioxidants in mechanically ventilated patients with severe sepsis and septic shock. *Crit Care Med* 2006;34:2325–2333.

14. Gadek JE, DeMichele SJ, Karlstad MD, et al. Effect of enteral feeding with eicosapentaenoic acid, gamma-linolenic acid, and antioxidants in patients with acute respiratory distress syndrome. *Crit Care Med* 1999;27:1409–1420.

15. Rice TW, Wheeler AP, Thompson BT, et al. Enteral omega-3 fatty acid, gamma-linolenic acid, and antioxidant supplementation in acute lung injury. Acute Respiratory Distress Syndrome Network of Investigators. *JAMA* 2011;306:1574–1581.

16. Stapleton RD, Martin TR, Weiss NS, et al. A phase II randomized placebo-controlled trial of omega-3 fatty acids for the treatment of acute lung injury. *Crit Care Med* 2011;39: 1655–1662.

17. O'Keefe SJD. A guide to enteral access procedures and enteral nutrition. *Nat Rev Gastroenterol Hepatol* 2009;6:207–215.

18. Szary N, Arif M, Matteson M, et al. Enteral feeding within three hours after percutaneous endoscopic gastrostomy placement: a meta-analysis. *J Clin Gastroenterol* 2011;54:e34–e38.

19. Niv E, Fireman Z, Vaisman N. Post-pyloric feeding. *World J Gastroenterol* 2009;15:1281–1288.

20. DiBaise J, Scolapio J. Home parenteral and enteral nutrition. *Gastroenterol Clin N Am* 2007;36:123–144.

21. Mirtallo JM, Canada T, Johnson D, et al. Safe practices for parenteral putrition. *J Parenter Enteral Nutr* 2004;28:S39–S70.

22. Rice TW, Mogan S, Hays MA, et al. Randomized trial of initial trophic versus full-energy enteral nutrition in mechanically ventilated patients with acute respiratory failure. *Crit Care Med* 2011;39:967–974.

23. DeLegge MH. Managing gastric residual volumes in the critically ill patient: an update. *Curr Op Clin Nutr Metab Care* 2011;14:193–196.

24. Braunschweig C, Levy P, Sheean P, et al. Enteral versus parenteral nutrition: a meta analysis. *Am J Clin Nutr* 2001;74:534–542.

25. Casaer MP, Mesotten D, Hermans G, et al. Early versus late parenteral nutrition in critically ill adults. *N Eng J Med* 2011;365:506–517.

26. Atkinson, M,Worthley LIG. Nutrition in the critically ill patient: Part II. *Parenteral Nutr Crit Care Resus* 2003;5:121–136.

27. Huckleberry Y. Nutrition support and the surgical patient. *Am Soc Health-System Pharm* 2004;61:671–682.

28. ASPEN Board of Directors. Guidelines for the use of parenteral and enteral nutrition in adults and pediatric patients. *J Parenter Enteral Nutr* 2002;26:1,9SA–138SA.

29. Harris JA, Benedict FG. *A biometric study of basal metabolism in man.* Publication No. 279. Carnegie Institute. Washington, DC, 919.

30. Frankenfield DC, Coleman A, Alam S, et al. Analysis of estimation methods for resting metabolic rate in critically ill adults. *J Parenter Enteral Nutr* 2009;33:27–36.

31. RxKinetics. Tutorial: http://www.rxkinetics.com/tpntutorial/13.thml. Accessed 2012.

32. Gines P. Parenteral nutrition in the critically ill patient. *N Eng J Med* 2010;362:81–84.

33. Mueller C. Parenteral nutrition order writing. *Support Line* 1999;21:3–7.

34. Trissel LA. *Handbook on Injectable Drugs*, 15th edition. American Society of Health System Pharmacy, Bethesda, 2008.

35. McCrae JD, O'Shea R, Udine ML. Parenteral nutrition: hospital to home. *J Am Diet Assoc* 1993;93:664–670, 673.

36. Bing C. *Extended Stability for Parenteral Drugs*, 4th edition. American Society of Health System Pharmacy, Bethesda, 2009.

37. Driscoll DF, Blackburn GL. Total parenteral nutrition: a review of its current status in hospitalized patients and the need for patient specific feeding. *Drugs* 1990;40:346–363.

38. Fogle P. Vitamin κ and lipid emulsions. *Support Line* 2001;23:3–8.

39. Jeejeebhoy KN, Anderson GH, Nakhooda AF, et al. Metabolic studies in total parenteral nutrition with lipid in man, comparison with glucose. *J Clin Invest* 1975;37:125–136.

40. van den Berghe G, Wouters P, Weekers F, et al. Intensive insulin therapy in the critically ill patients. *N Eng J Med* 2001;345:1359–1367.

41. Mirtallo JM, Dasta JF, Kleinschmidt KC. State of the art review: intravenous fat emulsions: current applications, safety profile, and clinical implications. *Ann Pharm* 2010;44:688–700.

42. Dickerson R. Guidelines for the intravenous management of hypophosphatemia, hypomagnesemia, hypokalemia, and hypocalcemia: 2001 fact comparisons. *Hosp Pharm* 2001;36:1201–1208.

43. Ziegler TR. Parenteral Nutrition in the Critically Ill Patient. *NEJM* 2009;10:1088–1097.

44. Taylor B, Krenitsky J. Nutrition in the intensive care unit: year in review 2008–2009. *J Parenter Enteral Nutr* 2010;34:21–31.

45. Parish CR. Much ado about refeeding. *Nutr Issues Gastroenterol* 2005;23:26–44.

46. Kraft MD, Btaiche IF, Sacks GS. Review of the refeeding syndrome. *Nutr Clin Prac* 2005;20:625–633.

47. Buchman AL. *Clinical Nutrition in Gastrointestinal Disease*. Slack Inc, Thorofare, 2006.

48. Vanek WV. The ins and outs of venous access: Part II. *Nutr Clin Prac* 2002;17:142–155.

49. Ireton-Jones CS, Robinson N. Peripheral parenteral nutrition: indications and guidelines. *Support Line* 1995;17:11–13.

50. Almuete VI. Osmolarity for peripheral parenteral nutrition formulas. *Medscape Pharmacists* 2005;5.

51. NICE-SUGAR study investigators. Intensive versus conventional glucose control in critically ill patients. *N Eng J Med* 2009;360:1283–1297.

52. Kumpf VJ. Parenteral nutrition associated liver disease in adult and pediatric patients. *Nutr Clin Prac* 2006;21:279–290.

53. Fuchs M, Sanyal A. Sepsis and cholestasis. *Clin Liver Dis* 2008;12:151–172.

54. Schiavone, PA, Stoner, NE, Compher, CW, et al. Management of catheter-related infection in patients receiving home parenteral nutrition. *Practical Gastroenterology* 2010;88:22–34.

55. Rogers KL, Fey PD, Rupp ME. Coagulase-negative staphylococcal infections. *Inf Dis Clin N Am* 2009;23:73–98.

56. Seipler J, Principles and strategies for monitoring home parenteral nutrition: invited review. *Nutr Clin Prac* 2007;22:340–350.

Appendices

The Nurse Practitioner's Guide to Nutrition, Second Edition. Edited by Lisa Hark, Kathleen Ashton and Darwin Deen.
© 2012 John Wiley & Sons, Inc. Published 2012 by John Wiley & Sons, Inc.

Appendix A

Food Sources of Vitamin A

Food, Standard Amount	Serving Size	Vitamin A (µg RE)
Margarine	1tbsp	
Liver (beef, veal, goose, and turkey)	3oz	13000–19000
Liver (chicken, lamb)	3oz	6000–10000
Various ready-to-eat cereals, with added vitamin A	1oz	180–376
Instant cooked cereals, fortified	1 packet	285–376
Beets	1 cup	3.4
Apricots, dried	1/2 cup	80
Broccoli, fresh, cooked	1 cup	120.2
Herring, Atlantic	3oz	219
Cantaloupe, raw	1/4 medium melon	233
Chinese cabbage, cooked	1 cup	360
Red sweet pepper, cooked	1 cup	371
Peppers, chili	1 cup	405
Mustard greens, cooked	1 cup	442
Milk, (all types) with added vitamin A	1 cup	478
Winter squash, cooked	1 cup	535
Turnip greens, cooked from frozen	1 cup	549
Collards, cooked from frozen	1 cup	771
Kale, cooked from frozen	1 cup	885
Spinach, cooked from frozen	1 cup	943
Mixed vegetables, canned	1 cup	949
Pumpkin, canned	1/2 cup	953
Carrots, raw	1 cup	1026
Sweet potato with peel, baked	1 medium	1096
Mango, raw	1 cup	1262
Carrot juice	3/4 cup	1692
Tomatoes and vegetable juice	1 cup	3770
Fish oil, cod liver	1 tbsp	4051

Source: www.nutritiondata.com

The Nurse Practitioner's Guide to Nutrition, Second Edition. Edited by Lisa Hark, Kathleen Ashton and Darwin Deen.
© 2012 John Wiley & Sons, Inc. Published 2012 by John Wiley & Sons, Inc.

Appendix B
Food Sources of Vitamin D

Food, Standard Amount	Serving Size	Vitamin D (IU)
Herring, Atlantic	3 oz	1384
Fish oil, cod liver	1 tbsp	1350
Fish, sardines, salmon, codfish	3 oz	649–71.4
Catfish	3 oz	425
Oysters	3 oz	268.8
Egg, yolk, raw, fresh	1 large	260
Milk (all types)	1 cup	299–97.6
Milk, whole	1 cup	100
Margarine	1 tbsp	60
Cereals ready-to-eat	1 cup	126–88
Butter, salted	1 tbsp	7.8
Cheddar cheese	1.5 oz	5.1

Source: www.nutritiondata.com

The Nurse Practitioner's Guide to Nutrition, Second Edition. Edited by Lisa Hark, Kathleen Ashton and Darwin Deen.
© 2012 John Wiley & Sons, Inc. Published 2012 by John Wiley & Sons, Inc.

Appendix C
Food Sources of Vitamin E

Food, Standard Amount	Serving Size	Alpha Tocopherol (mg)
Fortified ready-to-eat cereals	1 cup	33.8–13.5
Sunflower seeds, dry roasted	1 oz	7.4
Almonds	1 oz	7.3
Sunflower oil	1 tbsp	5.6
Tomato sauce	1 cup	5.0
Safflower oil	1 tbsp	4.6
Spinach, frozen, cooked	1 cup	3.7
Swiss chard, cooked	1 cup	3.3
Mixed nuts, dry roasted	1 oz	3.1
Turnip greens, frozen, cooked	1 cup	2.7
Pine nuts	1 oz	2.6
Peanut butter	2 tbsp	2.5
Canola oil	1 tbsp	2.4
Wheat germ, toasted, plain	2 tbsp	2.3
Peanuts	1 oz	2.2
Avocado, raw	1/2 avocado	2.1
Carrot juice, canned	3/4 cup	2.1
Corn oil and olive oil	1 tbsp	1.9
Mustard greens, frozen, cooked	1 cup	1.7
Sardine, Atlantic, in oil, drained	3 oz	1.7
Radicchio	1 cup	0.9
Herring, Atlantic	3 oz	0.9
Margarine	1 tbsp	0.8
Salad dressing (Italian)	1 tbsp	0.7

Source: www.nutritiondata.com

The Nurse Practitioner's Guide to Nutrition, Second Edition. Edited by Lisa Hark, Kathleen Ashton and Darwin Deen.
© 2012 John Wiley & Sons, Inc. Published 2012 by John Wiley & Sons, Inc.

Appendix D
Food Sources of Vitamin K

Food, Standard Amount	Serving Size	Phyloquinone per serving (µg)
Kale, frozen, cooked	1 cup	1062
Collard greens, frozen, cooked	1 cup	1060
Spinach, frozen, cooked	1 cup	889
Turnip greens, frozen, cooked	1 cup	529
Mustard greens, frozen, cooked	1 cup	419
Parsley, raw	1/4 cup	246
Brussels sprouts, fresh	1 cup	218
Broccoli, fresh	1 cup	110
Asparagus, fresh	1 cup	91
Okra, frozen, cooked	1 cup	88
Cabbage, fresh	1 cup	67.6
Green peas, frozen, cooked	1 cup	38.4
Cauliflower	1 cup	17.2
Celery, raw	1 medium stalk	17
Carrot, raw	1 cup	16.1
Grapes, red/green, seedless, raw	1 1/2 cup	12
Plums, raw	2 medium	11
Pear, raw	1 medium	8.1
Tomato juice, bottled	8 fluid oz	5.6
Tomato, red, raw	1 medium	4.4
Avocado, raw	1/5 medium	4.3
Apricot, raw	1/2 cup	2.5

Source: www.nutritiondata.com

The Nurse Practitioner's Guide to Nutrition, Second Edition. Edited by Lisa Hark, Kathleen Ashton and Darwin Deen.
© 2012 John Wiley & Sons, Inc. Published 2012 by John Wiley & Sons, Inc.

Appendix E
Food Sources of Vitamin C

Food, Standard Amount	Serving Size	Vitamin C (mg)
Guava, raw	1/2 cup	188
Peppers (all types), raw	1 cup	155
Peppers (all types) cooked	1 cup	150
Broccoli, cooked	1 cup	101.2
Strawberries, raw	1 cup	100
Brussels sprouts, cooked	1 cup	96.8
Kohlrabi, cooked	1 cup	90
Broccoli, raw	1 cup	81.2
Peas, Snowpeas, Sugar snap peas, cooked	1 cup	76.6
Kiwi fruit	1 medium	70
Orange, raw	1 medium	70
Orange juice	3/4 cup	61–93
Peas, edible-podded, raw (Snowpeas, Sugar snap peas)	1 cup	58.8
Tangerines (mandarin oranges), raw	1 cup	52.1
Green pepper, sweet, cooked	1/2 cup	51
Grapefruit juice	3/4 cup	50–70
Vegetable juice cocktail	3/4 cup	50
Cantaloupe	1/4 medium	47
Papaya, raw	1/4 medium	47
Tomato juice	3/4 cup	33
Raspberries, raw	1 cup	32.2
Melons, honeydew, raw	1 cup	31.9
Sweet potato, cooked	1 medium	22.3

Source: www.nutritiondata.com

The Nurse Practitioner's Guide to Nutrition, Second Edition. Edited by Lisa Hark, Kathleen Ashton and Darwin Deen.
© 2012 John Wiley & Sons, Inc. Published 2012 by John Wiley & Sons, Inc.

Appendix F
Food Sources of Folate

Food, Standard Amount	Serving Size	Folate (µg)
Ready-to-eat cereals	1 cup	1010
Chicken liver	3 oz	495
Beef liver	3 oz	243.6
Spinach, frozen, cooked	1 cup	230
Lentils, cooked	1/2 cup	180
Tomato	1 medium	75–97
Mustard and turnip greens, frozen, cooked	1 cup	170
Seaweed, kelp, raw	1 cup	144
Chickpeas, canned	1/2 cup	140
Okra, frozen, cooked	1 cup	134
Collard greens, frozen, cooked	1 cup	129
Asparagus, fresh, cooked	1 cup	121.2
Peas, green, boiled	1 cup	94.4
Brussels sprouts, raw	1 cup	93.6
Broccoli, fresh, cooked	1 cup	84.2
Lettuce, romaine	1 cup	63.9
Orange juice	6 oz	55.8
Cauliflower	1 cup	54.6
Potato, baked with skin	1 medium	40
Egg, boiled	1 large	24

Source: www.nutritiondata.com

The Nurse Practitioner's Guide to Nutrition, Second Edition. Edited by Lisa Hark, Kathleen Ashton and Darwin Deen.
© 2012 John Wiley & Sons, Inc. Published 2012 by John Wiley & Sons, Inc.

Appendix G
Food Sources of Calcium (Dairy)

Food, Standard Amount	Serving Size	Calcium (mg)
Lactose-free calcium fortified milk	1 cup	500
Plain yogurt, non-fat	8 oz	452
Romano cheese	1.5 oz	452
Plain yogurt, low-fat	8 oz	415
Soy milk, calcium fortified	1 cup	368
Fruit yogurt, low-fat	8 oz	345
Swiss cheese	1.5 oz	336
Ricotta cheese, part skim	1/2 cup	335
Pasteurized process Swiss cheese	1.5 oz	324
Provolone cheese	1.5 oz	321
Egg, yolk, raw, fresh	1 large	313
Mozzarella cheese, part-skim	1.5 oz	311
Cheddar cheese	1.5 oz	307
Fat-free (skim) milk	1 cup	306
Muenster cheese	1.5 oz	305
1% low-fat milk	1 cup	290
Low-fat chocolate milk (1%)	1 cup	288
2% reduced fat milk	1 cup	285
Reduced fat chocolate milk (2%)	1 cup	285
Buttermilk, low-fat	1 cup	284
Chocolate milk	1 cup	280
Whole milk	1 cup	276
Yogurt, plain, whole milk	8 oz	275
Ricotta cheese, whole milk	1/2 cup	255
Pasteurized process American cheese food	1.5 oz	232
Blue cheese	1.5 oz	225
Mozzarella cheese, whole milk	1.5 oz1	215
Feta cheese	1.5 oz	210

Source: www.nutritiondata.com

The Nurse Practitioner's Guide to Nutrition, Second Edition. Edited by Lisa Hark, Kathleen Ashton and Darwin Deen.
© 2012 John Wiley & Sons, Inc. Published 2012 by John Wiley & Sons, Inc.

Appendix H
Food Sources of Calcium (Non-dairy)

Food, Standard Amount	Serving Size	Calcium (mg)
Soy beverage, calcium fortified	1 cup	368
Collard greens, frozen, cooked	1 cup	357
Sardines, Atlantic, in oil, drained	3 oz	325
Tofu, firm, prepared with nigari	1/2 cup	253
Spinach, frozen, cooked	1 cup	245
Turnip greens, frozen, cooked	1 cup	197
Pink salmon, canned, with bone	3 oz	181
Okra, frozen, cooked	1 cup	176
Molasses, blackstrap	1 tbsp	172
Beet greens, fresh, cooked	1 cup	164
Pak-choi, Chinese cabbage, cooked from fresh	1 cup	158
Soybeans, green, cooked	1/2 cup	130
Ocean perch, Atlantic, cooked	3 oz	116
White beans, canned	1/2 cup	96
Kale, frozen, cooked	1 cup	93.6
Clams, canned	3 oz	78
Nuts, almonds, oil roasted	1 oz	74.5
Rainbow trout, farmed, cooked	3 oz	73
Oatmeal, plain and flavored, instant, fortified	1 packet prepared	99–110

Source: www.nutritiondata.com

The Nurse Practitioner's Guide to Nutrition, Second Edition. Edited by Lisa Hark, Kathleen Ashton and Darwin Deen.
© 2012 John Wiley & Sons, Inc. Published 2012 by John Wiley & Sons, Inc.

Appendix I
Food Sources of Sodium

Food, Standard Amount	Serving Size	Sodium (mg)
Salt (sodium chloride)	1 tsp	2325
Pickle relish, sweet	1 cup	1987
Soup, canned (all types)	1 cup	850–2500
Tomato sauce	1 cup	1284
Soy sauce made from soy (tamari)	1 tbsp	1006
Sauerkraut, canned	1 cup	939
Chicken pot pie, frozen entree	1 pie	841
Potato chips, regular and baked	1 bag (1 oz)	837
Pretzels, hard, plain, salted	10 twists	814
Cheese American	1.5 oz	670
Tomato juice, canned, with salt added	1 cup	654
Vegetable juice cocktail, canned	1 cup	653
Pickles, kosher dill	1 medium	569
Beef frankfurter, hot dog	1 frank	461
Olives, canned or bottled, green	1 oz	440
Scrapple, pork	2 oz	369
Gravy, canned	1/4 cup	352
Canned tuna	3 oz	320
Canned vegetables	1 cup	243
Lunch meats (turkey, ham, salami, pastrami)	3 slices	250–500
Barbeque sauce	1 tbsp	212
Noodles, Chinese, chow mein	1 cup	198
Cheese pizza	1 slice	194
Beef sausage, fresh, cooked	1 oz	184
Salad dressings	1 tbsp	147
Peanuts, oil-roasted, with salt	1 oz	121
Frozen dinner	1 dinner	360–768

Source: www.nutritiondata.com

The Nurse Practitioner's Guide to Nutrition, Second Edition. Edited by Lisa Hark, Kathleen Ashton and Darwin Deen.
© 2012 John Wiley & Sons, Inc. Published 2012 by John Wiley & Sons, Inc.

Appendix J
Food Sources of Potassium

Food, Standard Amount	Serving Size	Potassium (mg)
Beet greens, cooked	1 cup	1309
Spinach, cooked	1 cup	839
Tomato sauce	1 cup	810
Sweet potato, baked	1 medium	694
Potato, baked, flesh	1 medium	610
White beans, canned	1/2 cup	595
Yogurt, plain, non-fat	8 oz	579
Tomato puree	1/2 cup	549
Clams, canned	3 oz	534
Yogurt, plain, low-fat	8 oz	531
Prune juice	3/4 cup	530
Carrot juice	3/4 cup	517
Apricots, dried	1/2 cup	514
Blackstrap molasses	1 tbsp	498
Halibut, cooked	3 oz	490
Soybeans, green, cooked	1/2 cup	485
Tuna, yellow fin, cooked	3 oz	484
Lima beans, cooked	1/2 cup	484
Artichokes, (globe or French), raw	1 artichoke	474
Winter squash, cooked	1 cup	449
Soybeans, mature, cooked	1/2 cup	443
Rockfish, Pacific, cooked	3 oz	442
Cod, Pacific, cooked	3 oz	439
Bananas	1 medium	422
Tomato juice	3/4 cup	417
Peaches, fresh	1 medium	398
Prunes, stewed	1/2 cup	398
Milk, non-fat	1 cup	382
Pork chop, center loin, cooked	3 oz	382
Rainbow trout, farmed, cooked	3 oz	375
Pork loin, center rib (roasts), lean, roasted	3 oz	371
Buttermilk, cultured, low-fat	1 cup	370
Cantaloupe	1/4 medium	368
1%–2% milk	1 cup	366
Honeydew melon	1/8 medium	365
Lentils, cooked	1/2 cup	365
Plantains, cooked	1/2 cup slices	358
Kidney beans, cooked	1/2 cup	358
Orange juice	3/4 cup	355
Split peas, cooked	1/2 cup	355
Yogurt, plain, whole milk	8 oz container	352

Source: www.nutritiondata.com

The Nurse Practitioner's Guide to Nutrition, Second Edition. Edited by Lisa Hark, Kathleen Ashton and Darwin Deen.
© 2012 John Wiley & Sons, Inc. Published 2012 by John Wiley & Sons, Inc.

Appendix K
Food Sources of Magnesium

Food, Standard Amount	Serving Size	Magnesium (mg)
Beet greens, cooked	1 cup	97.9
Okra, cooked from frozen	1 cup	93.8
Halibut, cooked	3 oz	91
Quinoa, dry	1/4 cup	89
Almonds	1 oz	78
Soybeans, mature, cooked	1/2 cup	74
Nuts, (various types)	1 oz	70–107
White beans	1/2 cup	67
Pollock, walleye, cooked	3 oz	62
Black beans, cooked	1/2 cup	60
Oat bran, raw	1/4 cup	55
Soybeans, green, cooked	1/2 cup	54
Tuna, yellow fin, cooked	3 oz	54
Lima beans, baby, cooked from frozen	1/2 cup	50
Navy beans, cooked	1/2 cup	48
Tofu, firm, prepared with nigari	1/2 cup	47
Soy beverage	1 cup	47
Cowpeas, cooked	1/2 cup	46
Hazelnuts	1 oz	46
Great northern beans, cooked	1/2 cup	44
Oat bran, cooked	1/2 cup	44
Buckwheat groats, roasted, cooked	1/2 cup	43
Brown rice, cooked	1/2 cup	42
Haddock, cooked	3 oz	42
Spinach, frozen, cooked	1 cup	157
Pumpkin and squash seed kernels, roasted	1 oz	151
Bran ready-to-eat cereal (100%)	1 oz	103

Source: www.nutritiondata.com

The Nurse Practitioner's Guide to Nutrition, Second Edition. Edited by Lisa Hark, Kathleen Ashton and Darwin Deen.
© 2012 John Wiley & Sons, Inc. Published 2012 by John Wiley & Sons, Inc.

Appendix L
Food Sources of Iron

Food, Standard Amount	Serving Size	Iron (mg)
Spinach, frozen, cooked	1 cup	6.4
Liver (various types) cooked	3 oz	5.0–9.9
Fortified instant cooked cereals (various)	1 packet	5.0–8.1
Soybeans, mature, cooked	1/2 cup	4.4
Pumpkin and squash seed kernels, roasted	1 oz	4.2
White beans, canned	1/2 cup	3.9
Blackstrap molasses	1 tbsp	3.5
Lentils, cooked	1/2 cup	3.3
Fortified ready-to-eat cereals (various)	1 cup	19–28
Clams, canned, drained	3 oz	23.8
Clams, canned	3 oz	23.8
Kidney beans, cooked	1/2 cup	2.6
Sardines, canned in oil, drained	3 oz	2.5
Chickpeas, cooked	1/2 cup	2.4
Duck, meat only, roasted	3 oz	2.3
Prune juice	3/4 cup	2.3
Shrimp, canned	3 oz	2.3
Cowpeas, cooked	1/2 cup	2.2
Ground beef, 15% fat, cooked	3 oz	2.2
Tomato puree	1/2 cup	2.2
Lima beans, cooked	1/2 cup	2.2
Soybeans, green, cooked	1/2 cup	2.2
Navy beans, cooked	1/2 cup	2.1
Refried beans	1/2 cup	2.1
Tomato paste	1/4 cup	2.0
Oysters, eastern, wild, cooked	3 oz	10.2
Beef, lean ground, raw	3 oz	1.5
Beef, sirloin steak or filet mignon, raw	3 oz	1.2
Lamb, shoulder, arm, raw	3 oz	1.1

Source: www.nutritiondata.com

The Nurse Practitioner's Guide to Nutrition, Second Edition. Edited by Lisa Hark, Kathleen Ashton and Darwin Deen.
© 2012 John Wiley & Sons, Inc. Published 2012 by John Wiley & Sons, Inc.

Appendix M
Food Sources of Omega-3 Fatty Acids

Food, Standard Amount	Serving Size	Omega-3 Fatty Acids (g)
Flaxseed oil	1 tbsp	6.7
Salmon, Atlantic, wild, cooked	3.0 oz	2.198
Flaxseeds	1 tbsp	2.63
Walnuts	1 oz	2.5
Soybeans, cooked	1/2 cup	2.1
Canola oil	1 tbsp	1.4
Walnut oil	1 tbsp	1.3
Sardine	3.0 oz	1.2
Tuna, white, canned in water	3.0 oz	0.81
Wheat germ oil	1 tbsp	0.86

Source: www.nutritiondata.com

The Nurse Practitioner's Guide to Nutrition, Second Edition. Edited by Lisa Hark, Kathleen Ashton and Darwin Deen.
© 2012 John Wiley & Sons, Inc. Published 2012 by John Wiley & Sons, Inc.

Appendix N
Food Sources of Oxalic Acid

Food, Standard Amount	Serving Size	Oxalic acid (mg)
Spinach, frozen	1 cup	1230
Beans in tomato sauce	1 cup	1148
Beetroot, pickled	1 cup	1135
Chard, Swiss, boiled	1 cup	1129
Spinach, boiled	1 cup	420
Okra, boiled	1 cup	234
Chard, Swiss, raw	1 cup	232
Tea, Indian, 6 minute infusion	1 cup	185
Potato, sweet, boiled, mashed	1 cup	184
Peanuts, roasted	2 oz	137
Cocoa, dry powder	1/4 cup	134
Berries, green goose	1 cup	132
Crackers, soybean	2 oz	118
Pecans	2 oz	111
Leeks, raw, boiled	1 cup	110
Grits, white corn, cooked	1 cup	99
Collards, raw, boiled	1 cup	95
Chocolate, plain	2 oz	66
Raspberries, black	1 cup	65
Parsley, raw	1 cup	64
Grapes, concord	1 cup	40
Squash, summer	1 cup	40
Berries, black	1 cup	26
Celery	1 cup	24
Berries, blue	1 cup	22
Wheat germ	1 tbsp	19
Raspberries, red	1 cup	18
Eggplant, boiled	1 cup	17
Dandelion greens, raw	1 cup	14
Pepper, green	1 cup	12
Escarole, raw	1 cup	9

Source: www.nutritiondata.com

The Nurse Practitioner's Guide to Nutrition, Second Edition. Edited by Lisa Hark, Kathleen Ashton and Darwin Deen.
© 2012 John Wiley & Sons, Inc. Published 2012 by John Wiley & Sons, Inc.

Appendix O
Food Sources of Dietary Fiber

Food, Standard Amount	Serving Size	Dietary Fiber (g)
Cereal, All-Bran	1 cup	25.8
Wheat bran	1 cup	24.6
Cereal, Fiber One	1 cup	23.8
White beans, great-northern, canned	1 cup	14.4
Kidney beans, red, cooked	1 cup	13.8
Navy beans, cooked	1 cup	13.0
Black beans, cooked	1 cup	12.2
Pinto beans, cooked	1 cup	11.8
Lentils, cooked	1 cup	10.4
White beans, great northern beans, cooked	1 cup	10.0
Lima beans, canned	1 cup	8.6
Chickpeas, cooked	1 cup	8.6
Peas, cooked	1 cup	8.6
Peas, green, cooked	1 cup	8.6
Okra, frozen, cooked	1 cup	8.2
Brussels sprouts, cooked	1 cup	7.6
Split peas, cooked	1 cup	6.2
Pear, fresh with skin	1 small	6.0
Cracker, Matzo	6 crackers	6.0
Bread, pumpernickel	2 slices	5.4
Spaghetti, whole-wheat, cooked	1 cup	5.4
Figs, dried	3 pieces	4.6
Carrots, cooked	1 cup	4.0
Apple sauce, canned, unsweetened	1 cup	4.0
Prunes, dried, stewed	6 pieces	3.4
Raspberries, fresh	1 cup	3.3
Spinach, cooked	1 cup	3.2
Orange, fresh without skin	1 small	3.0
Carrots, canned	1 cup	3.0
Apple, fresh with skin	1 small	2.8

Source: www.nutritiondata.com

The Nurse Practitioner's Guide to Nutrition, Second Edition. Edited by Lisa Hark, Kathleen Ashton and Darwin Deen.
© 2012 John Wiley & Sons, Inc. Published 2012 by John Wiley & Sons, Inc.

Appendix P
Food Sources of Purine

Food, Standard Amount	Purine (mg/100 g)
Sweetbreads	825
Anchovies	363
Brains	363
Sardines	295
Scallops	295
Liver, calf/beef	233
Mackerel	233
Kidney, beef	200
Game meats	200
Herring	200
Asparagus	50–150
Bread and cereals, whole grain	50–150
Cauliflower	50–150
Fish, fresh and saltwater	50–150
Legumes, beans/lentils/peas	50–150
Meat-beef/lamb/pork/veal	50–150
Mushrooms	50–150
Oatmeal	50–150
Peas, green	50–150
Poultry, chicken/duck/turkey	50–150
Shellfish, crab/lobster/oysters	50–150
Spinach	50–150
Wheat germ and bran	50–150

Source: www.nutritiondata.com

The Nurse Practitioner's Guide to Nutrition, Second Edition. Edited by Lisa Hark, Kathleen Ashton and Darwin Deen.
© 2012 John Wiley & Sons, Inc. Published 2012 by John Wiley & Sons, Inc.

Appendix Q
Therapeutic Lifestyle Changes (TLC) Diet (Low-fat, Low-saturated Fat Diet)

Food Items to Choose More Often	Food Items to Choose Less Often
Breads and Cereals	
≥6 servings per day, adjusted to caloric needs Breads, cereals, especially whole grain; pasta; rice; potatoes; dry beans and peas; low fat crackers and cookies	Many bakery products, including doughnuts, biscuits, butter croissants, Danish, pies, cookies Many grain-based snacks, including chips, cheese puffs, snack mix, regular crackers, buttered popcorn
Vegetables and Fruits	
4–5 servings vegetables/day fresh, frozen, or canned, without added fat, sauce, or salt 3–4 servings fruits per day fresh, frozen, canned, dried	Vegetables fried or prepared with butter, cheese, or cream sauce Fruits fried or served with butter or cream
Dairy Foods	
3 servings/day fat-free, 1% low-fat milk, buttermilk, low-fat yogurt, 1% low-fat cottage cheese; fat-free, low-fat cheeses	Whole milk, 2% milk, whole-milk yogurt, ice cream, cream, full-fat cheese
Eggs	
≤2 egg yolks per week Egg whites or egg substitute	>3 egg yolks, whole eggs
Meat, Fish and Poultry	
≤6 oz per day Lean cuts: loin, leg, round; extra lean hamburger; cold cuts made with lean meat or soy protein; skinless poultry; fish, shellfish without butter	Higher fat meat cuts: ribs, t-bone steak, regular hamburger, bacon, sausage; cold cuts: salami, bologna, hot dogs; organ meats: liver, brains, sweetbreads; poultry with skin; fried meat; fried poultry; fried fish
Fats and Oils	
Amount adjusted to caloric level: unsaturated oils; soft tub or liquid margarines and vegetable oil spreads, salad dressings, seeds, nuts, nut butters	Butter, shortening, stick margarine, coconut and palm oil, trans fats, partially hydrogenated vegetable oils

Source: National Heart, Lung, and Blood Institute *Third Report of the National Cholesterol Education Program Expert Panel on Detection, Evaluation, and Treatment of High Blood Cholesterol in Adults (Adult Treatment Panel III). Executive Summary.* National Institutes of Health, Bethesda, MD, 2001. NIH publication 01-3670.

The Nurse Practitioner's Guide to Nutrition, Second Edition. Edited by Lisa Hark, Kathleen Ashton and Darwin Deen.
© 2012 John Wiley & Sons, Inc. Published 2012 by John Wiley & Sons, Inc.

Appendix R

DASH Diet. This DASH eating plan is based on 2000 calories daily. The number of servings may vary from those listed depending on caloric needs

Food Group	Daily Servings	Serving Sizes
Grains and grain products	7–8	1 slice bread 1 cup dry cereal* 1/2 cup cooked rice, pasta or cereal
Vegetables	4–5	1 cup raw leafy vegetables 1/2 cup cooked vegetables 6 oz low-sodium vegetable juice
Fruits	4–5	6 oz 100% fruit juice 1 medium fruit 1/4 cup dried fruit 1/2 cup fresh, frozen or canned fruit
Low-fat or fat free dairy foods	3	8 oz 1% low-fat or fat-free milk 1 cup low-fat yogurt 1 1/2 oz low-fat cheese
Meats, poultry, and fish	2 or less	3 oz cooked meats, poultry, or fish
Nuts, seeds, and dry beans	4–5/week	1/3 cup or 1 1/2 oz nuts 2 tbsp or 1/2 oz seeds 1/2 cup cooked dry beans
Fats and oils	2–3	1 tbsp soft tub "light" margarine 1 tbsp low-fat mayonnaise 2 tbsp "light" salad dressing 1 tsp vegetable oil
Sweets	5/week	1 tbsp sugar 1 tbsp jelly or jam 1/2 oz jelly beans 8 oz lemonade

*Serving sizes may vary between 1/2 and 1 1/4 cups. Source: Appel LJ, Brands MW, Daniels SR, Karanja N, Elmer PJ, Sacks FM. Dietary approaches to prevent and treat hypertension. A Scientific Statement from the American Heart Association. *Hypertension*. 2006;47:296–308.

The Nurse Practitioner's Guide to Nutrition, Second Edition. Edited by Lisa Hark, Kathleen Ashton and Darwin Deen.
© 2012 John Wiley & Sons, Inc. Published 2012 by John Wiley & Sons, Inc.

Appendix S

Dietary Reference Intakes (DRIs): Recommended Intakes for Individuals, Vitamins Food and Nutrition Board, Institute of Medicine, National Academies

Life Stage Group	Vitamin A (µg/d)[a]	Vitamin C (mg/d)	Vitamin D (µg/d)[b,c]	Vitamin E (mg/d)[d]	Vitamin K (µg/d)	Thiamin (mg/d)	Riboflavin (mg/d)	Niacin (mg/d)[e]	Vitamin B$_6$ (mg/d)	Folate (µg/d)[f]	Vitamin B$_{12}$ (µg/d)	Pantothenic Acid (mg/d)	Biotin (µg/d)	Choline[g] (mg/d)
Infants														
0–6 mo	400*	40*	5*	4*	2.0*	0.2*	0.3*	2*	0.1*	65*	0.4*	1.7*	5*	125*
7–12 mo	500*	50*	5*	5*	2.5*	0.3*	0.4*	4*	0.3*	80*	0.5*	1.8*	6*	150*
Children														
1–3 y	300	15	5*	6	30*	0.5	0.5	6	0.5	150	0.9	2*	8*	200*
4–8 y	400	25	5*	7	55*	0.6	0.6	8	0.6	200	1.2	3*	12*	250*
Males														
9–13 y	600	45	5*	11	60*	0.9	0.9	12	1.0	300	1.8	4*	20*	375*
14–18 y	900	75	5*	15	75*	1.2	1.3	16	1.3	400	2.4	5*	25*	550*
19–30 y	900	90	5*	15	120*	1.2	1.3	16	1.3	400	2.4	5*	30*	550*
31–50 y	900	90	5*	15	120*	1.2	1.3	16	1.3	400	2.4	5*	30*	550*
51–70 y	900	90	10*	15	120*	1.2	1.3	16	1.7	400	2.4[h]	5*	30*	550*
>70 y	900	90	15*	15	120*	1.2	1.3	16	1.7	400	2.4[h]	5*	30*	550*
Females														
9–13 y	600	45	5*	11	60*	0.9	0.9	12	1.0	300	1.8	4*	20*	375*
14–18 y	700	65	5*	15	75*	1.0	1.0	14	1.2	400[i]	2.4	5*	25*	400*
19–30 y	700	75	5*	15	90*	1.1	1.1	14	1.3	400[i]	2.4	5*	30*	425*
31–50 y	700	75	5*	15	90*	1.1	1.1	14	1.3	400[i]	2.4	5*	30*	425*
51–70 y	700	75	10*	15	90*	1.1	1.1	14	1.5	400	2.4[h]	5*	30*	425*
>70 y	700	75	15*	15	90*	1.1	1.1	14	1.5	400	2.4[h]	5*	30*	425*
Pregnancy														
≤18 y	750	80	5*	15	75*	1.4	1.4	18	1.9	600[j]	2.6	6*	30*	450*
19–30 y	770	85	5*	15	90*	1.4	1.4	18	1.9	600[j]	2.6	6*	30*	450*

(Continued)

Appendix S (*Continued*)

Life Stage Group	Vitamin A (µg/d)[a]	Vitamin C (mg/d)	Vitamin D (µg/d)[b,c]	Vitamin E (mg/d)[d]	Vitamin K (µg/d)	Thiamin (mg/d)	Riboflavin (mg/d)	Niacin (mg/d)[e]	Vitamin B$_6$ (mg/d)	Folate (µg/d)[f]	Vitamin B$_{12}$ (µg/d)	Pantothenic Acid (mg/d)	Biotin (µg/d)	Choline[g] (mg/d)
31–50 y	770	85	5*	15	90*	1.4	1.4	18	1.9	600[i]	2.6	6*	30*	450*
Lactation														
≤18 y	1200	115	5*	19	75*	1.4	1.6	17	2.0	500	2.8	7*	35*	550*
19–30 y	1300	120	5*	19	90*	1.4	1.6	17	2.0	500	2.8	7*	35*	550*
31–50 y	1300	120	5*	19	90*	1.4	1.6	17	2.0	500	2.8	7*	35*	550*

Note: This appendix (taken from the DRI reports; see www.nap.edu) presents Recommended Dietary Allowances (RDAs) in **bold type** and Adequate Intakes (AIs) in ordinary type followed by an asterisk (*). RDAs and AIs may both be used as goals for individual intake. RDAs are set to meet the needs of almost all (97–98%) individuals in a group. For healthy breast-fed infants, the AI is the mean intake. The AI for other life stage and gender groups is believed to cover needs of all individuals in the group, but lack of data or uncertainty in the data prevent being able to specify with confidence the percentage of individuals covered by this intake.

[a] As retinol activity equivalents (RAEs). 1 RAE I = 1 µg retinol, 12 µg β-carotene, 24 µg α-carotene, or 24 µg β-cryptoxanthin. The RAE for dietary provitamin A carotenoids is twofold greater than retinol equivalents (RE), whereas the RAE for preformed vitamin A is the same as RE.

[b] cholecalciferol. 1 µg cholecalciferol I = 40 IU vitamin D.

[c] In the absence of adequate exposure to sunlight.

[d] As α-tocopherol. α-Tocopherol includes RRR-α-tocopherol, the only form of α-tocopherol that occurs naturally in foods, and the 2R-stereoisomeric forms of α-tocopherol (RRR-, RSR-, RRS-, and RSS-α-tocopherol) that occur in fortified foods and supplements. It does not include the 2S-stereoisomeric forms of α-tocopherol (SRR-, SSR-, SRS-, and SSS-α-tocopherol), also found in fortified foods and supplements.

[e] As niacin equivalents (NE). 1 mg of niacin I = 60 mg of tryptophan; 0–6 months I = preformed niacin (not NE).

[f] As dietary folate equivalents (DFE). 1 DFE I = 1 µg food folate I = 0.6 µg of folic acid from fortified food or as a supplement consumed with food I = 0.5 µg of a supplement taken on an empty stomach.

[g] Although AIs have been set for choline, there are few data to assess whether a dietary supply of choline is needed at all stages of the life cycle, and it may be that the choline requirement can be met by endogenous synthesis at some of these stages.

[h] Because 10–30% of older people may malabsorb food-bound B12, it is advisable for those older than 50 years to meet their RDA mainly by consuming foods fortified with B12 or a supplement containing B12.

[i] In view of evidence linking folate intake with neural tube defects in the fetus, it is recommended that all women capable of becoming pregnant consume 400 µg from supplements or fortified foods in addition to intake of food folate from a varied diet.

[j] It is assumed that women will continue consuming 400 µg from supplements or fortified food until their pregnancy is confirmed and they enter prenatal care, which ordinarily occurs after the end of the periconceptional period — the critical time for formation of the neural tube.

Appendix T

Dietary Reference Intakes (DRIs): Recommended Intakes for Individuals, Elements Food and Nutrition Board, Institute of Medicine, National Academies

Life Stage Group	Calcium (mg/d)	Chromium (µg/d)	Copper (µg/d)	Fluoride (mg/d)	Iodine (µg/d)	Iron (mg/d)	Magnesium (mg/d)	Manganese (mg/d)	Molybdenum (µg/d)	Phosphorus (mg/d)	Selenium (µg/d)	Zinc (mg/d)
Infants												
0–6 mo	210*	0.2*	200*	0.01*	110*	0.27*	30*	0.003*	2*	100*	15*	2*
7–12 mo	270*	5.5*	220*	0.5*	130*	11*	75*	0.6*	3*	275*	20*	3
Children												
1–3 y	500*	11*	340	0.7*	90	7	80	1.2*	17	460	20	3
4–8 y	800*	15*	440	1*	90	10	130	1.5*	22	500	30	5
Males												
9–13 y	1300*	25*	700	2*	120	8	240	1.9*	34	1250	40	8
14–18 y	1300*	35*	890	3*	150	11	410	2.2*	43	1250	55	11
19–30 y	1000*	35*	900	4*	150	8	400	2.3*	45	700	55	11
31–50 y	1000*	35*	900	4*	150	8	420	2.3*	45	700	55	11
51–70 y	1200*	30*	900	4*	150	8	420	2.3*	45	700	55	11
>70 y	1200*	30*	900	4*	150	8	420	2.3*	45	700	55	11
Females												
9–13 y	1300*	21*	700	2*	120	8	240	1.6*	34	1250	40	8
14–18 y	1300*	24*	890	3*	150	15	360	1.6*	43	1250	55	9
19–30 y	1000*	25*	900	3*	150	18	310	1.8*	45	700	55	8
31–50 y	1000*	25*	900	3*	150	18	320	1.8*	45	700	55	8
51–70 y	1200*	20*	900	3*	150	8	320	1.8*	45	700	55	8
>70 y	1200*	20*	900	3*	150	8	320	1.8*	45	700	55	8

(Continued)

Appendix T (*Continued*)

Life Stage Group	Calcium (mg/d)	Chromium (µg/d)	Copper (µg/d)	Fluoride (mg/d)	Iodine (µg/d)	Iron (mg/d)	Magnesium (mg/d)	Manganese (mg/d)	Molybdenum (µg/d)	Phosphorus (mg/d)	Selenium (µg/d)	Zinc (mg/d)
Pregnancy												
≤18 y	1300*	29*	1000	3*	220	27	400	2.0*	50	1250	60	13
19–30 y	1000*	30*	1000	3*	220	27	350	2.0*	50	700	60	11
31–50 y	1000*	30*	1000	3*	220	27	360	2.0*	50	700	60	11
Lactation												
≤18 y	1300*	44*	1300	3*	290	10	360	2.6*	50	1250	70	14
19–30 y	1000*	45*	1300	3*	290	9	310	2.6*	50	700	70	12
31–50 y	1000*	45*	1300	3*	290	9	320	2.6*	50	700	70	12

Note: This table presents Recommended Dietary Allowances (RDAs) in **bold type** and Adequate Intakes (AIs) in ordinary type followed by an asterisk (*). RDAs and AIs may both be used as goals for individual intake. RDAs are set to meet the needs of almost all (97–98%) individuals in a group. For healthy breast-fed infants, the AI is the mean intake. The AI for other life stage and gender groups is believed to cover needs of all individuals in the group, but lack of data or uncertainty in the data prevent being able to specify with confidence the percentage of individuals covered by this intake.
Sources: *Dietary Reference Intakes for Calcium, Phosphorous, Magnesium, Vitamin D, and Fluoride* (1997); *Dietary Reference Intakes for Thiamin, Riboflavin, Niacin, Vitamin B₆, Folate, Vitamin B₁₂, Pantothenic Acid, Biotin, and Choline* (1998); *Dietary Reference Intakes for Vitamin C, Vitamine E, Selenium, and Carotenoids* (2000); and *Dietary Reference Intakes for Vitamin A, Vitamin K, Arsenic, Boron, Chromium, Copper, Iodine, Iron, Manganese, Molybdenum, Nickel, Silicon, Vanadium, and Zinc* (2001). These reports may be accessed via www.nap.edu

Appendix T (*Continued*) Dietary Reference Intakes (DRIs): Tolerable Upper Intake Levels (UL[a]), Elements Food and Nutrition Board, Institute of Medicine, National Academies

Life Stage Group	Vitamin A (µg/d)[b]	Vitamin C (mg/d)	Vitamin D (µg/d)	Vitamin E (mg/d)[c,d]	Vitamin K	Thiamin	Riboflavin	Niacin (mg/d)[d]	Vitamin B$_6$ (mg/d)	Folate (µg/d)[d]	Vitamin B$_{12}$	Pantothenic Acid	Biotin	Choline (g/d)	Carotenoids[e]
Infants															
0–6 mo	600	ND[f]	25	ND	ND	ND	ND	ND	ND	ND	ND	ND	ND	ND	ND
7–12 mo	600	ND	25	ND	ND	ND	ND	ND	ND	ND	ND	ND	ND	ND	ND
Children															
1–3 y	600	400	50	200	ND	ND	ND	10	30	300	ND	ND	ND	1.0	ND
4–8 y	900	650	50	300	ND	ND	ND	15	40	400	ND	ND	ND	1.0	ND
Males, Females															
9–13 y	1700	1200	50	600	ND	ND	ND	20	60	600	ND	ND	ND	2.0	ND
14–18 y	2800	1800	50	800	ND	ND	ND	30	80	800	ND	ND	ND	3.0	ND
19–70 y	3000	2000	50	1000	ND	ND	ND	35	100	1000	ND	ND	ND	3.5	ND
>70 y	3000	2000	50	1000	ND	ND	ND	35	100	1000	ND	ND	ND	3.5	ND
Pregnancy															
≤18 y	2800	1800	50	800	ND	ND	ND	30	80	800	ND	ND	ND	3.0	ND
19–50 y	3000	2000	50	1000	ND	ND	ND	35	100	1000	ND	ND	ND	3.5	ND
Lactation															
≤18 y	2800	1800	50	800	ND	ND	ND	30	80	800	ND	ND	ND	3.0	ND
19–50 y	3000	2000	50	1000	ND	ND	ND	35	100	1000	ND	ND	ND	3.5	ND

[a] UL = The maximum level of daily nutrient intake that is likely to pose no risk of adverse effects. Unless otherwise specified, the UL represents total intake from food, water, and supplements. Due to lack of suitable data, ULs could not be established for vitamin K, thiamin, riboflavin, vitamin B$_{12}$, pantothenic acid, biotin, or carotenoids. In the absence of ULs, extra caution may be warranted in consuming levels above recommended intakes.

[b] As preformed vitamin A only.

[c] As α-tocopherol; applies to any form of supplemental α-tocopherol.

[d] The ULs for vitamin E, niacin, and folate apply to synthetic forms obtained from supplements, fortified foods, or a combination of the two.

[e] β-Carotene supplements are advised only to serve as a provitamin A source for individuals at risk of vitamin A deficiency.

[f] ND = Not determinable due to lack of data of adverse effects in this age group and concern with regard to lack of ability to handle excess amounts. Source of intake should be from food only to prevent high levels of intake.

Appendix T (*Continued*) Dietary Reference Intakes (DRIs): Tolerable Upper Intake Levels (UL[a]), Elements Food and Nutrition Board, Institute of Medicine, National Academies

Life Stage Group	Arsenic[b] (mg/d)	Boron (mg/d)	Calcium (g/d)	Chromium	Copper (µg/d)	Fluoride (mg/d)	Iodine (µg/d)	Iron (mg/d)	Magnesium (mg/d)[c]	Manganese (mg/d)	Molybdenum (µg/d)	Nickel (mg/d)	Phosphorus (g/d)	Selenium (µg/d)	Silicon[d]	Vanadium (mg/d)[e]	Zinc (mg/d)
Infants																	
0–6 mo	ND[f]	ND	ND	ND	ND	0.7	ND	40	ND	ND	ND	ND	ND	45	ND	ND	4
7–12 mo	ND	ND	ND	ND	ND	0.9	ND	40	ND	ND	ND	ND	ND	60	ND	ND	5
Children																	
1–3 y	ND	3	2.5	ND	1000	1.3	200	40	65	2	300	0.2	3	90	ND	ND	7
4–8 y	ND	6	2.5	ND	3000	2.2	300	40	110	3	600	0.3	3	150	ND	ND	12
Males, Females																	
9–13 y	ND	11	2.5	ND	5000	10	600	40	350	6	1100	0.6	4	280	ND	ND	23
14–18 y	ND	17	2.5	ND	8000	10	900	45	350	9	1700	1.0	4	400	ND	ND	34
19–70 y	ND	20	2.5	ND	10000	10	1100	45	350	11	2000	1.0	4	400	ND	1.8	40
>70 y	ND	20	2.5	ND	10000	10	1100	45	350	11	2000	1.0	3	400	ND	1.8	40
Pregnancy																	
≤18 y	ND	17	2.5	ND	8000	10	900	45	350	9	1700	1.0	3.5	400	ND	ND	34
19–50 y	ND	20	2.5	ND	10000	10	1100	45	350	11	2000	1.0	3.5	400	ND	ND	40
Lactation																	
≤18 y	ND	17	2.5	ND	8000	10	900	45	350	9	1700	1.0	4	400	ND	ND	34
19–50 y	ND	20	2.5	ND	10000	10	1100	45	350	11	2000	1.0	4	400	ND	ND	40

[a]UL = The maximum level of daily nutrient intake that is likely to pose no risk of adverse effects. Unless otherwise specified, the UL represents total intake from food, water, and supplements. Due to lack of suitable data, ULs could not be established for arsenic, chromium, and silicon. In the absence of ULs, extra caution may be warranted in consuming levels above recommended intakes.

[b]Although the UL was not determined for arsenic, there is no justification for adding arsenic to food or supplements.

[c]The ULs for magnesium represent intake from a pharmacological agent only and do not include intake from food and water.

[d]Although silicon has not been shown to cause adverse effects in humans, there is no justification for adding silicon to supplements.

[e]Although vanadium in food has not been shown to cause adverse effects in humans, there is no justification for adding vanadium to food and vanadium supplements should be used with caution. The UL is based on adverse effects in laboratory animals and this data could be used to set a UL for adults but not children and adolescents.

[f]ND = Not determinable due to lack of data of adverse effects in this age group and concern with regard to lack of ability to handle excess amounts. Source of intake should be from food only to prevent high levels of intake.

Sources: *Dietary Reference Intakes for Calcium, Phosphorous, Magnesium, Vitamin D, and Fluoride* (1997); *Dietary Reference Intakes for Thiamin, Riboflavin, Niacin, Vitamin B₆, Folate, Vitamin B₁₂, Pantothenic Acid, Biotin, and Choline* (1998); *Dietary Reference Intakes for Vitamin C, Vitamine E, Selenium, and Carotenoids* (2000); and *Dietary Reference Intakes for Vitamin A, Vitamin K, Arsenic, Boron, Chromium, Copper, Iodine, Iron, Manganese, Molybdenum, Nickel, Silicon, Vanadium, and Zinc* (2001). These reports may be accessed via www.nap.edu

Review Questions

Chapter 1 The Role of Nurse Practitioners

1. *Healthy People 2020* nutrition objectives state that 75% of primary care clinician office visits should include nutrition counseling for hypertension, hyperlipidemia, and which of the following conditions?

a. Degenerative joint disease
b. Peripheral vascular disease
c. Alopecia
d. Diabetes

2. According to the *Dietary Guidelines for Americans*, adult patients should be advised to reduce consumption of which of the following?

a. Polyunsaturated fats
b. Sodium intake to less than 5000 mg per day
c. Cholesterol intake to less than 300 mg per day
d. Whole grains

3. According to data from NHANES III, what percentage of Americans *do not* get the recommended amount of fruits and vegetables in their diet?

a. 25%
b. 50%
c. 75%
d. 100%

4. According to the *Dietary Guidelines for Americans*, women capable of becoming pregnant should consume which of the following?

a. 1 serving of a low-fat dairy food per day
b. 4 to 6 servings of seafood per week
c. At least 400 µg of synthetic folic acid per day
d. At least 2000 mg of calcium per day

The Nurse Practitioner's Guide to Nutrition, Second Edition. Edited by Lisa Hark, Kathleen Ashton and Darwin Deen.
© 2012 John Wiley & Sons, Inc. Published 2012 by John Wiley & Sons, Inc.

5. According to a 2006 report from the Pew Research Center, 90% of Americans recognize that as a nation, we are obese. What percentage of respondents felt that this was a potential problem for them?

a. 30%
b. 40%
c. 50%
d. 60%

6. Some studies indicate that primary care clinicians lack the inclination to provide dietary advice to their patients because of several barriers. Which of the following barriers were cited in these studies for lack of nutrition counseling by primary care clinicians? (May be more than one correct answer)

a. Lack of nutrition knowledge and confidence to teach nutrition
b. Lack of office space
c. Lack of patient interest
d. Lack of support and commitment

Chapter 2 Nutrition Assessment for Nurse Practitioners

1. Dermatitis and easily pluckable hair may be signs of which of the following conditions?

a. Chronic infection
b. Hyperlipidemia
c. Vitamin D deficiency
d. Protein deficiency

2. Body mass index (BMI) may not accurately reflect body fat in which of the following individuals?

a. Underweight individuals
b. Normal weight individuals
c. Overweight individuals
d. Obese individuals

3. Why should waist circumference (WC) be measured only in patients with a BMI measurement less that $35 \, kg/m^2$?

a. WC measurement is not accurate in obese patients
b. WC measurement confers little additional information about risk
c. WC cutoff thresholds do not apply in obese patients
d. WC standards have not been developed for Class II/III obesity

4. Nutrition issues that can appear abnormal on the review of systems include which of the following?

a. Delayed reflexes
b. Kyphosis
c. Tetany
d. Changes in appetite

5. When interpreting serum albumin in hospitalized patients, levels may decrease irrespective of nutritional status in which of the following conditions?

a. Dehydration
b. Liver disease
c. Diabetes
d. Stroke

6. The energy and protein requirements of hospitalized and critically ill patients should be calculated separately. Which of the following value ranges is recommended to calculate the protein needs of post-surgical patients who are highly catabolic with burns, infection or fever?

a. 0.6–1.0 g/kg/day
b. 1.0–1.4 g/kg/day
c. 1.5–2.0 g/kg/day
d. 2.0–2.5 g/kg/day

7. Diagnosis of underweight patients includes assessment of their BMI. Which of the following BMI values would indicate a risk of malnutrition in a patient who is consistently underweight?

a. $<18.5 \, kg/m^2$
b. $<19.5 \, kg/m^2$
c. $<20.5 \, kg/m^2$
d. $<21.5 \, kg/m^2$

8. CT is a 48-year-old man who has recently been diagnosed with colon cancer. He has lost 15 lb over the past 3 months, which is a clinically significant weight loss. His usual weight is 170 lb and his current weight is 155 lb. Which of the following percent weight change accurately reflects this patient's weight history?

a. 2.5% weight change
b. 5.5% weight change
c. 8.8% weight change
d. 10% weight change

9. A patient with a BMI of $>40\,kg/m^2$ should be diagnosed as which class of obesity?

a. Class I
b. Class II
c. Class III
d. Class IV

10. DD is a 3-year-old boy from Africa who is admitted to the hospital and diagnosed with kwashiorkor. Which of the following macronutrients is believed to be deficient in patients with kwashiorkor?

a. Carbohydrates
b. Calories
c. Fat
d. Protein

Chapter 3 Nutrition Counseling for Effective Behavior Change

1. RP is a 50-year-old man who comes to see his Nurse Practitioner for a blood pressure check. He is 5′10″ and weighs 190 lb (BMI: $27\,kg/m^2$). His blood pressure is 140/90 mmHg. He works at a sedentary job and states that he has been planning to join a gym. Which of the following stages of change does RP exhibit in the Transtheoretical Model?

a. Pre-contemplation
b. Contemplation
c. Preparation
d. Action

2. An appropriate intervention for RP in question #1 would be to:

a. Refer him to a patient educator for more information about hypertension
b. Provide him with a list of community resources for exercise
c. Ask him to make a list of pros and cons to getting more exercise
d. Start him on a blood pressure medication

3. FM is a 48-year-old woman who makes an appointment with her Nurse Practitioner for help with weight loss. She says she has been avoiding fried foods and has switched to low-fat milk. Which of the following stages of change does FM exhibit in the Transtheoretical Model?

a. Pre-contemplation
b. Contemplation
c. Action
d. Regret

4. Which of the following healthcare provider behaviors has been shown to be the most effective counseling strategies for effective behavior change models?

a. Asking direct questions
b. Interrupting to clarify statements
c. Taking notes during the interview
d. Setting realistic goals

5. Which of the following statements best defines motivational interviewing?

a. A group approach that can be used to provide support to help patients make changes
b. A client-centered directive approach that helps patients explore and resolve ambivalence
c. A Socratic approach in which the counselor asks patients to make choices about changes
d. A counselor-centered approach that applies stages of change to help patients make changes

6. AD is a 37-year-old man who has followed a low-fat diet for the past 5 years after his father's cardiac bypass surgery. AD states that he recently went on a cruise for his honeymoon and has been having difficulty getting back on his low-fat dietary regimen. You identify his stage in the Transtheoretical Model as relapse. The most appropriate intervention at this point is to:

a. Ask him to bring his wife to the next visit so that you can speak with her about his difficulty
b. Recommend that he avoid cruises in the future
c. Acknowledge that dieting is hard and offer that when he is ready to resume, you will help him
d. Remind him that behavior change is a process of starts and stops and support his goal of getting back to his plan

7. Which of the following best describes activities that have been shown to influence self-efficacy?

a. Projecting into the future
b. Focusing on negative reinforcement
c. Modeling the behavior to attain
d. Listing to audio tapes

8. Which of the following healthcare provider behaviors has been shown to be the most effective counseling technique across all behavior change models?

a. Asking probing questions
b. Interrupting to clarify statements
c. Taking notes during the interview
d. Active listening

9. Current evidence suggests that behavior change is most effective when it is:

a. Initiated by a consultant
b. Reinforced by patient education materials
c. Reinforced by the primary care clinician
d. Discussed primarily by the registered dietitian

10. Motivational Interviewing is designed to elicit motivation from the patient. Which of the following is a key to the Motivational Interview process?

a. Resolving ambivalence
b. Agreeing with patients
c. Debating
d. Giving advice

Chapter 4 Nutrition from Pre-conception Through Lactation

1. BC is a 26-year-old woman who presents for her first prenatal visit at 12 weeks gestation. She has gained only a few pounds since she became pregnant. Based on her pre-pregnancy BMI ($22\,kg/m^2$) what is the total amount of recommended weight gain during pregnancy according to the Institute of Medicine?

a. 10–15 pounds
b. 15–20 pounds
c. 20–30 pounds
d. 25–35 pounds

2. TC is a 28-year-old woman who has just found out that she is pregnant and asks her obstetrician about caffeine intake during pregnancy. She has had two previous miscarriages. According to the March of Dimes what is the current recommendation for limiting caffeine intake during pregnancy?

a. <200 mg/day
b. <300 mg/day
c. <400 mg/day
d. <500 mg/day

3. CT is a 31-year-old pregnant woman who comes to see her obstetrician for a routine prenatal visit. She is complaining of fatigue and her hemoglobin and hematocrit results indicate that she is anemic. According to the CDC, which of the following hematocrit results should be used to diagnose anemia in the 3 rd trimester?

a. <30%
b. <33%
c. <35%
d. <37%

4. DW is a 32-year-old obese woman who is at 25 weeks gestation. She is being screened for gestational diabetes by her obstetrician since she has a family history of type 2 diabetes. Which of the following results for a 1-hour, 50 g glucose load would be considered a positive diagnosis for gestational diabetes?

a. ≥100 mg/dL
b. ≥110 mg/dL
c. ≥120 mg/dL
d. ≥130 mg/dL

5. Nutritional requirements for certain macronutrients and micronutrients increase significantly during pregnancy. Which of the following nutrient requirements increases the most during pregnancy?

a. Protein
b. Fat
c. Carbohydrates
d. Fiber

6. It is recommended that during the first 6 months of breastfeeding, lactating women should increase their energy intake by how many calories per day?

a. 150 kcal/day
b. 250 kcal/day
c. 350 kcal/day
d. 500 kcal/day

7. JH is a 23-year-old woman who recently delivered a healthy, full-term infant. She is breastfeeding her 2-month old and complains to her family doctor about sore nipples. Which of the following strategies could help JH prevent and treat sore nipples associated with breastfeeding?

a. Apply moisturizer to the breast after feeding
b. Clean the breasts with a washcloth and soap after breastfeeding
c. Apply heat to the nipple area after feeding
d. Make sure the infant is latching on properly and in the proper position

8. PR is a 29-year-old woman who has been successfully breastfeeding her infant since she gave birth 4 weeks ago. This week she notices a red mark on her right breast and she has flu-like symptoms. She is diagnosed with mastitis and prescribed an antibiotic. Which of the following is the most appropriate recommendation for breastfeeding women with mastitis?

a. Switch to infant formula until the mastitis is resolved
b. Discontinue breastfeeding
c. Continue breastfeeding and nurse frequently
d. Avoid breastfeeding with the infected breast

9. The US Public Health Service recommends that women of childbearing age take supplements containing folic acid (>400 µg/day) during which of the following time periods?

a. Before becoming pregnant and during the first trimester
b. During the second trimester of pregnancy
c. During the third trimester of pregnancy
d. Never, if they are consuming a high-folate diet

10. CJ asks how quickly after delivery she can return to her pre-pregnancy weight while she is breastfeeding. Which of the following would be considered a safe weight loss while breastfeeding?

a. 1–2 lb/week
b. 1–2 lb/month
c. 6–8 lb/month
d. Women should not lose weight during breastfeeding

Chapter 5 Nutrition from Infancy Through Adolescence

1. Head circumference measurements reflect brain growth in infants and children. Assessing head circumference is recommended for infants and children up to what age?

a. 6 months
b. 12 months
c. 24 months
d. 36 months

2. Pasteurized cow's milk is an important source of calories, protein, and calcium for children, but should not be introduced until a child is at what age?

a. 6 months
b. 9 months
c. 12 months
d. 18 months

3. According to the American Academy of Pediatrics (AAP), intake of 100% fruit juice should be limited in children. What is the AAP's recommendation for daily juice intake for children aged 1–5 years of age?

a. <3 oz/day
b. <6 oz/day
c. <8 oz/day
d. <10 oz/day

4. Children under the age of two should not follow a low-fat diet because normal fat intake is required to maintain the development of which of the following systems?

a. Central nervous system
b. Respiratory system
c. Musculoskeletal system
d. Digestive system

5. JK is a 16-year-old boy who has been diagnosed as obese because his BMI is greater than the 95th percentile. Obesity intervention for children and adolescents has been found to be most effective when:

a. The provider/program, child, and parents have a high degree
   of contact
b. The parents have group therapy
c. The program is fairly unstructured
d. The parents are not involved at all

6. Anemia is a common problem in infants, toddlers and preschool children. Which of the following age groups has the highest prevalence of anemia?

a. Birth to 12 months old
b. 1–2 year olds
c. 2–3 year olds
d. 3–4 year olds

7. According to the CDC and AAP, the maximum amount of time a child should spend engaging in sedentary activities, such as watching TV and/or playing computer/video games, on a daily basis is:

a. <1.0 hour/day
b. <1.5 hours/day
c. <2.0 hours/day
d. <2.5 hours/day

8. DF is an 18-year-old woman parents suspect she has an eating disorder. Her symptoms include esophagitis and electrolyte abnormalities, suggesting which of the following?

a. DF is using laxatives in an effort to keep her weight down
b. DF is vomiting in an effort to keep her weight down
c. DF has amenorrhea
d. DF has been taking mega doses of vitamins.

9. JD is a 16-year-old teenager who has informed his parents that he is now a vegan and will be eating a strict vegetarian diet. At his most recent physical, JD's mother asks his Nurse Practitioner for nutrition advice. Which of the following nutrients is of greatest concern for deficiency in any patient following a vegan diet?

a. Vitamin C
b. Vitamin B$_{12}$
c. Folate
d. Magnesium

10. TK is a 16-year-old teenager who is brought to her doctor by her parents for a sports physical. Her BMI is 17 kg/m^2 and she has missed her period several times this year. She is very active, running almost every day. What is the most appropriate next step in the management of this patient?

a. Ask the patient to drink more milk
b. Refer the patient to a behavioral therapist
c. Give the patient a prescription for a multivitamin
d. Tell the parents she is fine and schedule a 1-year follow-up appointment

Chapter 6 Nutrition for Older Adults

1. It is important for Nurse Practitioners to take an active role in assessing patients' nutritional status, especially in older adults because they are less likely to complain about their diet or changes in appetite. Which of the following best explains this behavior in older adults?

a. Lack of interest
b. Unwillingness to express themselves
c. Fear of traveling
d. Shame associated with having a chronic disease

2. Which of the following groups in the US are at increased risk of malnutrition due to inadequate funds to purchase food?

a. Men
b. Asians
c. Individuals living in an urban setting
d. Individuals living with a relative

3. JN is an 88-year-old man who is living in a nursing home. He has experienced a 10% weight loss over the past 6 months. This unintentional weight loss in older adults is most likely related to which of the following factors?

a. Normal age-related changes
b. Underlying disease processes
c. Increased metabolic rate
d. Changes in fat-to-lean ratio

4. Malnutrition in older adults is associated with which of the following factors?

a. Moderate alcohol intake
b. Problems with chewing and swallowing
c. Reduced gait
d. Glaucoma

5. CJ is an 81-year-old woman who lives in an assisted living facility. Her daughters visit frequently and determine that she is having a bowel movement only once or twice a week. Which of the following dietary interventions should be prescribed for CJ to manage her constipation?

a. Increased consumption of garlic
b. Decreased consumption of fried foods
c. Increased consumption of whole grains
d. Decreased consumption of dairy foods

6. Dehydration in older adults has been linked to impaired cognition, kidney stones, and constipation. This population is less likely to experience signs and symptoms of dehydration because of which of the following physiological changes associated with aging?

a. Increased total body water
b. Decline in thirst perception
c. Reduced tolerance to fluid
d. Increased taste sensation

7. RF is an 83-year-old woman who is living in an assisted living facility. Her recent blood tests results show a low serum vitamin B_{12} level even though her dietary intake of vitamin B_{12} is adequate. Which of the following mechanisms most likely explains the cause of RF's low vitamin B_{12} levels?

a. Decreased ability to absorb protein-bound vitamin B_{12}
b. Increased conversion of vitamin B_{12} to the inactive form
c. Increased HCL production
d. Decreased vitamin C intake which is required for vitamin B_{12} absorption

8. Dimensions of nutritional frailty in older adults includes which of the following factors:

a. Albumin $< 2.5\,mg/dL$
b. Oral health problems which change appetite
c. Sarcopenia and rapid, unintentional weight loss
d. Complaints of food tasting bland

9. Body composition changes are a normal consequence of aging. Which of the following age-related physiological changes results in a reduced caloric need in older adults?

a. Lean body mass declines, fat mass increases
b. Bone mineral density increases
c. Vitamin and mineral absorption declines
d. Fat mass is reduced

10. BMI is used in older adults to assess nutritional status. Which of the following BMI cut-off points should be used as a red flag to signal the patient is underweight and further assessment is warranted?

a. $BMI < 16 \, kg/m^2$
b. $BMI < 18.5 \, kg/m^2$
c. $BMI < 22 \, kg/m^2$
d. $BMI < 25 \, kg/m^2$

Chapter 7 Obesity and Bariatric Surgery Care

1. JJ is a 55-year-old woman who comes to see her Nurse Practitioner for a yearly physical and requests a drug to help treat her obesity. Assuming JJ meets the criteria for prescribing an obesity medication, approximately how much weight can she expect to lose on this medication when combined with diet and exercise?

a. 1–3% of her body weight
b. 5–10% of her body weight
c. 12–15% of her body weight
d. 20–22% of her body weight

2. MJ is a 35-year-old man who comes to his Nurse Practitioner requesting a referral for gastric bypass surgery. Which of the following criteria must he meet to be considered for this surgery?

a. Patient has a $BMI > 40 \, kg/m^2$
b. Patient has diabetes
c. Patient can not exercise
d. Patient is able to take 1 month off from work

3. Which of the following medical conditions is most commonly associated with obesity?

a. Type 1 diabetes
b. Polycystic ovarian syndrome
c. Multiple sclerosis
d. Reduced bone density

4. AB is a 55-year-old overweight woman who is interested in losing weight. Her waist circumference measures 39 inches. Which of the following waist circumference result is considered a risk factor for chronic disease in this patient?

a. >32 inches
b. >34 inches
c. >35 inches
d. >37 inches

5. A version of Orlistat has been approved for over-the-counter use. Which of the following dietary recommendation is indicated in order to minimize the side-effects associated with Orlistat?

a. Low fat
b. High fiber
c. Low carbohydrate
d. Low protein

6. According to the Centers for Disease Control (CDC), how many Americans are considered to be obese?

a. 23 million
b. 55 million
c. 72 million
d. 98 million

7. Over the past decade overweight and obesity has increased dramatically in both adults and children in the US. Which of the following hypotheses offers the best explanation for the increased prevalence in overweight and obesity?

a. Change in the gene pool
b. Decrease in sedentary behavior
c. Increase in calorie intake
d. Increase in whole grain intake

8. FL is a 48-year-old obese man who questions his Nurse Practitioner about the side effects and benefits of bariatric surgery. Which of the following procedures has been shown to have the least amount of post-operative side effects?

a. Gastric banding
b. Gastric bypass
c. Roux-en-Y procedure
d. Whipple procedure

9. Side effects associated with Roux-en-Y bariatric surgery frequently include the GI tract. Which of the following GI side effects occurs in approximately 70% of patients following this type of procedure?

a. Inflammatory bowel disease
b. Irritable bowel syndrome
c. Dumping syndrome
d. Lactose intolerance

10. JT is a 39-year-old woman who recently underwent gastric bypass surgery. She presents to her primary care Nurse Practitioner 6 months post-operatively complaining of headaches, fatigue, and being cold all the time. Which of the following deficiencies is most likely associated with these symptoms in patients who have undergone gastric bypass surgery?

a. Vitamin C
b. Riboflavin
c. Zinc
d. Iron

Chapter 8 Cardiology Care

1. Which of the following risk factors for metabolic syndrome has different criteria among various ethnic groups?

a. Blood pressure levels
b. Fasting plasma glucose levels
c. Waist circumference measurements
d. HDL levels

2. Omega-3 fatty acids (eicosapentanoic acid and docosahexenoic acid) are effective at reducing serum levels of which of the following lipids?

a. Triglycerides
b. LDL-cholesterol
c. Lp(a)
d. Total cholesterol

3. JK is a 45-year-old man who presents for a routine physical examination. He is 5'8" and 210 lb (BMI: 32 kg/m²). Waist circumference: 41 inches. Fasting glucose: 109 mg/dL, triglycerides: 360 mg/dL. In addition to adhering to the TLC diet, which of the following dietary intervention should be prescribed?

a. Reduce saturated fat intake
b. Reduce added sugars and fructose intake
c. Reduce trans fat intake
d. Increase monounsaturated fat intake

4. The metabolic syndrome, which is targeted by the National Cholesterol Education Program ATP III guidelines for intensive lifestyle change, includes low HDL-C cholesterol and waist circumference defined in *women* as which of the following?

a. HDL < 50 mg/dL and waist circumference 35 inches
b. HDL < 40 mg/dL and waist circumference 40 inches
c. HDL < 35 mg/dL and waist circumference 40 inches
d. HDL < 35 mg/dl and waist circumference 35 inches

5. The *US Dietary Guidelines* advises eating as little trans fats as possible. Which of the following statement is true regarding trans fats?

a. Trans fats are saturated fats found in animal products
b. Trans fats raise both LDL and HDL cholesterol levels
c. Trans fats raise LDL-C and lower HDL-C levels
d. Trans fats are polyunsaturated fats found in liquid vegetable oils

6. The Dietary Approaches to Stop Hypertension (DASH) initial trial produced reductions in diastolic blood pressure levels by how many mmHg?

a. 2 mmHg
b. 5 mmHg
c. 8 mmHg
d. 10 mmHg

7. Which of the following daily combined number of fruit and vegetable servings were included in the DASH diet?

a. 2–4 servings of fruits and vegetables
b. 3–6 servings of fruits and vegetables
c. 6–7 servings of fruits and vegetables
d. 8–10 servings of fruits and vegetables

8. Which of the following statements is correct regarding the relationship between an individual's alcohol consumption, blood pressure (BP) and lifestyle?

a. The relationship between alcohol and BP is dependent on both the amount and type of alcohol consumed
b. The relationship between alcohol and BP is dependent on the amount of alcohol consumed, not the type of alcohol
c. The relationship between alcohol and BP is dependent on the effects of obesity and sodium intake
d. There is no relationship between alcohol and BP

9. MG is a 55-year-old woman who has been overweight most of her adult life. She comes to her Nurse Practitioner for her annual physical examination and laboratory data reveal the following results:

Blood pressure: 133/86 mmHg   Waist Circumference: 36"

Triglycerides: 230 mg/dL   HDL-C: 60 mg/dL   Glucose: 98 mg/dL

She is diagnosed with metabolic syndrome. How many of the metabolic syndrome criteria does she meet based on these results?

a. 1
b. 2
c. 3
d. 4

10. Heart failure affects approximately 5 million adults in the US. Which of the following medical nutrition therapies should be prescribed for patients with heart failure?

a. Reduce sodium intake
b. Reduce protein intake
c. Increase fiber intake
d. Increase vitamin C intake

Chapter 9 Endocrinology Care of the Diabetic Patient
1. Which of the following statements best describes the expected outcome of nutrition therapy for patients with type 2 diabetes?

a. 15% increase in HDL-cholesterol
b. 1–2% decrease in A1C
c. 15 mmHg decrease in systolic blood pressure
d. 10% increase in serum creatinine

2. Which of the following statements summarizes the first priority of nutrition therapy for patients with type 2 diabetes?

a. Weight loss
b. Correct dyslipidemia
c. Improve glycemia, lipid profiles, and blood pressure
d. Eliminate sugars and white foods from the diet

3. Which of the following statements is correct regarding carbohydrate intake in patients with type 2 diabetes who are taking insulin?

a. The total amount of carbohydrate ingested is most important
b. Any increase in dietary fiber will improve glycemic control
c. Varied amounts of carbohydrate intake are important
d. Any change in dietary protein will improve glycemic control

4. Two major studies showed a 58% reduction in the onset of diabetes in a population of people with pre-diabetes. What percentage weight loss was necessary to achieve diabetes risk reduction?

a. 5–7%
b. 10–12%
c. 15–17%
d. 20–22%

5. Which of the following are appropriate guidelines for treating hypoglycemia in a patient taking insulin?

a. Treat with 20 g of protein
b. Treat with 10 g of fiber
c. Treat with 5 g of omega-3 fatty acids
d. Treat with 15 g of carbohydrate

6. Excessive amounts of alcohol intake in patients with diabetes who are taking insulin can lead to which of the following medical conditions?

a. Diabetic retinopathy
b. Increased BUN
c. Alopecia
d. Hypoglycemia

7. The United Kingdom Prospective Diabetes Study demonstrated that reducing elevated blood glucose levels with diet and insulin results in which of the following?

a. Alteration in C-reactive protein production
b. Increased neurological symptoms
c. Increased insulin secretion
d. Decreased microvascular complication rates

8. What is the target pre-meal plasma glucose range for non-pregnant adults with diabetes mellitus?

a. 90–130 mg/dL
b. 100–140 mg/dL
c. 150–180 mg/dL
d. 180–200 mg/dL

9. What is considered an optimal HgbA1C target for younger patients with diabetes with few complications?

a. <7%
b. <8%
c. <9%
d. <10%

10. Which of the following increases a patient's likelihood of developing insulin resistance?

a. History of liver disease
b. Having a distant cousin with type 2 diabetes
c. Obesity, especially abdominal or central obesity
d. Active lifestyle

Chapter 10 Digestive Disorders and Gastrointestinal Care

1. ST is a 24-year-old woman with unintentional weight loss of 30 lb (13.6 kg) over the past 4 months despite a normal intake. ST also complains of foul-smelling stools and after several days of work-up, she is diagnosed with Crohn's disease. Which of the following is the most likely cause of her weight loss?

a. Bowel obstruction
b. Malabsorption
c. Perforated colon
d. Vitamin deficiency

2. JF is a 48-year-old man recently diagnosed with peptic ulcer disease. Nutrition therapy for patients with peptic ulcer disease includes which of the following?

a. Reducing carbohydrate intake
b. Reducing protein intake
c. Reducing caffeine, tobacco and alcohol intake
d. Reducing omega-3 fatty acid intake

3. Individuals who are lactose intolerant may not meet their daily calcium requirements if they choose to avoid dairy products. Which of the following are good non-dairy source of calcium to recommend to patients who are lactose intolerant?

a. Almond milk
b. Ice cream
c. Fortified whole-wheat bread
d. Whole grains

4. SS is a 60-year-old man with chronic liver disease and ascites. He has lost a significant amount of weight and is at risk of malnutrition. Which of the following is most likely contributing to his poor dietary intake?

a. Hyperkalemia
b. Hypoglycemia
c. Dehydration
d. Early satiety

5. DE is a 35-year-old obese woman, recently diagnosed with gastroesophogeal reflux disease (GERD). She states that her symptoms mostly occur in the middle of the night. Which of the following recommendations may be most helpful in alleviating her symptoms?

a. Avoid eating at least 2 hours before bedtime
b. Sleep with at least two pillows at night
c. Drink warm milk before bed
d. Take an over-the-counter sleeping pill

6. LD is a 45-year-old man who presents to the emergency department after falling. LD admits to drinking at least five alcoholic drinks daily and having failed several rehab attempts. Lab data indicates an elevated mean corpuscular volume (MCV), a characteristic finding in megaloblastic anemia. Which of the following is the most likely cause of this type of anemia in alcoholic patients?

a. Vitamin B_{12} deficiency
b. Iron deficiency
c. Zinc deficiency
d. Calcium deficiency

7. LK is a 30-year-old woman with severe Crohn's disease. She recently required an intestinal resection of her ileum. Which of the following is the most likely cause of fat malabsorption in patients with Crohn's disease?

a. Decreased hepatic synthesis of albumin
b. Poor liver function
c. Inability to reabsorb bile salts
d. Decreased protein intake

8. Individuals with celiac disease are advised to avoid all foods containing rye, wheat, and barley because they are especially sensitive to which of the following proteins?

a. Albumin
b. Gluten
c. Transferrin
d. Casein

9. FC is a 28-year-old obese woman diagnosed with gallstones. Her BMI is 37 kg/ m². Her Nurse Practitioner recommends that she try to lose weight to help control her gallstone formation. What would be the maximum amount of weight that she should lose each week to prevent additional gallstones?

a. 0.5–1 lb per week
b. 1–2 lb per week
c. 3–4 lb per week
d. 5 lb per week

10. DM is a 30-year-old woman with ulcerative colitis who has been prescribed sulfasalazine. Which of the following vitamins should be prescribed to patients who are being treated with sulfasalazine?

a. Folate
b. Vitamin A
c. Vitamin C
d. Thiamin

Chapter 11 Renal Care

1. SS is a 24-year-old woman with acute renal failure who is admitted to the hospital. A nutrition support service consultation is requested to determine the patient's calorie requirements. Which of the following calorie requirements should be used for individuals with acute kidney injury?

a. 10–20 kcal/kg/day
b. 20–30 kcal/kg/day
c. 30–50 kcal/kg/day
d. 50–60 kcal/kg/day

2. RE is a 65-year-old man with Stage 4 chronic kidney disease. He is scheduled to go on dialysis in a few months. Nutrition therapy for patients prior to initiating dialysis restricts protein for which of the following reasons?

a. To slow the progression of renal disease
b. To compensate for an increase in excretion of nitrogenous waste products
c. To better control hypertension
d. To promote weight loss

3. PR is a 45-year-old man who recently passed a kidney stone. Which of the following foods contains the highest amount of oxalate and should be limited in patients with calcium oxalate kidney stones?

a. Apples
b. Yogurt
c. Tomatoes
d. Dark green leafy vegetables

4. NH is a 45-year-old woman who has recently undergone renal transplantation due to kidney failure. Side effects related to some immunosuppressive agents that would require dietary recommendations include which of the following?

a. Hyperlipidemia
b. Hypermagnesemia
c. Hypoglycemia
d. Hypokalemia

5. Restricting dietary phosphate intake for individuals with chronic kidney disease to maintain proper calcium/phosphorus balance may decrease the severity of which of the following medical problems?

a. Primary hyperparathyroidism
b. Vascular and soft tissue calcifications
c. Rheumatoid arthritis
d. Hypertension

6. BG is a 46-year-old woman receiving hemodialysis (HD). She is 5'3" (160 cm) and weighs 110 lb (50 kg). Her lab data are BUN: 65 mg/dL, albumin: 3.7 g/dL, creatinine: 9.2 mg/dL. Considering BG is receiving HD three times per week, how much protein should BG be consuming daily?

a. <50 g protein/day
b. 60–65 g protein/day
c. 75–90 g protein/day
d. >90 g protein/day

7. The kidney plays an essential role in which of the following metabolic conversions, which is why supplementation may be needed in patients with chronic kidney disease?

a. Beta-carotene → vitamin A
b. Oxalic acid → ascorbic acid
c. Ferrous sulfate → ferric sulfate
d. 25(OH) vitamin D → 1,25(OH)$_2$ vitamin D

8. PF is a 56-year-old man with nephrotic syndrome. In addition to reducing dietary fat intake, protein intake should also be limited to 0.8–1.0 g/kg per day. Which of the following mechanisms explains why moderate protein intake is advised for patients with nephrotic syndrome?

a. To reduce the amino acid load in the glomerulus
b. To increase albumin excretion
c. To reduce nitrogen balance
d. To increase hepatic protein synthesis

9. TD is a 56-year-old man with chronic kidney disease and normocytic, normochromic anemia. Which of the following mechanisms most likely explains the associated anemia in a patient with chronic kidney disease?

a. Blood loss due to dialysis procedure
b. Vitamin B$_{12}$ deficiency
c. Decreased erythropoietin production
d. Folate deficiency

10. When assessing the nutritional status of a patient with chronic kidney disease it is important to use the patient's dry weight for all calculations. Which of the following is the best definition of "dry weight"?

a. The weight when the patient is dehydrated
b. The weight when the patient has not drank any fluids in 12 hours
c. The weight when the patient has taken diuretics for several days
d. The weight of the patient minus the estimated amount of fluid retention

Chapter 12 Cancer Prevention and Oncology Care

1. According to research on the link between obesity and cancer risk, which of the following women have the highest risk of developing breast cancer?

a. Pre-menopausal woman with a BMI of $30\,\text{kg/m}^2$
b. Pre-menopausal woman with a BMI of $25\,\text{kg/m}^2$
c. Post-menopausal woman with a BMI of $30\,\text{kg/m}^2$
d. Post-menopausal woman with a BMI of $40\,\text{kg/m}^2$

2. According to the National Cancer Institute, what is the strongest and most consistent predictor of breast cancer risk?

a. Amount of physical activity
b. Weight gain during adulthood
c. High intake of saturated fat
d. Irregular menstruation

3. Weight gain in which area of the body poses the highest risk for colon cancer?

a. Hips
b. Buttocks
c. Abdomen
d. Thighs

4. According to the American Institute for Cancer Research, dietary recommendations to reduce the risk of colorectal cancer include which of the following statements about red meat intake?

a. A maximum of 18 oz of cooked red meat per week with no processed meat consumption
b. Avoidance of all processed meats
c. Avoid both cooked red meat and processed meats as much as possible
d. Red meat consumption has no relation to cancer

5. Flavonoids are a class of phytochemicals that have been shown to protect against certain types of cancer. What is the mechanism of actions of flavonoids related to cancer prevention?

a. Increase tyrosine protein kinases
b. Act as an antioxidant and absorb free radicals
c. Reduce phytoestrogen absorption
d. Enhance growth factor receptors

6. CR is a 51-year-old woman who questions her gynecologist about the pros and cons of eating more foods with soy. Consumption of foods made with soy may contribute to protection against which type of cancer?

a. Breast
b. Colon
c. Stomach
d. Liver

7. CH is an 84-year-old man who was admitted to the hospital with dehydration and pneumonia. At what point should cancer cachexia first be suspected?

a. Immediately upon diagnosis
b. If the patient is intubated
c. If he had experienced an unintentional weight loss greater than 10% of his weight over the previous year
d. Only if nausea and fatigue are present

8. EC is an 86-year-old man who is receiving daily radiation treatment for colon cancer. Which of the following side effects of radiation treatment is most likely to affect a patient's nutritional status?

a. Alopecia
b. Radiation pneumonitis
c. Nausea and vomiting
d. Oral mucositis

9. NT is a 59-year-old woman who is receiving weekly chemotherapy following surgery for breast cancer. Which of the following nutritional recommendations can help control her complaints of nausea after treatment?

a. Consuming warm or hot drinks
b. Eating smaller, more frequent meals
c. Eating larger meals in the middle of the day
d. Adequate fiber intake

10. EP is a 45-year-old man with a family history of cancer. He recently quit smoking and is eating more healthy foods. Which of the following lifestyle changes should be recommended to help reduce EP's risk of developing cancer?

a. Eat only organic foods
b. Begin a regular physical activity program for 30 minutes every day
c. Eliminate all dairy foods
d. Take 1000 mg of vitamin C daily

Chapter 13 Enteral and Parenteral Nutrition Support

1. A patient with which of the following condition is considered a candidate for enteral nutrition support?

a. Paralytic ileus
b. High output proximal fistula
c. Short bowel syndrome
d. Intestinal obstruction

2. What formula density is appropriate for a patient with normal fluid requirements?

a. 0.5–0.8 kcal/mL
b. 0.8–1.0 kcal/mL
c. 1.0–1.2 kcal/mL
d. 1.5–2.0 kcal/mL

3. Which of the following is recommended for home infusion of an enteral formula via a jejunostomy?

a. Cycled over 12 hours at night
b. Continuous over 24 hours
c. Bolus feedings over 20 minutes, 6 times/day
d. Intermittent feedings over 30 minutes, 6 times/day

4. Which of the following ranges is recommended for protein needs for parenteral nutrition in severely stressed patients?

a. 0.8–1.0 g/kg/day
b. 1.0–1.5 g/kg/day
c. 1.5–2.0 g/kg/day
d. >2.0 g/kg/day

5. Patients receiving parenteral nutrition support may experience complications that include a sudden change in body temperature, new onset shaking chills, leukocytosis, or unexplained hyperglycemia. Which of the following is most likely to cause these complications?

a. Intra-abdominal infection
b. Urinary tract infection
c. Catheter-related blood stream infection
d. Dehydration

6. According to the American Society for Parenteral and Enteral Nutrition, enteral nutrition should be initiated in non-ICU patients who are expected to not receive adequate oral intake for at least how many days?

a. 7 days
b. 10 days
c. 12 days
d. 15 days

7. Enteral nutrition offers many benefits over parenteral nutrition support. These benefits are due in part to which of the following?

a. Preservation of gut integrity
b. Lower rates of hypoglycemia
c. Suppressed thyroid function
d. Reduced risk of bleeding

8. When using peripheral parenteral nutrition (PPN) solutions, what is the maximum allowable concentration to prevent vascular damage?

a. 700 mOsm/L
b. 900 mOsm/L
c. 1000 mOsm/L
d. This is not a concern with parenteral nutrition

9. According to the American Society for Parenteral and Enteral Nutrition, which of the following ranges is most commonly recommended when determining energy needs for parenteral nutrition in adults?

a. 10–15 kcal/kg daily
b. 20–30 kcal/kg daily
c. 30–45 kcal/kg daily
d. 45–60 kcal/kg daily

10. Refeeding syndrome is an imbalance that may lead to cardiac, neuromuscular, hepatic, hematologic, and respiratory dysfunction, and ultimately organ failure. Which of the following are typically added to PN to prevent this problem?

a. Potassium, sodium, iron, biotin
b. Phosphate, magnesium, calcium, potassium
c. Magnesium, niacin, folate, zinc
d. Calcium, zinc, iron, pyridoxine

Review Answers

Chapter 1 The Role of Nurse Practitioners

1. D
2. C
3. C
4. C
5. B
6. A

Chapter 2 Nutrition Assessment for Nurse Practitioners

1. D
2. A
3. B
4. D
5. B
6. D
7. A
8. C
9. C
10. D

Chapter 3 Nutrition Counseling for Effective Behavior Change

1. B
2. C
3. C
4. D
5. B
6. D
7. C
8. D
9. C
10. A

Chapter 4 Nutrition from Pre-conception Through Lactation

1. D
2. A
3. B
4. D
5. A
6. D
7. D
8. C
9. A
10. B

Chapter 5 Nutrition from Infancy Through Adolescence

1. D
2. C
3. B
4. A
5. A
6. D
7. C
8. B
9. B
10. B

The Nurse Practitioner's Guide to Nutrition, Second Edition. Edited by Lisa Hark, Kathleen Ashton and Darwin Deen.
© 2012 John Wiley & Sons, Inc. Published 2012 by John Wiley & Sons, Inc.

Chapter 6 Nutrition for Older Adults

1. D
2. C
3. B
4. B
5. C
6. B
7. A
8. C
9. A
10. C

Chapter 7 Obesity and Bariatric Surgery Care

1. B
2. A
3. B
4. C
5. A
6. C
7. C
8. A
9. C
10. D

Chapter 8 Cardiology Care

1. C
2. A
3. B
4. A
5. C
6. B
7. D
8. B
9. C
10. A

Chapter 9 Endocrinology Care of the Diabetic Patient

1. B
2. C
3. A
4. A
5. D
6. D
7. D
8. A
9. A
10. C

Chapter 10 Digestive Disorders and Gastrointestinal Care

1. B
2. C
3. A
4. D
5. A
6. A
7. C
8. B
9. B
10. A

Chapter 11 Renal Care

1. B
2. A
3. D
4. A
5. B
6. B
7. D
8. A
9. C
10. D

Chapter 12 Cancer Prevention and Oncology Care

1. D
2. B
3. C
4. A
5. B
6. A
7. B
8. C
9. B
10. B

Chapter 13 Enteral and Parenteral Nutrition Support

1. B
2. C
3. A
4. C
5. C
6. A
7. A
8. B
9. B
10. B

Index

absorption, 208
  see also malabsorption
acetate in parenteral nutrition, 303
acute kidney injury (AKI), 239–41
acute tubular necrosis, 254
adipose tissue breakdown in cancer, 276
adjustable gastric banding (AGB), 58
adolescence, 105–9
  athletes, 107
  binge eating, 108
  bone mineral density, 106
  calcium deficiency risk, 106
  eating disorders, 107–8
  iron deficiency risk, 106
  physical activity, 106–7
  pregnancy, 56–7, **68,** 106
  specific needs, 105
  vegetarianism, 108–9
albumin, serum levels, **26**
alcohol consumption
  breastfeeding, 71
  cancer risk, 271–2
  cardiovascular disease, 171
  diabetes mellitus, 201
  hypertension, 174–5
  inflammatory bowel disease, 219
  pregnancy, 53
allergies, 95, 98, **98**
allium vegetables, 268–9
Alzheimer's disease, 126
amino acids
  parenteral feeding formula, 300–301
  see also essential amino acids
anemia
  iron-deficiency, 84

inflammatory bowel disease, 218, 221
  Roux-en-Y procedure, **153**
  older people, 119
  pregnancy, 52
anencephaly, 50–51, **51**
anorexia, 18
  cancer cachexia, 275
anorexia nervosa, 107–8
antacids, pregnancy, 63
anthocyanidins, 267
anthropometric measures, 19, **20–21,** 21, *22, 23*
antidepressants, malnutrition interventions, 128
antioxidants, 266
  enteral formula content, **292,** 293
appetite
  improvement in older adults, 127
  loss, 18
appetite stimulants, 128–9
arachidonic acid, breast milk content, 90
ascites, 230
assessment of individual, 7–8, **7**
  physical examination, 18–19, **20–21,** 21, *22, 23*
  see also nutrition assessment
asthma, risk with smoking, 53
atherogenesis, 161
atherosclerotic vascular disease (AV), 83
athletes, adolescent, 107

bariatric surgery, 145–54
  biliopancreatic diversion, 148
  BMI criteria, 146
  contraindications, 146

The Nurse Practitioner's Guide to Nutrition, Second Edition. Edited by Lisa Hark, Kathleen Ashton and Darwin Deen.
© 2012 John Wiley & Sons, Inc. Published 2012 by John Wiley & Sons, Inc.

ENROLLMENT FORM/ANSWER SHEET

The Nurse Practitioner's Guide to Nutrition
Edited by Lisa Hark, PhD, RD, Kathleen Ashton, PhD, RN, ACNS-BC
and Darwin Deen, MD, MS

This Independent Study activity has been approved for 35 nursing continuing education contact hours through the Temple University College of Health Professions and Social Work Department of Nursing Provider Unit, an approved provider of continuing nursing education by the Pennsylvania State Nurses Association, itself an accredited approver by the American Nurses Credentialing Center's Commission on Accreditation.

1. Read *The Nurse Practitioner's Guide to Nutrition* and complete the test questions in the back of the book after completing each chapter (pages 339–364).

2. Write the correct answers on the answer sheet (reverse side).

3. Please note how long each chapter and questions took to complete on answer sheet.

4. Grade yourself using the answers in *The Nurse Practitioner's Guide to Nutrition* (page 365). Successful completion of this independent study requires that you attain at least 80% correct. If you do not attain this score, retest yourself again and indicate the corrected score on the form. Please note, credits are awarded for completion of the entire book only.

5. Complete the Evaluation Form and return this Enrollment Form, Answer Sheet, Evaluation form, and $40 fee to:

Temple University
Chairperson, Department of Nursing
College of Health Professions and Social Work
3307 North Broad Street
Philadelphia, PA 19140

Make check payable to the Temple University Department of Nursing
Approved for: 35 CE Credit Units Beginning September 1, 2012 to November 1, 2015

Name_____ Credentials_____

Date completed_____

Address_____

_____

City_____ State_____ Zip_____

Email (PRINT CLEARLY)_____

Daytime Telephone_____

Provider questions contact Dr. Lisa Hark (610) 659-1834 or email to hark@Lisahark.com

ANSWER SHEET

The Nurse Practitioner's Guide to Nutrition

Fill in the correct answers and grade yourself when finished.
Complete the other side. No additional self-reporting form is needed.
Activity Title: *The Nurse Practitioner's Guide to Nutrition*
Activity Type: Independent-Study Print
Approved for: 35 CE Credits Valid September 1, 2012 to November 1, 2015

Credits are awarded for completion of the entire book only, not for individual chapters.

Chapter 1	Chapter 2	Chapter 3	Chapter 4	Chapter 5
1)	1)	1)	1)	1)
2)	2)	2)	2)	2)
3)	3)	3)	3)	3)
4)	4)	4)	4)	4)
5)	5)	5)	5)	5)
6)	6)	6)	6)	6)
	7)	7)	7)	7)
	8)	8)	8)	8)
	9)	9)	9)	9)
	10)	10)	10)	10)

Chapter 6	Chapter 7	Chapter 8	Chapter 9	Chapter 10
1)	1)	1)	1)	1)
2)	2)	2)	2)	2)
3)	3)	3)	3)	3)
4)	4)	4)	4)	4)
5)	5)	5)	5)	5)
6)	6)	6)	6)	6)
7)	7)	7)	7)	7)
8)	8)	8)	8)	8)
9)	9)	9)	9)	9)
10)	10)	10)	10)	10)

Chapter 11	Chapter 12	Chapter 13
1)	1)	1)
2)	2)	2)
3)	3)	3)
4)	4)	4)
5)	5)	5)
6)	6)	6)
7)	7)	7)
8)	8)	8)
9)	9)	9)
10)	10)	10)

Correct_____/ 126

Answers to these questions are located in *The Nurse Practitioner's Guide to Nutrition*
Completion of this independent learning activity requires that you attain at least 80% correct
(>100 correct).
If not, retest yourself and indicate the corrected score on the form.

Questions, please call Lisa Hark, PhD, RD at 610-659-1834, hark@Lisahark.com

Continuing Education Activity Evaluation Form

In order to help the Temple Nursing Continuing Education Committee evaluate and plan future programs, please complete the following evaluation form.

Title of Activity: The Nurse Practitioner's Guide to Nutrition   **Date:**

Purpose: To improve the knowledge and skills of Nurse Practitioners regarding the role of nutrition in the prevention and management of acute and chronic diseases.

1.   Did the educational activity achieve the overall purpose stated above?   Yes   No

2.   Did the Educational Activity meet each of the overall objectives stated below?

Objectives:

i.   Identify key nutrition history and concepts within the physical examination.

                    Yes   No

ii. Explain nutrition-related changes and appropriate nutrition interventions through the lifespan.

                    Yes   No

iii. List the appropriate nutrition therapy for patients with a variety of acute and chronic medical problems

                    Yes   No

3.   How well were the following objectives met for each chapter? Please check and rate the following using the scale:

   1 – Not Applicable,   **2** – Poor,   **3** – Fair,   **4** – Good,   **5** – Excellent

Chapter	Title and Page of Objectives	Rating
Chapter 1	The Role of Nursing Practitioners (page 3)	
Chapter 2	Nurtrition Assessment for Nurse Practitioners (page 12)	
Chapter 3	Nutrition Counseling for Effective Behavior Change (page 31)	
Chapter 4	Nutrition from Pre-conception through Lactation (page 45)	
Chapter 5	Nutrition from Infancy through Adolescence (page 79)	
Chapter 6	Nutrition for Older Adults (page 113)	
Chapter 7	Obesity and Bariatric Surgery Care (page 137)	
Chapter 8	Cardiology Care (page 160)	
Chapter 9	Endocrinology Care of the Diabetic Patient (page 184)	
Chapter 10	Digestive Disorders and Gastrointestinal Care (page 207)	
Chapter 11	Renal Care (page 235)	
Chapter 12	Cancer Prevention and Oncology Care (page 261)	
Chapter 13	Enteral and Parenteral Nutrition Support (page 289)	

4. Please Rate the following using the same 1–5 Scale.

Criteria	Rating	Criteria	Rating
Learner satisfaction		Skills and attitude change	
Knowledge enhancement		Change in practice/ performance	

5. Were the materials in this activity: ____new ____review ____new and review

6. Was the material clearly written?   Yes   No
   Comments:

7. Using the Answer Key, total up the time you spent on each chapter and indicate how many hours/minutes you spent to complete the entire book, including both reading the chapters and completing the test questions.

                    _____hours _____minutes

To receive 35 CE credits return the graded Answer Sheet, Enrollment Form, Evaluation Form, and $40 made payable to Temple University Department of Nursing. You will receive a certificate in the mail.

Temple University
Chairperson, Department of Nursing
College of Health Professions and Social Work
3307 North Broad Street
Philadelphia, PA 19140
215-707-8327

Approved for 35 CE Credits
Valid September 1, 2012 to November 1, 2015